Neurological Emergencies

Fourth edition

Edited by

RAC Hughes

Head, Department of Clinical Neurosciences,
Guy's, King's and St Thomas' School of Medicine,
London, UK

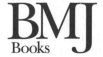

First published in 1994
by BMJ Books, BMA House, Tavistock Square,
London WC1H 9JR

www.bmjbooks.com

First edition 1994
Second edition 1997
Third edition 2000
Fourth edition 2003

British Library Cataloguing in Publication Data

A catalogue record for this book is available from the British Library

ISBN 0 7279 1774 9

Typeset by SIVA Math Setters, Chennai, India
Printed and bound in Spain by GraphyCems, Ltd

Contents

Contributors

Peter JD Andrews
Reader in Anaesthesia, Critical Care and Pain Medicine, University of Edinburgh, Clinical and Surgical Sciences (Anaesthetics) and Western General Hospital, Edinburgh, UK

David Bates
Professor of Clinical Neurology, Department of Neurology, University of Newcastle-upon-Tyne, Newcastle-upon-Tyne, UK

J Brown
Consultant Neurosurgeon, Institute of Neurosurgical Sciences, Southern General Hospital, Glasgow, UK

Carol Croft
Associate Professor of Internal Medicine, University of Texas Southwestern Medical Center, Dallas, Texas, USA

M Czosnyka
Director of Neurophysics, Academic Neurosurgery Unit, Addenbrooke's Hospital, Cambridge, UK

R Davenport
Consultant Neurologist, Department of Clinical Neurosciences, Western General Hospital, Edinburgh, UK

M Dennis
Consultant Physician, Department of Clinical Neurosciences, Western General Hospital, Edinburgh, UK

J Greig
Specialist Registrar, Department of Infection and Tropical Medicine, Birmingham Heartlands Hospital, UK

RAC Hughes
Head, Department of Clinical Neurosciences, Guy's, King's and St Thomas' School of Medicine, London, UK

RA Johnston
Consultant Neurosurgeon, Institute of Neurosurgical Sciences, Queen Elizabeth National Spinal Injuries Unit, Southern General Hospital, Glasgow, UK

Thomas A Kopitnik
Professor of Neurological Surgery, Director of Cerebrovascular Surgery, University of Texas Southwestern Medical Center, Dallas, Texas, USA

S Lewis
Professor of Adult Psychiatry, University of Manchester, Withington Hospital, Manchester, UK

GG Lloyd
Consultant Liaison Psychiatrist, Royal Free Hospital, London, UK

A McLuckie
Consultant Intensive Care Physician, Intensive Care Unit, St Thomas' Hospital, London, UK

Shawn Moore
Resident in Neurological Surgery, University of Texas Southwestern Medical Center, Dallas, Texas, USA

MD O'Brien
Consultant Neurologist, Department of Neurology, Guy's Hospital, London, UK

JD Pickard
Professor of Neurosurgery, Academic Neurosurgery Unit, Addenbrooke's Hospital, Cambridge, UK

J Pimm
Lecturer in Psychiatry, Royal Free and University College Medical School, London, UK

Simon Shorvon
Professor in Clinical Neurology, Institute of Neurology, University College London, London, UK

LA Steiner
Department of Anaesthesia, Kantonsspital, Basel, Switzerland

S Turner
Consultant in Old Age Psychiatry, Carleton Clinic, Carlisle, UK

Matthew Walker
Honorary Consultant and Senior Lecturer in Neurology, Department of Clinical and Experimental Epilepsy, Institute of Neurology, London, UK

Jonathan A White
Assistant Proffessor of Neurological Surgery, University of Texas Southwestern Medical Center, Dallas, Texas, USA

MJ Wood
Late Consultant Physician, Department of Infection and Tropical Medicine, Birmingham Heartlands Hospital, Birmingham, UK

Shirley H Wray
Professor of Neurology, Department of Neurology, Harvard Medical School and Director, Unit for Neurovisual Disorders, Massachusetts Hospital, Boston, Massachusetts, USA

Preface

This popular book is designed for every doctor who deals with neurological emergencies. Each chapter reviews current management and the evidence for its efficacy, and concludes with a brief summary of recommendations that should be a useful *aide-mémoire* in an emergency.

The fourth edition of the book, which was first published as a series in 1993 in the *Journal of Neurology, Neurosurgery and Psychiatry*, has been thoroughly revised and based on the latest evidence. The first-time reader will find succinct reviews of the pathogenesis and especially management of all the common neurological emergencies. "Neurological" is used in the broadest sense to include neurosurgery (head injury, compression, subarachnoid haemorrhage, raised intracranial pressure), psychiatry (delirium, acute behaviour disturbances), neuro-ophthalmology (acute visual failure), infectious disease (cerebral infections), and intensive care (acute neuromuscular respiratory paralysis). Old lags can quickly bring themselves up to date because each chapter has taken advantage of the increasing collection of relevant Cochrane reviews to provide the best evidence on which to base practice. Are you confident that you know the latest guidelines for head injury, raised intracranial pressure and acute spinal cord compression, the best antibiotics for meningitis, and the best antiepileptic drug regimen for status epilepticus?

Although a book like this is inevitably targeted at the doctor in training, especially residents in internal medicine, accident and emergency medicine, and neurology (including neurosurgery and psychiatry), we are all perpetual students of medicine. We hope therefore that this work will help the whole profession improve the care of neurological patients when they most need it, in an emergency.

We regret to report the death of Dr Martin Wood shortly after submitting the fine chapter on cerebral infections, of which he was co-author.

RAC HUGHES

1: Medical coma

DAVID BATES

The patient in coma who is brought to the hospital casualty department, or seen on the intensive care unit, though not having been exposed to evident trauma, may be harbouring delayed effects of head injury such as a subdural haematoma or meningitis arising from a basal skull fracture. The possibilities of raised intracranial pressure following a parenchymal haematoma in a hypertensive patient, the decompensation of a cerebral tumour, or the collection of pus means that all possible causes of loss of consciousness must be considered in coma. In the diagnosis of medical coma it is not easy to exclude the possibility of head injury.

If patients with a transient loss of consciousness following seizure, syncope, cardiac dysrhythmia or hypoglycaemia, and those unresponsive due to impending death are excluded, then, once a patient has been unconscious for 5–6 hours, about 40% of such patients seen in medical practice will have taken some form of sedative drug with or without alcohol.[1] Of the remainder just over 40% will have suffered a hypoxic-ischaemic insult as a result of cardiac arrest or anaesthetic accident, a third will be unconscious as a result of cerebrovascular accident, either haemorrhage or infarction, and about a quarter as a result of metabolic coma, including infection, renal or hepatic failure, and complications of diabetes mellitus. If one considers only those cases which are initially regarded as of "unknown aetiology" the proportion of drug overdoses is about 30%, mass lesions 35%, and diffuse metabolic causes 35%.[2]

Few problems are more difficult to manage than the unconscious patient because the potential causes of loss of consciousness are considerable and because the time for diagnosis and effective intervention is relatively short. All alterations in arousal should be regarded as acute and potentially life threatening emergencies until vital functions are stabilised, the underlying cause of the coma is diagnosed, and reversible causes are corrected. Delay in instituting treatment for a patient with raised intracranial pressure may have obvious consequences in terms of pressure coning but, similarly, the unnecessary investigation by imaging techniques of patients in metabolic coma may delay the initiation of appropriate therapy. It is therefore essential for the physician in charge to adopt a systematic approach, initially to ensure resuscitation then to direct further tests towards producing the most rapid diagnosis and the most appropriate therapy. The development of such a systematic approach demands an understanding of the pathophysiology of consciousness and the ways in which it may be deranged.

Causes of coma

Consciousness depends upon an intact ascending reticular activating substance (ARAS) in the brain stem acting as the alerting or awakening element of consciousness, together with a functioning cerebral cortex of both hemispheres which determines the content of that consciousness. The ARAS is a continuous isodendritic core, extending from the medulla through the pons to the midbrain which is continuous caudally with the reticular intermediate grey lamina of the spinal cord and rostrally with the subthalamus, the hypothalamus, and the thalamus (Figure 1.1).[3] The functions and interconnections of the ARAS are considerable and its role greater than that of a simple cortical arousal system. There are named nuclei throughout the reticular formation. Although it was originally considered that cortical arousal depended upon projections from the reticular formation via the midline thalamic nuclei to the thalamic reticular nucleus and cortex, it now seems unlikely that the thalamic reticular nucleus is the final relay. The specific role of the various links from the reticular formation to the thalamus has yet to be identified.

Similarly the neurotransmitters involved in this arousal system are not fully determined though it seems likely that, in addition to cholinergic and monoaminergic systems, gamma aminobutyric acid (GABA) may be important in controlling consciousness.[4-6]

It follows from the anatomy and pharmacology of the ARAS that structural damage to this pathway or chemical

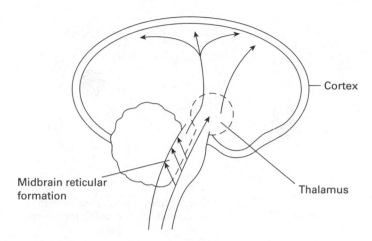

Figure 1.1 The anatomy of consciousness

derangement of the neurotransmitters involved are mechanisms whereby consciousness may be impaired. Such conditions will occur with focal lesions in the brain stem, mass lesions in the posterior fossa impinging directly on the brain stem, or mass lesions involving the cerebral hemispheres causing tentorial pressure coning and consequently compromising the ARAS either by direct pressure or by ischaemia (Figure 1.2). In addition toxins, including most commonly ingested drugs, may have a significant depressant effect upon the brain stem ARAS and thereby result in loss of consciousness.

The content of consciousness resides in the cerebral cortex of both hemispheres. Unlike those discrete cortical functions such as language or vision which are focally located within the cortex, the content of consciousness can best be regarded as the amalgam of all cognitive functions. Coma arising from disruption of cortical activity requires a diffuse pathology such as generalised anoxia or ischaemia, commonly seen after cardiac arrest or anaesthetic accidents, or cortical vasospasm seen in infective meningitis, or subarachnoid haemorrhage, where generalised cortical ischaemia is believed to be the cause of disruption of function.

The physician attempting to diagnose the cause of coma should consider the following.

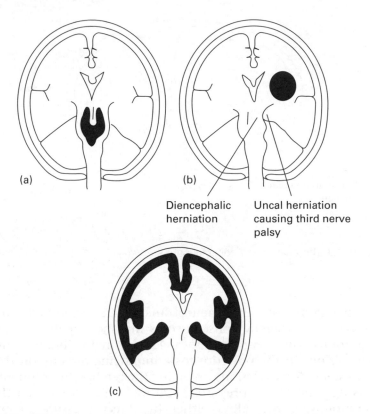

Diencephalic   Uncal herniation
herniation   causing third nerve
                palsy

Figure 1.2 Causes of coma. (a) Focal brain stem lesions; (b) mass lesions; (c) diffuse cortical pathology

1. *Supratentorial or infratentorial mass lesions.* Typically these will provide evidence of raised intracranial pressure and commonly produce focal signs. Processes such as neoplasm or haematoma, infarction with cerebral oedema, abscess, focal encephalitis, and venous sinus thrombosis must all be considered.
2. *Subtentorial destructive lesions or the local effect of toxin.* These processes will directly damage the ARAS in brain stem infarction, rhombencephalitis, brain stem demyelination, and the more common effects of self-poisoning with sedative drugs.
3. *Diffuse damage to the cerebral cortex.* Bilateral cortical injury is most commonly seen following hypoxia and ischaemia

but may be mimicked by hypoglycaemia, ketoacidosis, electrolyte abnormalities, bacterial meningitis, viral encephalitis, and diffuse postinfective encephalomyelitis. It is also the likely pathology of coma following subarachnoid haemorrhage.

Definitions

There is a continuum from the individual in full consciousness to the patient in deep coma. The terminology which is most usually employed derives from the Brain Injuries Committee of the Medical Research Council (MRC).[7]

1. *Confusion*. "Disturbance of consciousness characterised by impaired capacity to think clearly and to perceive, respond to and remember current stimuli; there is also disorientation." Confusion involves a generalised disturbance of cortical cerebral function which is usually associated with considerable electroencephalographic (EEG) abnormality. Some authors describe an intervening state between normal consciousness and confusion, that of "clouding of consciousness".[2]
2. *Delirium*. "A state of much disturbed consciousness with motor restlessness, transient hallucinations, disorientation and delusions."
3. *Obtundation*. "A disturbance of alertness associated with psychomotor retardation."
4. *Stupor*. "A state in which the patient, though not unconscious, exhibits little or no spontaneous activity." Although the individual appears to be asleep he or she will awaken to vigorous stimulation but show limited motor activities and usually fail to speak.
5. *Coma*. "A state of unrousable psychologic unresponsiveness in which the subject lies with eyes closed and shows no psychologically understandable response to external stimulus or inner need." This may be shortened to "a state of unrousable unresponsiveness" which implies both the defect in arousal and in awareness of self or environment manifest as an inability to respond. A more useful assessment of coma is that derived from the hierarchical Glasgow Coma Scale.[8] Patients who fail to show eye

opening in response to voice, perform no better than weak flexion in response to pain, and make, at best, only unrecognisable grunting noises in response to pain, are regarded as being in coma. This allows the patient to have an eye opening response of two or fewer, a motor response of four or fewer, and a verbal response of two or fewer. The sum Glasgow Score of eight should not be regarded as being definitive of coma since the total score can be achieved in several different ways (see below).

6. *Vegetative state.* "A clinical condition of unawareness of self and environment in which the patient breathes spontaneously, has a stable circulation and shows cycles of eye closure and eye opening which may simulate sleep and waking. This may be a transient stage in the recovery from coma or it may persist until death."[9] When the cortex of the cerebral hemispheres of the brain recovers more slowly than the brain stem or when the cortex is irreversibly damaged there will arise a situation in which the patient enters a vegetative state without cognitive function. This may be a transient phase through which patients in coma pass as they recover or deteriorate but, commonly after anoxic injuries to the brain, a state develops in which the brain stem recovers function but the cerebral hemispheres are not capable of recovery. This is the "persistent vegetative state" described by Jennett and Plum.[10] Such patients may survive for long periods, on occasion for decades, but never recover outward manifestations of higher mental activity and the condition, which is comparatively newly recognised, relates to the development of modern resuscitative techniques. Other terms have, in the past, been used to identify similar conditions including coma vigile, the apallic syndrome, cerebral death, neocortical death, and total dementia.

7. *Akinetic mutism.* This term has been used to define a similar condition of unresponsiveness but apparent alertness together with reactive alpha and theta EEG rhythms in response to stimuli. The major difference from the vegetative state, in which there is tone in the muscles and extensor or flexor responses, is that patients with akinetic mutism have flaccid tone and are unresponsive to peripheral pain. It is thought that this state is due to

bilateral frontal lobe lesions, diffuse cortical lesions, or lesions of the deep grey matter.[11]

8. *The locked-in syndrome.* Feldman[12] described a de-efferented state caused by a bilateral ventral pontine lesion involving damage to the cortico-spinal, cortico-pontine, and cortico-bulbar tracts. The patient has total paralysis below the level of the third nerve nuclei and, although able to open, elevate and depress the eyes, has no horizontal eye movements and no other voluntary movements. The diagnosis depends upon the clinician being able to recognise that the patient can open the eyes voluntarily and allow them to close and can signal assent or dissent, responding numerically by allowing the eyelids to fall. Similar states are occasionally seen in patients with severe polyneuropathy, myasthenia gravis, and after the use of neuromuscular blocking agents.

9. *Pseudo-coma.* Rarely, patients who appear in coma without structural, metabolic, toxic, or psychiatric disorder being apparent can be shown by tests of brain stem function to have intact brain stem activity and corticopontine projections and not to be in coma.

Resuscitation

Although resuscitation is commonly performed by the casualty officer or the anaesthetist in the intensive care unit rather than by the neurologist, it is appropriate that the neurologist remembers that in patients who are unconscious, protection of the airway, respiration, support of the circulation, and provision of an adequate supply of glucose are all important in stabilising the patient. It is frequently necessary to intubate the trachea in a patient in coma, not only to ensure an adequate airway but also to prevent the aspiration of vomit. It is also important to note the respiratory rate and pattern before intubation and certainly before instituting mechanical ventilation; because depressed respiration may be a clue to drug overdose or metabolic disturbance, increasing respiration to hypoxia, hypercapnia, or acidosis and fluctuating respiration to a brain stem lesion. The possibility that respiratory failure is the cause of a coma should always be considered in a patient with disordered respiration.

Once adequate oxygenation and circulation are ensured and monitored, blood should be withdrawn for the determination of blood glucose, biochemical estimations, and toxicology. It is reasonable to give a bolus of 25–50 g of dextrose despite the present controversy about the use of intravenous glucose in patients with ischaemic or anoxic brain damage. It could be argued that extra glucose in this situation might augment local lactic acid production by anaerobic glycolysis and eventually worsen ischaemic or anoxic damage. In practice, with ischaemic or anoxic brain damage and even in the presence of a diabetic ketoacidosis the administration of such a quantity of glucose will not be immediately harmful and in the hypoglycaemic patient it may well be life saving. A reasonable compromise would be to obtain an early assessment of the level of blood glucose by Dextrostix testing, but these are not sufficiently accurate to preclude the need for formal laboratory assessment. When glucose is given in this situation an argument can be made for giving a bolus of thiamine at the same time to prevent the precipitation of Wernicke's encephalopathy.[13]

An essential part of resuscitation includes the establishment of baseline blood pressure, pulse, temperature, the insertion of an intravenous line, and the stabilisation of the neck, together with an examination for meningitis. It may be difficult in those patients who sustain some degree of trauma in their collapse to assess the stability of the neck, but the establishment of an adequate airway certainly takes precedence and the identification of meningism in a febrile patient probably takes precedence over the stabilisation of neck movements. In a comatose, febrile patient with meningism seen outside the hospital environment, the intramuscular injection of penicillin before transfer is now recognised to carry a significant advantage.

History

Once the patient is stable it is important to obtain as much information as possible from those who accompanied the patient to hospital or who watched the onset of coma. The circumstances in which consciousness is lost are of vital importance in helping to identify the diagnosis. Generally, coma is likely to present in one of three ways: as the predictable progression of an underlying illness; as an unpredictable event in a patient with a previously known disease; or as a totally unexpected event. Distinctions between these presentations are often achieved by the history of the circumstances in which consciousness was lost. In the first category are patients following focal brain stem infarction who deteriorate or those with known intracranial mass lesions who show similar deterioration. In the second category are patients with recognised cardiac arrhythmia or the known risk factor of sepsis from an intravenous line. In the final category it is important to determine whether there has been a previous history of seizures, trauma, febrile illness, or focal neurological disturbances. The history of a sudden collapse in the midst of a busy street or office indicates the need for different investigations from those necessary for the patient discovered at home in bed surrounded by empty bottles which previously contained sedative tablets.

Examination and monitoring

The third phase of the management of the patient in coma involves a rapid but systemic examination to identify possible causes of coma.

Temperature

Fever usually indicates infection and, rarely, a brain stem or diencephalic lesion affecting the temperature centres.[14] Most commonly the combination of fever and coma indicates systemic infection such as pneumonia or septicaemia, or a cerebral cause such as meningitis, encephalitis, or abscess. When seizures occur together with fever, the possibility of encephalitis or cerebral abscess is greatly increased. Heat stroke may present as febrile coma when the clue to the diagnosis is in the environment. Hypothermia is most commonly seen as a complication of an accident or cerebrovascular disease when an elderly patient is discovered, having lain for hours or days in an underheated room. This may also be seen following intoxication with alcohol or barbiturates, with peripheral circulatory failure and, rarely, with profound myxoedema.

Heart rate

A tachyarrhythmia or bradyarrhythmia may be significant in identifying the cause of cerebral hypoperfusion. Irregularity of the pulse always raises the question of atrial fibrillation and associated embolic disease.

Blood pressure

Hypotension might indicate shock, myocardial infarction, septicaemia, or intoxication. It may also indicate diabetes mellitus or Addison's disease. Hypertension is of less help in the diagnosis of coma as it may be the cause, as in cerebral haemorrhage or hypertensive encephalopathy, or the result of the cerebral lesion.

Respiration

For those reasons already given assessment of respiration may be compromised by the need to give sedation but, generally, slow and shallow breathing raises the question of drug intoxication. Deep rapid respiration suggests pneumonia or acidosis but may also occur in brain stem lesions causing central neurogenic hyperventilation.

Integument

The appearance of the skin and mucous membranes may identify anaemia, jaundice, cyanosis, or carbon monoxide poisoning. Bruising over the scalp or mastoids, or the presence of blood in the external auditory meatus or nostrils, raises the possibility of basal skull fracture, and bruising elsewhere in the body raises the question of trauma. An exanthem may indicate the presence of a viral infection causing meningoencephalitis or of meningococcal septicaemia, or raise the question of haemorrhagic disease. Hyperpigmentation raises the possibility of Addison's disease. Bullous skin lesions are frequently seen in barbiturate intoxication. Kaposi's sarcoma, anogenital herpetic lesions, or oral candidiasis would raise the question of the acquired immune deficiency syndrome (AIDS) with a consequent plethora of possible central nervous system disease.

Breath

The odour of the breath of an unconscious patient may indicate intoxication with alcohol, raise the question of diabetes, or suggest uraemic or hepatic coma.

Cardiovascular

Auscultation and examination of the heart may indicate valvular disease and raise the possibility of endocarditis. Bruits over the carotid vessels may indicate the presence of cerebrovascular disease, and splinter haemorrhages seen in the nail beds raise the possibility of subacute bacterial endocarditis or collagen vascular diseases.

Abdomen

Examination of the abdomen may reveal signs of trauma or rupture of viscera; hepatomegaly or splenomegaly raises the possibility of a portocaval shunt, and the finding of polycystic kidneys raises the possibility of subarachnoid haemorrhage.

Meningism

Examination of the skull and spine is important and the physician should always look for neck stiffness. Kernig's test in which the resistance to flexion of the thigh with the leg extended is examined, or Brudzinski's test in which the flexion of one thigh is noted to cause flexion of the other, should be performed to help in differentiating neck stiffness due to meningeal irritation from that due to a developing tonsillar pressure cone. Positive Kernig's and Brudzinski's tests together with neck stiffness imply inflammation in the lumbar theca and suggest a diffuse meningitic process. If these tests are negative, however, then the neck stiffness alone is more suggestive of a foraminal pressure cone.[15]

Fundal examination

The presence of papilloedema or fundal haemorrhage or emboli, together with the findings of hypertensive vascular or

Table 1.1 Neurological assessment of coma

Function	Response/reaction
Glasgow Coma Scale	Eye opening Motor response Verbal response
Brain stem function	Pupillary reactions Corneal responses Spontaneous eye movements Oculocephalic responses Oculovestibular responses Respiratory pattern
Motor function	Motor response Muscle tone Tendon reflexes Seizures

diabetic retinopathy, is important. The fundal appearances may be diagnostic as in subhyaloid haemorrhage but more commonly only help to confirm or refute evidence of raised intracranial pressure. The absence of papilloedema does not necessarily mean that there is no raised intracranial pressure.

Neurological examination

The position, posture and spontaneous movements of the unconscious patient should be noted. A formal neurological examination consists of the elicitation of various reflex responses[14]; the most important aspects are those that define the level of consciousness, identify the activity of the brain stem, and search for evidence of lateralisation (Table 1.1).

Level of consciousness

The Glasgow Coma Scale[8] provides the most useful hierarchical assessment of the level of consciousness. The responses to commands, calling the patient's name, and painful stimuli are observed for eye opening, limb movement, and voice. Painful stimuli such as supraorbital pressure for central stimulation and nail bed pressure for peripheral stimulation are useful and reproducible. Eye opening is relatively easy to assess, though the fixed and unresponsive opening of the eyes sometimes seen in deep coma must not be confused with the volitional or reflex opening of the eyes from a closed position in response to stimuli. All four limbs are tested individually for movement and the best response is recorded in assessing the Glasgow Coma Scale. An asymmetry between the responses may be of importance in the overall assessment (see below). Patients in lighter grades of coma still retain the ability to vocalise and may grimace and withdraw their limbs from pain. These responses are progressively lost as the coma deepens. It is important to test pain bilaterally in the periphery and cranially as patients may only vocalise or respond to painful stimuli on one side, raising the possibility of hemi-anaesthesia and providing evidence for a focal lesion. A grimace response to painful stimulation is believed to indicate intact cortical bulbar function,[2] but there are patients in coma, particularly after hypoxic-ischaemic insults, who show grimace in response to minor peripheral stimulation yet have no associated peripheral motor response. When this situation is seen it always raises the question of a ventral pontine lesion or a cervical cord injury, but more commonly it evolves into a vegetative state and is, generally, a poor prognostic sign.

The level of coma should be documented serially and is one of the most important indicators of the need for further investigation. When the level of consciousness can be seen to be improving there is no need to make urgent decisions. When deterioration occurs then management decisions must be made. It may of course be correct, when the prognosis is recognised to be hopeless, to make the decision not to undertake further investigation or therapy.

Brain stem function

The brain stem reflexes are particularly important in helping to identify those lesions that may affect the ARAS, explain the reason for coma, and potentially help in assessing the prognosis. The following reflexes are predominantly related to the eyes and the pattern of respiration.

1. *Pupillary reactions.* The size, equality, and reaction of the pupils to light is recorded. Unilateral dilatation of the pupil with loss of the light response suggests uncal

herniation or a posterior communicating artery aneurysm. Midbrain lesions typically cause loss of the light reflex with mid-position pupils, whereas pontine lesions cause miosis but a retained light response. Fixed dilatation of the pupils is an indication of central diencephalic herniation and may be differentiated from the fixed dilatation due to atropine-like agents by the use of pilocarpine eye drops which cause miosis if the dilatation is as a result of loss of parasympathetic innervation but are ineffective if it is pharmacological. A Horner's syndrome may be seen ipsilateral to a lesion in the hypothalamus, thalamus, or brain stem, when it will be associated with anhydrosis of the ipsilateral side of the body. It can also be due to disease affecting the wall of the carotid artery when anhydrosis will only affect the face.[15] Hepatic or renal failure and other forms of metabolic coma may make the light reflexes appear unduly brisk and the pupils therefore relatively small. Most drug intoxications tend to cause small and sluggishly reactive pupils, and pontine haemorrhage will cause pinpoint pupils due to parasympathetic stimulation (Figure 1.3).[16]

2. *Corneal responses.* The corneal reflexes are usually retained until coma is very deep. If these responses are absent in the patient who is otherwise in a light coma then the possibility of a drug induced coma or of local causes of anaesthesia to the cornea should be considered. The loss of the corneal response when drug overdose is excluded is a poor prognostic sign.

3. *Eye movement.* The resting position of the eyes and the presence of spontaneous eye movements should be noted. Conjugate deviation of the eyes raises the question of an ipsilateral hemisphere or contralateral brain stem lesion. Abnormalities of vertical gaze are less common with patients in coma but depression of the eyes below the meridian may be seen with damage at the level of the midbrain tectum and in states of metabolic coma. The resting position of the eyes is normally conjugate and central but it may be dysconjugate when there is damage to the oculomotor or abducens nerves within the brain stem or along their paths.

Roving eye movements seen in light coma are similar to those of sleep. They cannot be mimicked and their

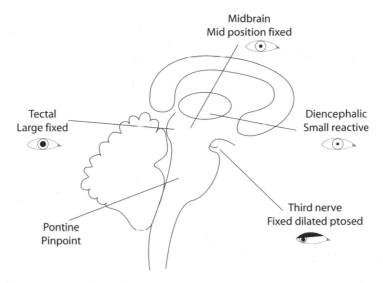

Figure 1.3 Pupillary changes

presence excludes psychogenic unresponsiveness.[14] Periodic alternating gaze or "ping-pong" gaze is a repetitive conjugate horizontal ocular deviation of uncertain aetiology.[17] Spontaneous nystagmus is rare in coma as it reflects interaction between the oculovestibular system and the cerebral cortex. Retractory nystagmus in which the eyes jerk irregularly back into the orbits and convergent nystagmus may be seen with midbrain lesions.[18] Ocular bobbing, an intermittent jerking of downward eye movement, is seen with destructive lesions in the low pons and with cerebellar haematoma or hydrocephalus.[19]

4. *Reflex eye movements*. These are tested by the oculocephalic and oculovestibular responses (Figure 1.4). The oculocephalic, or "doll's head", response is tested by rotating the patient's head from side to side and observing the eyes. In coma with an intact brain stem the eyes will move conjugately and in a direction opposite to the head movement. In a conscious patient such a response can be imitated by deliberate fixation of the eyes but is not common. In patients with pontine depression the

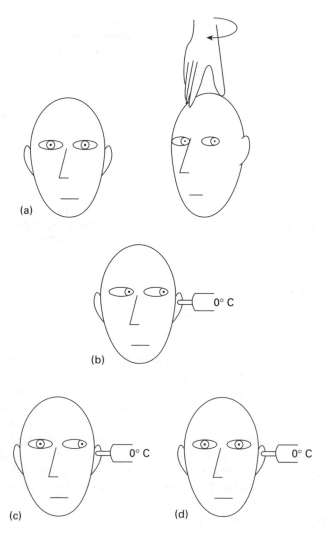

Figure 1.4 Reflex eye movements. (a) Normal doll's eye; (b) tonic oculovestibular response; (c) dysconjugate oculovestibular response; (d) absent oculovestibular response

oculocephalic response is lost and the eyes remain in the mid-position of the head when turned. The oculovestibular response is more accurate and useful. It is elicited by instilling between 50 and 200 ml of ice cold water into the external auditory meatus. The normal response in the conscious patient is the development of nystagmus with a quick phase away from the side of stimulation. A tonic response with conjugate movements of the eyes towards the stimulated side indicates an intact pons and suggests a supratentorial cause for the coma. A dysconjugate response or no response at all indicates brain stem damage or depression. Both ears should be stimulated separately. If unilateral irrigation causes vertical eye movements the possibility of drug overdose arises because many drugs affect lateral eye movement.

The value of oculovestibular testing in patients without lateralising eye signs is considerable because it identifies not only the intactness of the brain stem and corticopontine connections but also may reveal the presence of an intrinsic brain stem lesion by causing dysconjugate eye posturing. In addition, it is the definitive way of identifying patients in psychogenic coma who will show normal nystagmus and frequently be distressed by the manoeuvre.

5. *Respiration.* Modern techniques of assisted respiration and the need to examine patients in intensive care units where respiration is controlled complicates the assessment of normal respiratory function. If the patient is seen before respiration is controlled, the presence of long cycle periodic respiration suggests a relatively high brain stem lesion; central neurogenic hyperventilation implies a lesion at the level of the upper pons; and short cycle periodic respiration, which carries a poor prognosis, is seen with lesions lower in the brain stem. In general the presence of regular, rapid breathing correlates with pulmonary complications and a poor prognosis rather than with site of neurological disease in patients in coma.[20]

Motor function

As part of the assessment of Glasgow Coma Scale it may have been appreciated that there is lateralisation in the individual patient which implies a focal cause for the coma. The observation of involuntary movement affecting the face or limbs and asymmetry of reflexes will help to support this possibility. Focal seizures are an important indicator for a focal cause for the coma, and the observation of more generalised

---

Box 1.1 Clinico-anatomical correlation in coma

Bilateral hemisphere damage
  Symmetrical signs
  Fits or myoclonus
  Normal brain stem reflexes
  Normal oculocephalic and oculovestibular responses
  Normal pupils

Supertentorial mass lesion with brain stem compression
  Ipsilateral third nerve palsy
  Contralateral hemiplegia

Brain stem lesion
  Early eye movement disturbance
  Abnormal oculocephalic or vestibular responses
  Asymmetrical motor responses

Toxic/metabolic
  Reactive pupils
  Random eye movements until late in coma
  Absent oculocephalic and oculovestibular responses
  Extensor or flexor posturing
  Hypertonicity
  Hypotonicity
  Multifocal myoclonus.

---

seizure or of multifocal myoclonus raises the possibility of a metabolic or ischaemic-anoxic cause for coma with diffuse cortical irritation. The testing of tone as part of the assessment of muscle function can be useful in the comatose patient where it is possible to detect asymmetry of tone, not only in the limbs but also in the face. There are recognisable patterns of signs associated with the site of pathology (Box 1.1).[21]

By this stage it should be possible to identify those patients who are unconscious with focal signs, those who are unconscious without focal signs but with meningism, and those who have loss of consciousness without either focal signs or meningism (Box 1.2).

Investigation of the patient in coma

The relevant investigations to be undertaken in the individual patient will be determined by the differential

---

Box 1.2 Classification of differential diagnosis of coma

Coma without focal or lateralising signs and without meningism
 Anoxic-ischaemic conditions
 Metabolic disturbances
 Intoxications
 Systemic infections
 Hyperthermia/hypothermia
 Epilepsy

Coma without focal or lateralising signs but with meningeal irritation
 Subarachnoid haemorrhage
 Meningitis
 Encephalitis

Coma with focal brain stem or lateralising cerebral signs
 Cerebral tumour
 Cerebral haemorrhage
 Cerebral infarction
 Cerebral abscess.

---

diagnosis. In general the role of the investigation in the patient in coma is to help establish the aetiology of the coma and will vary from simple blood tests through more complex blood tests, examination of the cerebrospinal fluid, electrophysiological tests, and imaging. Although the EEG has shown hierarchical value in the assessment of depth of coma and has been used, to an extent, to identify the prognosis in coma,[21,22] its major role is in identifying patients who are in a subclinical status epilepticus or who have complex partial seizures, because this will significantly alter their management.[23] It may also be useful in distinguishing between feigned or psychiatric coma, in which it will be normal, and genuine cerebral disease, when it shows diffuse abnormalities, or to help identify a focal lesion. The prognostic value of the EEG is probably not as great as that obtained from careful observation of clinical signs,[21] though there are suggestions that a combination of clinical assessment and EEG may improve prediction.[24]

Evoked potentials, predominantly brain stem evoked potentials, and somatosensory evoked potentials may give information relating to the intactness of brain stem pathways and to the existence of a cortical component. Theoretically the use of brain stem evoked responses could provide evidence for the presence and site of the brain stem disease and, as they are relatively unaffected by drug coma, they may provide evidence on the aetiology.[24-26] Regrettably there is as yet little correlation between evoked response studies and coma and prognosis, but it seems that the use of somatosensory evoked potentials and brain stem auditory evoked potentials will become of value in identifying the prognosis of patients in coma. One technical problem is the need to undertake these recordings in the busy premises of an intensive care unit where considerable other electrical interference may occur.

Brain imaging techniques, including computerised tomography (CT) and magnetic resonance imaging (MRI), are important in coma in providing evidence of diagnosis.[27] CT has a very significant role to play in identifying those patients who have a structural cause for coma. MRI can be even more informative, though there are inevitable problems in inserting the patient in coma, together with the necessary life support systems, into the field of the magnet. Other, more complex techniques, such as intracranial pressure monitoring and cerebral blood flow studies are rarely of help in the diagnosis of medical coma; their role in prognosis is not fully evaluated, and their usefulness is likely to be limited by their invasiveness.[28] Measures of biochemical parameters in coma are predominantly diagnostic but some measures, such as brain type creatine kinase and neuron specific enolase in the cerebrospinal fluid (CSF), may help in determining prognosis.[29,30]

Diagnostic classification

On clinical grounds patients can be allocated to one of the following three varieties of coma.[31]

Coma with focal signs

Except in those patients in whom an underlying and irreversible terminal disease is recognised, it is obligatory that CT or MRI be undertaken to identify the cause of the coma. This will define whether or not structural abnormality is present and in many instances give a clue to the underlying cause. If the CT scan is normal then the possibility of a non-structural focal abnormality antedating the onset of coma or being part of the coma, as occasionally happens with hypoglycaemic or hepatic encephalopathy, must be considered. If there is no focal structural abnormality on the CT scan then other investigations including metabolic and CSF examination should be carried out. Once the image has been obtained the question of more definitive therapy, be it neurosurgical, a reduction of intracranial pressure by the use of steroids and mannitol, the application of a specific antibacterial or antiviral agent, or the use of chemotherapy may be considered.

Coma with meningeal irritation but without physical signs

Patients in this group will usually be suffering from subarachnoid haemorrhage, acute bacterial meningitis, or viral meningoencephalitis. The distinction between infective and non-infective causes can usually be made on the basis of fever and a lumbar puncture which would be expected to reveal the cause. It is a counsel of perfection that because of the theoretical potential of a collection of pus or of identifying the site of a subarachnoid haemorrhage, CT should be undertaken before lumbar puncture. In practice in many hospitals throughout the United Kingdom, CT of the head is not easily available, especially in the emergency situation, and the presence of meningism, particularly if associated with fever, raises the possibility of meningitis and indicates the need for an assessment of CSF. When CSF examination is undertaken by lumbar puncture it is important to remember that an inadequate lumbar puncture does not preclude the possibility of a pressure cone but may prevent proper assessment of the CSF. Although some authorities still recommend that only a few millilitres of fluid needs to be obtained for bacterial culture and cell count,[13] in practice once the dura and arachnoid are breached by a lumbar puncture needle the possibility of herniation does not depend solely upon the fluid which is collected but rather upon that which leaks out during subsequent hours; it is therefore important that when a decision to undertake a lumbar puncture is made, sufficient CSF is obtained to enable an adequate assessment of the cell count and a gram stain and to provide fluid for culture and antibody analyses, measurement of the total protein and sugar, and possibly polymerised chain reaction (PCR) testing.

In those centres where a CT is available the detection of blood in the subarachnoid space at CT avoids the need for a lumbar puncture. Whether or not lumbar puncture has been carried out to identify the presence of subarachnoid haemorrhage, the patient should then be transferred to a neurosurgical unit, probably be given intravenous nimodipine, and be subjected to angiography and surgery if indicated. In general those patients who are in coma from subarachnoid haemorrhage are less of a surgical emergency than those who have higher states of consciousness.

The presence of coma without focal signs or meningism

These patients are likely to have a metabolic or anoxic cause for the coma; one of the commonest causes remains that of drug overdose and it is appropriate to withdraw blood to send to the toxicology laboratories from patients presenting in this way. In general there will be a clue from the circumstances in which the patient was discovered and from the previous history. Reliance is placed upon the assessment of metabolic and toxic metabolites in the blood and evidence should be sought for hepatic failure, renal failure, hyperglycaemia, hypoglycaemia, and disturbances of electrolytes or acidosis. Most commonly available drugs can now be assayed within the blood and serum enzymes should also be estimated. Problems inevitably arise when patients who are conscious have been consuming alcohol and an assessment of the relevant importance of this in causing the unconsciousness may be difficult. Again the problem may be helped by the expedient of measuring the blood alcohol level.

Perhaps the most important single cause of unresponsiveness, which is directly treatable and correctable, is that of hypoglycaemia. This should have already been corrected during initial resuscitation of the patient. By this time in management the formal level of blood sugar will have been estimated and appropriate treatment for hypo- and hyperglycaemia may be instituted. The treatment of acid–base abnormalities will require not only routine biochemistry but also arterial blood gas analyses to monitor progress. Usually a patient who has suffered from hypoxia or ischaemia will have been identified by the mode of presentation and by the normality of investigations thus far. The possibility of poisoning with carbon monoxide should be considered and excluded by measurement of carboxyhaemoglobin. In general patients who have suffered from anoxic and ischaemic insults should be given 100% oxygen and the monitoring of Pao_2 will be important together with the maintenance of adequate circulation and oxygenation. Patients who are in shock or hypertensive encephalopathy will be diagnosed by the level of blood pressure and those with disturbed temperature regulation by the use of a thermometer. A rectal thermometer may be required. These causes can be corrected.

In patients with drug overdose the possibility of using specific antidotes should be considered: naloxone in patients in whom there is a high index of suspicion of opiate poisoning and benzodiazepine antagonists in self-poisoning with benzodiazepines. The use of analeptic agents in barbiturate poisoning cannot now be supported.[32] Consideration should also be given to clearing the ingested toxin from the stomach. The passage of a nasogastric tube should usually be considered and this is one indication for intubation of the trachea to prevent the risk of aspiration. The importance of the diagnosis of drug overdose coma is that such patients have a good prognosis provided that they are given adequate respiratory and circulatory support during their unconsciousness. They are, however, particularly liable to show sudden depression of brain stem responses and if the possibility of drug overdose is not considered their level of coma may be misinterpreted and their prognosis might be thought to be unduly pessimistic.

Prediction of outcome in coma

Having made an assessment of the cause of coma, established its severity, and introduced appropriate treatment, the physician should be able to prognosticate the likely outcome to colleagues and to friends and relatives of the patient. Sedative drugs or alcohol overdose is not usually lethal and carries a good prognosis provided that circulation and respiration are protected. The physician can reasonably give a good prognosis in patients suffering from self-poisoning with sedative drugs provided that the complications of cardiac dysrhythmia, aspiration pneumonia and respiratory arrest are avoided or corrected. In non-traumatic coma other than that which is drug induced, those factors that determine the outcome have been defined[33] and include the cause of coma, the depth of coma, the duration of coma, and certain clinical signs, among the most relevant of which are brain stem reflexes. Overall only 15% of patients with non-traumatic coma for more than 6 hours will make a good or moderate recovery; the other 85% will die, remain vegetative, or reach a state of severe disability in which they remain dependent.

Patients whose coma is due to metabolic factors, including infections, organ failure, and biochemical disturbances, have a better prognosis. Thirty-five per cent of patients will achieve moderate or good recovery; of those whose coma follows hypoxic-ischaemic insult only 11% will make such a recovery; of those in coma due to cerebrovascular disease only 7% can be expected to make such a recovery. Twenty per cent of patients in coma following a hypoxic-ischaemic injury will enter the vegetative state due to the likelihood of hypoxic ischaemia resulting in bihemispheric damage with relative sparing of the brain stem.

Apart from the diagnosis, the depth of coma affects the individual prognosis. Those patients not showing eye opening after 6 hours of coma have only a 10% chance of making a good or moderate recovery whereas those who eye open in response to painful stimuli have a 20% chance of making a good recovery. The longer the coma persists the less likely there is to be recovery; 15% of patients in coma for 6 hours make a good or moderate recovery, compared with only 3% who remain unconscious for one week.[34]

A study of 500 patients reported by Levy *et al.*[34] using prospective data from patients with clearly defined levels of coma, diagnoses, and outcomes showed that some clinical signs are significantly associated with poor prognosis: in the total cohort of 500 patients, corneal reflexes were absent 24 hours after the onset of coma in 90 patients and this sign was incompatible with survival. In a more uniform group who suffered anoxic injury there were 210 patients: 52 of these had no pupillary reflex for 24 hours, all of whom died by the third day; 70 were left with a motor response poorer than withdrawal and all died by the seventh day; the absence of roving eye movements was seen in 16 patients, all of whom died. The 95% confidence intervals for all of these criteria are given in Table 1.2.

Table 1.2 Clinical signs and prognosis

Time	Sign	Cohort	Patients with the sign	False-positive survivors	95% confidence interval (%)
24 hours	Absent corneal response	500	90	0	0–5
24 hours	Absent pupillary response	210	52	0	0–5
3 days	Motor poorer than withdrawal	210	70	0	0–5
7 days	Absent roving eye movements	210	16	0	0–5

Summarised from Levy et al.[34]

At the opposite end of the scale more than 25% of patients who show roving conjugate eye movements within 6 hours of the onset of coma or who show withdrawal responses to pain or eye opening to pain, will recover independence and make a moderate or good recovery. The use of combinations of clinical signs helps to improve the accuracy of prognosis: at 24 hours the absence of corneal responses, pupillary light reaction, or caloric or doll's eye response is not compatible with recovery to independence. Patients who are able to speak words within 24 hours or who show nystagmus on caloric testing are likely to make a good recovery (Table 1.3).[35]

A recent reassessment of this data to present the individual signs with their sensitivity and specificity may be helpful in aiding prognosis in the individual patient (Table 1.4).[36]

The most accurate prediction of outcome in a patient in medical coma is still that which is obtained from the use of clinical signs. There is little to be added by more sophisticated testing other than identifying the cause of the coma. It is possible to predict those patients who will not make a recovery and who will die in coma or who will enter a vegetative state within the first week of coma. It is rare for patients in medical coma who are in a vegetative state at one month to show any form of recovery.[37]

Table 1.3 Prediction of outcome of coma at 24 hours by a combination of clinical signs

	No. of patients	Percentage of patients with different outcomes		
		D/PVS	SD	MD/GR
500 patients				
Any two reacting: Pupils Corneals Oculovestibular — No	120	97	2	1
Motor better than flaccid — No	83	80	8	12
Motor withdrawal — No	135	69	14	17
Verbal moans — No	106	58	19	23
Verbal moans — Yes	56	46	13	41

Summarised from Levy et al.[34]
D/PVS = death or vegetative; SD = severe disability; MD/GR = moderate or good recovery.

Continuation of care

The long term care of patients in coma may be undertaken in an intensive care unit, on a specialist ward, or in a rehabilitation unit or long stay hospital. It is important that those patients in whom prognosis is hopeless should not be permanently exposed to the rigors of intensive care medicine,

Table 1.4 Sensitivity and specificity of individual signs

	Severe disability or worse	Moderate or good recovery	Sensitivity	Specificity	Positive predictive value	Negative predictive value	Likelihood ratio (positive test)	Likelihood ratio (negative test)
Verbal response								
Incomprehensible or none	187	45	0·96	0·26	0·81	0·67	1·30	0·16
Orientated, confused, or inappropriate	8	16						
Eye opening response								
To pain/none	270	42	0·89	0·48	0·87	0·53	1·69	0·24
Spontaneous/to noise	34	38						
Pupillary light reflex								
Absent	78	1	C·26	0·99	0·99	0·26	20·59	0·75
Present	225	79						
Corneal reflex								
Absent	90	0	0·32	1·00	1·00	0·29	20*	0·68
Present	190	77						
Spontaneous eye movements								
Roving dysconjugate, other or none	210	19	0·69	0·77	0·92	0·40	2·94	0·40
Orienting or roving conjugate	94	62						

(Continued)

Table 1.4 (Continued)

	Severe disability or worse	Moderate or good recovery	Sensitivity	Specificity	Positive predictive value	Negative predictive value	Likelihood ratio (positive test)	Likelihood ratio (negative test)
Oculocephalic responses								
Abnormal/absent	292	61	0·96	0·24	0·83	0·59	1·26	0·18
Normal	13	19						
Oculovestibular responses								
Abnormal	265	45	0·96	0·32	0·85	0·64	1·40	0·14
Normal	12	21						
Motor responses (best limb)								
Flexion, extension or none	206	15	0·68	0·81	0·93	0·40	3·66	0·40
Obeying, localising or withdrawing	98	66						
Deep tendon reflexes								
Absent	67	4	0·24	0·95	0·94	0·26	4·67	0·80
Present	213	74						
Skeletal muscle tone								
Absent	120	8	0·44	0·89	0·94	0·30	3·98	0·63
Present	155	65						

*Not able to calculate exactly.

but should continue to receive basic care within routine hospital wards or a more long stay environment. So long as patients are considered to have a potential for recovery they should be looked after in intensive care units or in specialist wards. Their respiration, skin, circulation, and bladder and bowel function need attention, seizures must be controlled, and the level of consciousness should be regularly assessed and monitored. It is important that the mobility of joints and circulation to pressure areas are maintained during the long term care of the patient and the possibility of aspiration pneumonia, peptic ulceration, and other complications of long term intensive care need to be considered. Techniques such as mechanical ventilation and steroid therapy are not to be used routinely in the management of a comatose patient as they do not improve prognosis and may compromise recovery.[36]

Persistent vegetative state

The relative resilience of the brain stem allows it to survive injuries that may create irreversible damage to the cerebral hemispheres – then the patient will enter that state defined as "vegetative". Retrospectively, after post-mortem examination, it may be possible to identify massive neocortical damage which will indicate that the patient was permanently in the vegetative state,[37] but there are no clinical or laboratory means of confirming this before post-mortem examination and therefore the term "persistent vegetative state" has been used clinically. Specialists in rehabilitation are concerned that physicians may take the attitude that there is no point in treating such patients, therefore creating a self-fulfilling prophecy of poor prognosis, no treatment, and poor outcome.[38]

There is continuing debate as to the potential for recovery for patients who are in a vegetative state. In patients who have suffered non-traumatic injuries such as anoxia and ischaemia, the prognosis for recovery from the vegetative state is poor after the first few weeks and almost negligible after 6 months.[39,40] There are some reports of patients who suffered coma as a result of head trauma and in whom an improvement from the vegetative state has been recognised after months, but these anecdotal cases of recovery are difficult to validate and it seems possible that such patients were not truly vegetative but rather in a state of profound disability with cognition at the beginning of the observation.[41–43]

Investigations are of little help in identifying the vegetative state because many types of EEG pattern have been recorded from near normality to a flat record. CT scans usually show considerable cortical atrophy with ventricular dilatation after the disease has been present for some time. Somatosensory evoked responses are said to show loss of the cortical component, and positron emission tomography (PET) shows cortical metabolic underactivity. None is diagnostic in its results.[44]

Patients in a persisting vegetative state will often have received artificial ventilation at some time during their initial coma or resuscitation but they are not truly respirator dependent and, as they are able to breathe, are only dependent upon carers for the supply of liquid and nutrients, and the prevention of complications. The management of individual patients will depend upon circumstances, other aspects of the diagnosis, and consideration of prognosis.[45] There is recent advice from the Royal Colleges in the UK[9] and an international working party[46] on the diagnosis and management of the permanent vegetative state and the involvement of the courts in the withdrawal of artificial hydration and nutrition. A recent review of the diagnosis of the permanent vegetative state and the law foresees potential problems in relation to human rights legislation.[47–49]

Management of medical coma

- The initial care for a patient in coma must be resuscitation by ensuring adequate oxygenation and circulation. A sample of blood should be withdrawn to estimate glucose and other parameters and, once stability is ensured, it is imperative to obtain an adequate history from those who brought the patient to the accident and emergency department or those who are responsible for the previous care.
- An assessment of the level of coma follows with an evaluation of those other features that may give clues to aetiology, including temperature, heart rate, blood pressure, pattern of respiration, abnormalities in the skin, and focal signs in the chest, abdomen, or limbs.
- Neurological examination must include a search for evidence of trauma, tests for meningism, examination of the fundi, assessment of the brain stem reflexes, and the identification of any focal abnormality in face or limbs.

- The relevant investigations may then be considered, including biochemical and serological assessments, drug levels, radiological imaging, and the possibility of EEG. Lumbar puncture will be indicated in certain circumstances and, with these investigations, the diagnosis of the aetiology of the coma should be established, corrective therapies instituted, and continuation of care and protection established.
- Most patients presenting to hospital in coma or lapsing into coma are ideally treated on an intensive care unit or a high dependency unit. The cause of the coma and the prognosis of the patient will determine their further follow up and the site of continuing care.
- After 6 hours of coma patients who do not show eye opening have only a 10% chance of making a good or moderate recovery.
- After one week of coma only 3% make a good or moderate recovery.

References

1   Bates C, Cartlidge NEF. The prognosis of medical coma. In: Tunbridge WMG, ed. *Advanced medicine*. London: Pitman Medical, 1981.
2   Plum F, Posner JB. *The diagnosis of stupor and coma*, 2nd edn. Philadelphia: Davis, 1980.
3   Brodal A. *Neurological anatomy in relation to clinical medicine*, 3rd edn. Oxford: Oxford University Press, 1981.
4   Jouvet M. The role of monoamines and acetyl choline containing neurones in the regulation of the sleep/wake cycle. *Rev Physiol* 1972;**64**:166–307.
5   Defedudis FV. Cholinergic roles in consciousness. In: Defedudis FV, ed. *Central cholinergic systems and behaviour*. London: Academic Press, 1974.
6   Tinuper P. Idiopathic recurring stupor: a case with possible involvement of the gamma amniobutric acid (GABA) ergic system. *Ann Neurol* 1992;**31**:503–6.
7   Medical Research Council Brain Injuries Committee. *A glossary of psychological terms commonly used in cases of head injury. MRC War Memorandum*. London: HMSO, 1941.
8   Teasdale G, Jennett WB. Assessment of coma and impaired consciousness: a practical scale. *Lancet* 1974;**ii**:81–4.
9   Working group of the Royal Colleges. The permanent vegetative state. *J R Coll Phys* 1996;**30**:119–21.
10 Jennett WB, Plum F. The persistent vegetative state: a syndrome in search of a name. *Lancet* 1972;**i**:734–7.
11 Cairns H. Disturbances of consciousness with lesions of the brain stem and diencephalon. *Brain* 1952;**75**:109–46.
12 Feldman MH. Physiological observations in a chronic case of locked-in syndrome. *Neurology* 1971;**21**:459–78.
13 Harris JO, Berger JR. Clinical approach to stupor and coma. In: Bradley WG, Daroff RB, Fenichel GM, Marsden CD, eds. *Neurology in clinical practice*. London: Butterworth, 1991.
14 Fisher CM. The neurological examination of the comatose patient. *Acta Neurol Scand* 1969;**45**(suppl 46):1–56.
15 Crill WE. Horner's syndrome secondary to deep cerebral lesions. *Neurology* 1966;**16**:325–7.

16 Walsh FB, Hoyt WF. *Clinical neuro-ophthalmology*, 3rd edn. Baltimore: Williams and Wilkins, 1969.

17 Stewart JD, Kirkham TH, Matthieson G. Periodic alternating gaze. *Neurology* 1979;**29**:222–4.

18 Daroff RB, Hoyt FB. Supranuclear disorders of ocular control systems in man. In: Bach-y-rita P, Collins CC, Hyde G, eds. *The control of eye movements*. New York: Academic Press, 1971.

19 Fisher CM. Ocular bobbing. *Arch Neurol* 1964;**11**:543–6.

20 Lee RJ, Shaw DA. Rapid regular breathing in unconscious patients. *Arch Neurol* 1967;**33**:356–61.

21 Bateman DE. Neurology assessment of coma. *J Neurol Neurosurg Psychiatry* 2001;**71**(suppl 1):13–17.

22 Jorgensen EO, Malcohw-Moller A. Natural history of global and critical brain ischaemia. *Resuscitation* 1981;**9**:133–91.

23 Synec VM. EEG abnormality grades and sub-divisions of prognostic importance in traumatic and anoxic coma in adults. *Clin Electroencephalograph* 199;**19**:160–6.

24 Engle J, Ludwig BI, Fetell M. Prolonged partial complex status epilepticus: EEG and behavioural observations. *Neurology* 1978;**28**:863–9.

25 Bassetti C, Bomeo F, Mathis J, Hess CW. Early prognosis in coma after cardiac arrest: a prospective clinical, electrophysiological and biochemical study of 60 patients. *J Neurol Neurosurg Psychiatry* 1996;**61**: 610–15.

26 Papanicolou AC, Loring CW, Eisenberg HM, *et al.* Auditory brain stem evoked responses in comatose head injury patients. *Neurosurgery* 1986;**18**:173–5.

27 Walser H, Emry M, Jenzer R. Somato sensory evoked potentials in comatosed patients: correlation with outcome and neuropathological findings. *J Neurol* 1968;**233**:34–40.

28 Tasker RC, Matthew DJ, Kendal B. Computed tomograph in the assessment of raised intracranial pressure in non-traumatic coma. *Neuro Paediatrics* 1990;**21**:91–4.

29 Jaggi JL, Obrist WD, Jennarelli TA, Langfitt TW. Relationship of early cerebral flow and metabolism to outcome in acute head injury. *J Neurosurg* 1990;**72**:176–182.

30 Rone RO, Somer H, Cast EM, *et al.* Neurological outcome after out of hospital cardiac arrest: prediction by cerebro-spinal fluid enzyme analysis. *Arch Neurol* 1989;**46**:753–6.

31 Hans P, Albert A, Fransen C, Born J. Improved outcome prediction based on CSF extrapolated creatine kinase BB isoenzyme activity and other risk factors in severe head injury. *J Neurosurg* 1989;**71**:54–8.

32 Adams RD, Victor M. *Principles of neurology*, 4th edn. New York: McGraw Hill, 1989.

33 Schwartz GB. Emergency toxicology and general principles of medical management of the poisoned patient. In Schwartz GB, Safar P, Stone N, Kayten CG, Birch NG, eds. *Principles and Practice of Emergency Medicine*. London: WB Saunders, 1978.

34 Levy DE, Bates D, Carona JJ, et al. Prognosis in non-traumatic coma. *Ann Intern Med* 1981;**94**:293–301.

35 Bates D. Coma. In: Swash M, Oxberry J, eds. *Clinical neurology*. Edinburgh: Churchill Livingstone, 1991.

36 Overell J, Bone I, Fuller GN. An aid to predicting the prognosis in patients with non-traumatic coma for one day. *J Neurol Neurosurg Psychiatry* 2001;**71**(suppl 1):24–5.

37 Bates D. Defining prognosis in medical coma. *J Neurol Neurosurg Psychiatry* 1991;**54**:569–71.

38 Teasdale G. Prognosis of coma after head injury. In: Tunbridge WMG, ed. *Advanced Medicine*. London: Pitman Medical, 1981.

39 Dougherty JH, Donald MD, Rawlinson DG, et al. Hypoxic-ischaemic brain injury in the vegetative state. *Neurology* 1981;**31**:991–7.

40 Andrews K. Managing the persistent vegetative state. *Br Med J* 1992;**305**: 486–7.

41 The Multi-society Task Force on PVS. Medical aspects of the persistent vegetative state. *N Engl J Med* 1994;**330**:1499–1508.

42 The Multi-society Task Force on PVS. Medical aspects of the persistent vegetative state. *N Engl J Med* 1994;**330**:1572–9.

43 May PG, Kailbing R. Coma of over a year's duration with favourable outcome. *Dis Nerv Syst* 1968;**29**:837–40.

44 Rosenberg GA, Johnson SF, Brenner RP. Recovery of cognition after prolonged vegetative state. *Ann Neurol* 1977;**2**:167–8.

45 Snyder BD, Cranford RE, Reubens AB. Delayed recovery from post-anoxic persistent vegetative state. *Ann Neurol* 1993;**14**:152–3.

46 Hansotia TI. Persistent vegetative state. *Arch Neurol* 1985;**42**:1048–52.

47 ANA Committee on Ethical Affairs. Persistent vegetative state: report of the American Neurology Association Committee on Ethical Affairs. *Ann Neurol* 1993;**33**:386–90.

48 *The international Working Party Report on the Vegetative State*. London: The Royal Hospital for Neuro-Disability, 1996.

49 McLean SAM. Permanent vegetative state and the law. *J Neurol Neurosurg Psychiatry*. 2001;**71**(suppl 1):26–27.

2: Traumatic brain injury

PETER JD ANDREWS

As widely appreciated, outcome after traumatic brain injury depends upon the initial severity of the injury, age, the extent of any subsequent complications, and how these are managed. Much of the early management of traumatic brain injury falls upon emergency room staff, primary care and ambulance services being involved prior to hospital admission. Of the many patients who attend hospital after a traumatic brain injury, most do not develop life threatening complications in the acute stage. However, in a small but important subgroup, outcome is made worse by failure to detect promptly and deal adequately with complications.

There is of course no debate about the effectiveness of surgical removal of an acute compressive intracranial haematoma, nor the interventions required to correct hypotension or hypoxia. Much of the debate surrounding management of patients with traumatic brain injury is instead focused on methods used to identify the patients at risk and provision of appropriate care, including utilisation of investigations, clinical observations required, and determination of the most appropriate site(s) of such care.

There has clearly been an improvement in the outcome of patients who have sustained a traumatic brain injury (TBI) in recent years. None the less, many clinicians still believe that there has been little real progress in this area. It should be emphasised that mortality after severe (coma inducing) TBI has fallen from around 50% to 25% over the past 20 years. Further those who survive are less likely to remain severely disabled than in the past.

Epidemiology

Traumatic brain injury severe enough to necessitate hospital admission has an incidence of between 100 and 400 per 100 000 population per year in both Europe and North America.[1] Head injuries are among the most common types of trauma seen in North American emergency departments, with an estimated one million cases seen annually.[2] "Minor" head injury (sometimes known as "mild") is defined by a history of loss of consciousness, amnesia, or disorientation in a patient who is conscious and talking, that is, with a Glasgow Coma Scale score of 13–15 (Table 2.1). The most common causes are road traffic accidents, falls,[3] assaults, sports injuries,[4] and domestic accidents.[5] Legislation and public health measures have helped reduce the incidence, by restricting blood alcohol levels while driving, mandating the wearing of seat belts, demanding protective helmets for construction workers and motor and pedal cyclists,[6] limiting traffic speeds, and encouraging increasing use of SRS (Supplementary Restraint System) airbags in modern cars. Males are affected by TBI twice as often as females, with a peak incidence between the ages of 15 and 35, with lesser peaks in children and the elderly.

The importance of injury as a major public health problem worldwide was highlighted in the seminal report "The Global Burden of Disease". Worldwide, injuries account for approximately one in eight deaths among males and one in 14 deaths among females. Motor vehicle injuries alone constitute the ninth leading cause of disease burden as measured by the number of associated disability-adjusted life years. By the year 2020, motor vehicle injuries are projected to increase in rank to third in the global burden.[7]

Since this population of patients is largely made up of young males, the economic cost of survival of dependent patients is great. Up to half of all head-injured patients admitted to hospital remain disabled at one year. The combination of this factor and young age make the economic burden greater than in, for example, stroke.

Mechanisms of brain injury

Haematomas occur in association with primary injury of varying severity, and can present in an alert, oriented patient, or in a deeply unconscious patient with a life threatening primary injury. They are a consequence of the primary impact but are often delayed in development.

Extradural haematoma

An extradural haematoma is formed when the inner layer of dura is stripped from the skull, with tearing of the meningeal artery, as a result of deformation or fracture of the skull. Seventy per cent of such haematomas occur in the temporal or parietal regions, as this is where the fracture crosses the path of the middle meningeal artery. Ten per cent occur in less obvious locations, such as the posterior fossa, where the fracture tears the sinus producing a venous haemorrhage, or the frontal region, from a small meningeal arterial haemorrhage. The clinical presentation may be abrupt in the former instance, associated with sudden loss of consciousness and respiratory arrest, or in the latter, insidious over 72 hours. One in five patients present with a "lucid interval", that is, improvement in conscious level following a TBI severe enough to cause concussion. Early surgical evacuation generally leads to a good recovery (Figure 2.1a).

Acute subdural haematoma

Acute subdural haematomas appear after high speed road traffic accidents, falls, or assaults. They occur experimentally after angular acceleration/deceleration, concentrating injury on vascular elements on the brain surface. They are commonly associated with other parenchymal injuries, which may affect outcome as much as the haematoma itself (Figure 2.1b). Ipsilateral and contralateral skull fractures are common. The haematoma often occurs over the temporal pole, either from tearing of bridging veins or from laceration of the brain and disruption of surface arteries. Arterial bleeding can occasionally produce the clinical picture of lucid interval before deterioration into coma. The common combination of temporal lobe laceration and contusion with an associated subdural haematoma is known as "burst temporal lobe". The typical clinical presentation is one of a focal neurological deficit with or without lowered level of consciousness but with deterioration a few days after injury. Such deterioration is often due to temporal lobe swelling rather than to increase in the size of the haematoma itself.

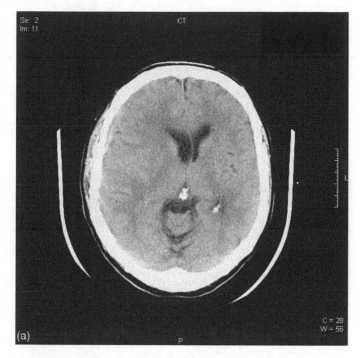

Figure 2.1 (a) An extradural haematoma is formed when the inner layer of dura is stripped from the skull, tearing the meningeal artery, and results from deformation or fracture of the skull.

Seventy per cent of haematomas occur in the temporal or parietal regions, as this is where the fracture crosses the path of the middle meningeal artery. One in five patients presents with a "lucid interval"; that is, a traumatic brain injury severe enough to cause concussion, followed by improvement in conscious level. Early evacuation leads to good recovery

Intraparenchymal injury: haematomas and contusions

Intraparenchymal haematomas result from disruption of vascular elements within the brain. They may be focal, as from a penetrating injury, or diffuse from rotational acceleration, which may produce widespread haemorrhage and axonal disruption (Figure 2.1c). Severe diffuse axonal injury may be associated with haemorrhage into the basal ganglia and

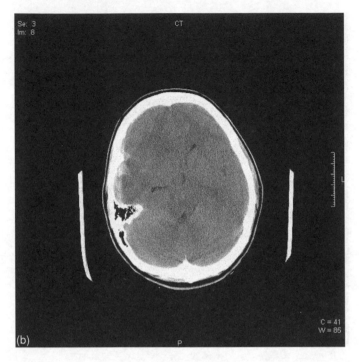

Figure 2.1 (b) Patients with an acute subdural haematoma are seen after high speed road traffic accidents, falls, or assaults. They are commonly associated with other parenchymal injuries, which may affect outcome as much as the haematoma itself.

The haematoma often occurs over the temporal pole either from tearing of bridging veins, or from laceration of the brain and disruption of surface arteries. The common combination of temporal lobe laceration and contusion with an associated subdural haematoma is known as "burst temporal lobe"

disruption of autoregulation of blood flow. Penetrating injury may be clinically silent, or produce focal neurological deficit, due either to the haematoma or to the underlying neuronal injury. Focal contusions occur both ipsilateral and contralateral to a fracture, as for example bifrontal contusions complicating an occipital fracture. As with subdural haematoma, delayed deterioration may occur in a patient with a brain contusion or intraparenchymal haematoma days after the injury.

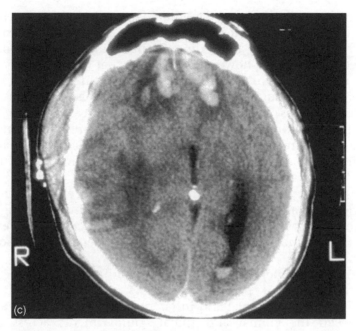

Figure 2.1 (c) Intraparenchymal haematomas occur from disruption of vascular elements.

This may be focal from a penetrating injury, or diffuse from rotational acceleration, producing widespread haemorrhage and axonal disruption. Penetrating injury may be clinically silent, or produce focal neurological deficit, due either to the haematoma or the underlying neuronal injury. Focal contusions occur both ipsilateral and contralateral to a fracture, for example, bifrontal contusions complicating an occipital fracture

Brain swelling and raised intracranial pressure

Intracranial pressure increases as a consequence of a rapidly developing intracranial mass lesion, hypoxia, hypercarbia, during an epileptic seizure, and in acute hydrocephalus. Brain oedema is defined as an increase in brain volume due to increase in brain water content. Klatzo defined it as "vasogenic"[8] because of disruption of the blood–brain barrier and escape of water and plasma into the extracellular compartment, in contrast to "cytotoxic oedema" in which a noxious factor produces intracellular swelling without increased vascular permeability.[9,10] The oedema around a contusion or haematoma was initially thought to be vasogenic; protein rich fluid leaking into the extracellular space, increasing the water and sodium in the brain to produce "mass effect". Marmarou, however, has shown that most of the water in areas of brain contusion is in fact intracellular and represents "cellular" oedema, caused by ischaemia.[11] This in turn produces astrocytic swelling and increased release of excitatory amino acids and a consequent failure of membrane ion pumps and cellular ionic homoeostasis. This is recognisable radiographically as an increase in the signal on T2 weighted MRI and as radiolucent areas on CT.

Alternatively, brain injury may lead to cerebrovascular congestion and an excess cerebral blood volume, resulting in cerebral hyperaemia, that is, an absolute or relative increase in the cerebral blood flow in relation to cerebral metabolic demand.

The consequence of raised intracranial pressure is the development of pressure gradients across the midline, between supratentorial and infratentorial compartments, and between the cranial and spinal compartments across the foramen magnum. In 1965 Langfitt showed how raised supratentorial pressure produces a rise in infratentorial pressure which subsequently plateaus and falls as the cisterna ambiens becomes blocked by tentorial herniation. The brain is shifted away from the region of higher pressure, so midline structures are pushed laterally, causing the cingulate gyrus to herniate under the fixed free edge of the falx. This distorts the pericallosal arteries, and may occlude the foramen of Munro. The cerebrospinal fluid (CSF) drainage of the contralateral ventricle is obstructed, so the ventricle dilates; the ipsilateral ventricle may become compressed, giving characteristic features suggesting raised intracranial pressure (ICP) on cross-sectional imaging. Further increases in ICP produce tentorial herniation, with a temporal or parietal lesion compression of the ipsilateral oculomotor nerve and midbrain. Further distortion leads to posterior cerebral artery compression. Bilateral or frontal lesions produce posterior herniation, compressing the tectal plate, resulting in failure of upward gaze and bilateral pupillary abnormalities. Infratentorial masses or further herniation of a supratentorial mass results in herniation through the foramen magnum. As the medulla and cerebellar tonsils are pushed inferiorly, distortion of the vasomotor and respiratory centres leads to circulatory collapse and respiratory arrest.

Pathophysiology

Mechanisms of primary brain injury after trauma

The primary injury, which can be correlated with prolonged coma and impaired motor response, was recognised by Strich in 1961 as a diffuse degeneration of the subcortical matter, subsequently termed diffuse axonal injury (DAI). Experimental work with primates confirms this to be a consequence of inertial loading of the head, with prolonged coronal angular acceleration. Microscopic pathological findings consist of small haemorrhages in the corpus callosum, septum pellucidum, deep grey matter of the cerebral hemisphere, and dorsilateral quadrant of midbrain and pons. Disrupted and swollen axons with globular ends known as "retraction balls of Cajal" are observed at an early stage. After a few weeks clusters of neuroglia form around the severed axons and wallerian degeneration of fibre tracts occurs.[12] Clinically, diffuse axonal injury is thought to be responsible for a broad spectrum of injury from mild concussion in which no structural lesion can be demonstrated and complete clinical recovery ensues, to prolonged coma and death in instances of much greater angular acceleration.

The events leading to axonal disruption have recently been examined. Povlishock and others have shown that this is a process requiring several hours to complete and may be reversible before frank axonal disruption occurs, at least in some axons.[13]

It should of course be stressed that not all primary injury is diffuse. Focal contusions and lacerations are seen, especially after falls and blows to the head, often involving the inferior (orbital) surface of the frontal lobes and the anterior poles of the temporal lobes. Brain oedema around contusions may lead to late clinical deterioration as a result of mass effect and brain shift.

Mechanisms of secondary brain injury after trauma

Secondary brain injury follows after primary damage, either as a consequence of the TBI itself, or due to systemic injury or "insult". TBI can be responsible for the development of an intracranial haematoma, brain swelling, raised intracranial pressure, and ischaemia, all of which may be worsened by systemic hypoxia, hypotension, or pyrexia.

Ischaemia

Since Douglas Miller[14,15] and others showed the strong relationship between deranged physiology, which would likely reduce brain oxygen delivery, and outcome, and the autopsy evidence of near universal, widespread, ischaemic brain damage after fatal head injury, investigators have sought to determine the causal pathophysiological mechanisms involved.

Cerebral perfusion pressure

Cerebral blood flow has been found to change passively with cerebral perfusion pressures (CPP) after head injuries of differing severity, suggesting that autoregulation is impaired. However, the cerebrovascular response to changes in arterial Pa_{CO_2} is often preserved. One explanation of pressure passive changes is that the autoregulatory curve has been shifted to the right, so that the minimum acceptable CPP needs to be higher than normal to ensure cerebral blood flow. Jugular venous oxygen saturation data and transcranial Doppler middle cerebral artery flow velocity studies suggest this threshold is a CPP of 70 mmHg, whether due to raised ICP or reduced arterial pressure. A shift of the autoregulatory curve due to a generalised increase in cerebral vascular resistance after TBI may be due to artificial ventilation or spontaneous hyperventilation. Alternatively, the absence or overproduction of luminal and abluminal modulators, such as endothelin and nitric oxide, may contribute to an autoregulatory threshold shift.[16,17]

Arterial hypotension

Arterial hypotension can occur immediately after trauma due to other injuries such as haemorrhage, cardiac tamponade, haemopneumothorax, myocardial or spinal cord injury. Experimental models of diffuse brain injury such as the impact acceleration model[18] produce transient hypotension for minutes after severe injury. Intrinsic myocardial disease, inadequate fluid replacement after osmotic diuretics, aggressive hyperventilation, and anaesthetic drugs (such as barbiturates and proprofol) can all contribute. Sepsis may further conspire to lower the blood pressure.

Pyrexia

Pyrexia is defined as a body temperature of greater than 37°C and is common following TBI. There has been much recent interest in the incidence, associations, pathogenesis, affect on outcome, and management. The incidence of pyrexia of greater than 38°C in the first 72 hours following TBI has been reported to be as high as 68% in closed head injury.[19] Fever most commonly occurs in patients with closed head injury and intracranial haemorrhage, with the risk increasing with prolonged hospital stay (93% of patients staying longer than 14 days).[20]

In many patients it is difficult to determine whether an increase in temperature is a consequence of their brain injury, coexisting conditions, or their treatment. Evidence for infection was found in 74% of the febrile patients and 50% of the afebrile patients. This makes it difficult to determine whether there is a causative relationship between hyperthermia and poor outcome, or purely an association.[21] Indeed, previously published TBI data showed pyrexia to be prognostically important, but limitations of the modelling process failed to highlight that pyrexia was associated with a *favourable* outcome.[22,23]

Several early studies demonstrated an association between fever and a poorer outcome following TBI. More recently there have been attempts to quantify the impact of hyperthermia on outcome. In the paediatric population early hyperthermia was found to be an independent predictor of poor outcome (OR 4·7) and prolonged ICU admission.

Pilot studies supported the view that hypothermia would be beneficial.[24] However, a well constructed randomised controlled trial has recently disproved this promising intervention. Patients in the hypothermia group showed no benefit in functional recovery[25] and required more interventions to support their systemic circulation. Treatment with hypothermia, with the body temperature reaching 33°C within eight hours after injury, is not effective in improving outcomes in patients with severe brain injury.[26–28]

Hypoxia

Finally, pulmonary disorders (atelectasis, contusion, infection, or acute respiratory distress syndrome) and a reduced haemoglobin oxygen carrying capacity (anaemia) may compromise tissue oxygen delivery. Reduced oxygen delivery to regions where cerebral blood flow is already compromised may of course worsen ischaemia.

Recently, researchers have combined microdialysis, which continuously monitors the chemistry of a small focal volume of the cerebral extracellular space, and positron emission tomography (PET), which conversely establishes metabolism of the whole brain for the duration of the scan. Both techniques were applied to head-injured patients simultaneously to assess the relationship between microdialysis (measures of oxygen dependent metabolism and glutamate) and PET (oxygen delivery and consumption) parameters. Hyperventilation resulted in a significant increase in oxygen extraction, in association with a reduction in glucose, but no significant change in glutamate.[29] The same researchers have reported an estimated ischaemic brain volume of up to 20% of the brain volume (DK Menon, personal communication). Therefore it is surprising that none of the microdialysis probes were able to detect changes associated with ischaemia. One reason might be that the pathology is not a simple failure of oxygen delivery, but rather a failure of oxygen utilisation.[30,31]

After traumatic brain injury it is hypothesised that there are a number of secondary biochemical processes that result in worsening of neurological damage. Excitotoxicity, free radicals, pro-inflammatory cytokines, and ecosanoids have all been shown in animal models, and some in human studies, to be involved in the processes that occur after traumatic injury to the brain.

Excitotoxicity

The excitatory amino acids aspartate and glutamate are released in a threshold manner in response to a reduction in cerebral blood flow (CBF < 20 ml 100 g^{-1}/min^{-1}) and produce rapid cell death (3–5 minutes) via activation of the N-methyl D-aspartate (NMDA) receptor and associated Ca^{2+} ion channel. Excitotoxicity may be mediated by an increase in inducible nitric oxide synthase (iNOS) in astrocytes and microglia, NO then forming a "super-radical" after interaction with O$_2$ free radicals.[32]

The use of antagonists at the NMDA receptor complex has been the subject of extensive investigation; these have failed to show a significant improvement (>10%) in the primary end point for each study. Explanations for such results include: poor study design; confounding influence of systemic secondary insults; and sensitivity of outcome measures.[33] As excitatory amino acids may have a role in hyperglycolysis after TBI, interest in this potential mechanism of neuronal injury persists.

Inflammation

Following acute brain injury there is increased intracranial production of cytokines, with activation of inflammatory cascades. McKeating *et al.* have shown a transcranial 11 : 1 cytokine gradient in the sera of TBI patients requiring intensive care after acute brain injury.[34,35]

Adhesion molecules control the migration of leucocytes into tissue after injury and this process may result in still further cellular damage. After TBI altered serum concentrations of soluble intercellular adhesion molecule (sICAM)-1 and soluble L-selectin (sL-selectin) can be correlated with injury severity and neurological outcome.[36–38]

Despite the strong association demonstrated between these soluble adhesion molecule concentrations in serum and severity of injury and outcome, there have been no successful attempts to beneficially modify this complex process. A phase III trial is recruiting patients to receive Dexanabinol (HU-211).[39] This is a cannabinoid with a diffuse range of actions, including anti-inflammatory effects. The intracranial pressure data from the phase II trial support further investigation of this compound. The treatment group (phase II)[40] had significantly less intracranial pressure problems on the second and third postinjury days, suggesting that the agent may have modified oedema formation. However, the outcome data were confounded by imbalanced randomisation, resulting in more patients having motor score 2 (extension) in the placebo group. The Glasgow Coma Scale (GCS) is not linear and such patients are much less likely to improve than patients who have motor score 3 or better. Therefore, the randomisation resulted in bias that cannot be "balanced" by more GCS 7 patients.

Free radicals

Direct biochemical evidence for free radical damage and lipid peroxidation in human injury of the central nervous system (CNS) is hampered by methodological difficulties. However, indirect evidence suggests a key role for oxygen radicals. CNS injury results in decompartmentalisation of iron from ferritin, transferrin, and haemoglobin, and Fe^{2+} catalyses reactions to give free radicals.

Eicosanoids

Normal cellular function relies upon transitory activation of enzymes by Ca^{2+}. If this Ca^{2+} signal is excessive, dysfunctional activation of phospholipases, non-lysomal proteases, protein kinases and phosphatases, endonucleases, and NO synthase will ensue. The activation of phospholipases releases free fatty acids which, in excess, cause increased mitochondrial membrane permeability to protons and uncouple oxidative phosphorylation. Activation of phospholipase A_2 produces excess arachadonic acid (AA), inducing endothelial dysfunction and derangement of the blood–brain barrier. Moreover, the oxidation of AA by cyclo-oxygenase and lipoxygenase pathways results in excess production of eicosanoids with free radical properties and adverse effects upon the microvasculature. The resultant effect is vasoderegulation, worsening ischaemia, and microvascular thrombosis.

Indirect evidence for the role of failure of calcium homoeostasis after head injury comes from the prospective randomised controlled trials of nimodipine.[41] A trend toward more favourable outcomes was noted in patients with traumatic subarachnoid haemorrhage.[42,43]

Hyperglycolysis

Experimental studies of TBI have shown that cerebral hyperglycolysis is a pathophysiological response to ionic and neurochemical cascades induced by injury.[44,45] This observation has important implications regarding cellular viability, vulnerability to secondary insults, and the functional capability of affected regions. Post-traumatic hyperglycolysis has also been shown in humans. Hyperglycolysis was documented in six of the 28 patients in whom both flucrodeoxyglucose positron emission tomography (FDG-PET) and cerebral metabolic rate for oxygen ($CMRO_2$) determinations were made within 8 days of injury. Five additional patients were found to have localised areas of hyperglycolysis adjacent to focal mass lesions.[46]

These clinical data support the experimental results, but unfortunately do not indicate which specific cell types are responsible. It is possible that the cells exhibiting hyperglycolysis are actually peripheral immune cells which have migrated into the brain, the observed metabolic pattern being typical of polymorphonuclear cells.

Hyperglycaemia

There is increasing evidence that hyperglycaemia may aggravate ischaemic injury of the CNS, including spinal cord injury. Glucose solutions should therefore not be used during the acute phase of resuscitation and blood glucose must be closely monitored (hourly); serum glucose above 11 mmolL should be treated by insulin infusion.[47] Evaluation of the combined effect of hypotension and hyperglycaemia occurring in the first 24 hours after severe head injury showed that mean arterial pressure (MAP) and blood glucose are linearly related to mortality. Regression analysis shows that each has an independent effect. Moreover, the relationship between blood glucose and mortality is stronger than the relationship between MAP and mortality.[48] Further studies on the combined effect of hyperglycaemia and hypotension on mortality after head injury are needed because this study suggests, but does not prove, an additive, causal association.

Apolipoprotein E ε4

This protein, synthesised by reactive astrocytes, is responsible for transporting lipids to regenerating neurons, promoting repair, and construction of new cell membranes and synapses.

Experimental data have suggested that apolipoprotein E (apoE) is important in the response of the nervous system to trauma. There are three common alleles of the apoE gene, ε2, ε3, and ε4; there is evidence of substantial variation in behaviour of these isoforms. As is now widely recognised, apoE genotype is the most important genetic determinant of susceptibility to Alzheimer's disease, and acts synergistically with a previous history of TBI. A recent study by Teasdale et al. demonstrated a significant genetic association between apoE polymorphism and outcome, supporting the notion of a genetically determined influence. In fact, patients with ε4 are more than twice as likely to have an unfavourable outcome as those without.[49,50]

Principles of care

Assessing the patient

The management of individual brain-injured patients, and the formulation and application of guidelines, depends upon the use of a widely accepted and applicable method of assessment and classification of the level of consciousness. The Glasgow Coma Scale, and its derivative the Glasgow Coma Score, are widely used for assessing patients before and after arrival at hospital (Table 2.1). Many studies support their repeatability, validity, and clinimetric properties.[51]

The Glasgow Coma Scale provides a framework for describing the state of the patient in terms of three aspects of responsiveness: eye opening, best motor response, and verbal response, each stratified according to increasing impairment. The distinction between normal and abnormal flexion can be difficult to make consistently and is rarely useful in monitoring the individual patient; it is, however, relevant to prognosis and is therefore used to classify severity in groups of patients. The Glasgow Coma Score can provide a single summary figure and a basis for systems of classification but contains less information than a description separately of the three responses. The three responses of the original scale, not

Table 2.1 The Glasgow Coma Scale and Score		
Feature	**Scale**	**Score**
Eye opening	Spontaneous	4
	To speech	3
	To pain	2
	None	1
Verbal response	Orientated	5
	Confused conversation	4
	Words (inappropriate)	3
	Sounds (incomprehensible)	2
	None	1
Best motor response	Obeys commands	6
	Localises to pain	5
	Flexion	
	Normal	4
	Abnormal	3
	Extension	2
	None	1
Total Coma Score (sum score)		3–15

Data from Teasdale et al.[77]

the total score, should be used in describing, monitoring, and exchanging information about individual patients.

Investigation

Intracranial lesions can be detected radiologically before they produce clinical changes. Rather than awaiting neurological deterioration, early imaging reduces the delay in detection and treatment of acute traumatic intracranial injury and is reflected in better outcomes. Exclusion or demonstration of intracranial injury can also guide decisions about the intensity and duration of observation in less severe injuries.

There has been a progressive shift away from simple skull radiography as a source of circumstantial evidence of intracranial damage towards CT scanning to provide definitive data. In the absence of randomised comparisons of different investigative strategies, indications for imaging at presentation after TBI depend upon the likely yield in different categories of patient. Although most patients with minor head injury can be discharged without sequelae after a period of observation, in a small proportion their neurological condition deteriorates and requires neurosurgical intervention for intracranial haematoma. The objective of the Canadian CT Head Rule Study was to develop an accurate and reliable decision rule for the use of computed tomography (CT) in patients with minor head injury. Such a decision rule would allow physicians to be more selective in their use of CT without compromising the care of patients with minor head injury (Table 2.2).[52]

Referral

The speed with which patients who would benefit from neurological and neurosurgical care are identified, referred, and transferred may critically influence their outcome. There is evidence that delays and errors in early management have occurred in those with unfavourable outcome even after transfer to neurosurgical centres. The benefits of specialist neurological care include the availability of skills and facilities for intracranial surgery, expertise for patient assessment, and capability for sophisticated monitoring and management of intracranial pathologies that constitute neurological intensive care (NICU) (Box 2.1). There are also benefits to be accrued in the access to enhanced knowledge and expertise resulting from the concentration of experience.

Transfer

It is important to consider the effects of the structure of the trauma service on the care of patients with severe TBI. In the United Kingdom, this was addressed in the recent Working Party Report from the Royal College of Surgeons of England. Neurosurgical services are structured on a regional basis, with one tertiary referral centre serving many hospitals that admit patients with traumatic injuries. The trauma service is structured on a district basis; this means that many patients are managed by clinicians without neurosurgical centres who have little experience or expertise in this field. As a result, management is often discussed by telephone, many patients are transferred between hospitals with the additional risks involved, and some are actually managed outside neurosurgical centres for the duration of their hospital stay.[53] It must be admitted, however, that management often varies even

Table 2.2 (a) Risk of an operable intracranial haematoma in brain-injured patients

GCS	Risk	Other features	Risk
15	1 in 3615	None	1 in 31 300
		Post-traumatic amnesia (PTA)	1 in 6700
		Skull fracture	1 in 81
		Skull fracture and PTA	1 in 29
9–14	1 in 51	No fracture	1 in 180
		Skull fracture	1 in 5
3–8	1 in 7	No fracture	1 in 27
		Skull fracture	1 in 4

Table 2.2(b) Canadian CT head rule – minor head Injury*

Five high-risk factors:
1. Failure to reach GCS of 15 within 2 hours
2. Suspected open skull fracture
3. Sign of basal skull fracture
4. Vomiting >2 episodes
5. Age >65 years

Two additional medium-risk factors:
1. Amnesia before impact >30 minutes
2. Dangerous mechanism of injury

The 3121 patients had the following characteristics: mean age 38·7 years; GCS scores of 13 (3·5%), 14 (16·7%), 15 (79·8%); 8% had clinically important brain injury; and 1% required neurological intervention.[52]

The high-risk factors were 100% sensitive (95% CI 92–100%) for predicting need for neurological intervention, and would require only 32% of patients to undergo CT. The medium-risk factors were 98·4% sensitive (95% CI 96–99%) and 49·6% specific for predicting clinically important brain injury, and would require only 54% of patients to undergo CT.

*Data from Stiell et al.[52]

between neurosurgical centres.[54,55] The publication of guidelines will hopefully standardise and improve care.[56]

Patients with an impaired level of consciousness have physiological instability that can result in secondary insults during transport and a worse outcome. These adverse events

Box 2.1 A patient with a traumatic brain injury should be discussed with neurosurgery

- When a CT scan in a general hospital shows a recent intracranial lesion
- When a patient fulfils the criteria for CT scanning but this cannot be done within an appropriate period
- Whatever the result of any CT scan, when the patient has clinical features that suggest that specialist neurological assessment, monitoring, or management are appropriate. These reasons include:
  - Persisting coma (GCS <9, no eye opening) after initial resuscitation
  - Confusion persists for more than 4 hours
  - Deterioration in conscious level after admission (a sustained decrease in one point in the motor or verbal GCS subscores, or 2 points on the eye opening subscale of the GCS)
  - Persistent focal neurological signs
  - A seizure without full recovery
  - Compound depressed fracture
  - Definite or suspected penetrating injury
  - A CSF leak or other sign of base of skull fracture

can be minimised by resuscitation before transfer, invasive monitoring, and care by appropriately trained staff, before, during and after transport.

Intensive care

Historically the role of the neurosurgical intensive care unit has been to prevent secondary brain damage following a TBI. The mainstay of this approach has been to correct macroscopic, measurable, physiological variables, such as blood pressure, oxygenation, and intracerebral pressure to "normal" or "supranormal" levels. The assumption is that manipulation of the physiological response to injury will improve outcome.

It is thought that the final common pathway in all acute brain injury is failure of oxygen delivery (Do_2), that is, ischaemia. Specialised monitors have been developed to alert the clinician to critical reductions in Do_2.

The fundamental aim of intensive care management is to avoid secondary insults and to optimise cerebral oxygenation by ensuring a normal arterial oxygen content, and by maintaining cerebral perfusion pressure (CPP) at a level greater than 70 mmHg. This figure may be modified depending on jugular bulb oxygen saturation (Sjo_2) measurement. While the actual level of ICP may be less important, in general it should be maintained at less than 25 mmHg.[57-60] Most ICP reducing therapies are double-edged swords and, it should be noted, have not been subject to large prospective randomised trials. The Cochrane Injuries Group has highlighted the lack of evidence[61,62] for much of the therapies used in TBI[63] and are coordinating the largest ever, randomised controlled trial in head injury, evaluating the effect of corticosteroids (www.crash.lshtm.ac.uk/Newsletter00No29-Oct01.htm).

Intracranial pressure monitoring

Even though ventricular fluid pressure is still regarded as the gold standard, most centres now use solid-state intraparenchymal monitors that are usually placed into the right (non-dominant) frontal region through a small burrhole. While the ICP level is important (normal 10 mmHg, acceptable upper limit 25 mmHg), more significant is the CPP, calculated as the difference between mean arterial pressure and intracranial pressure, since CPP is the principal determinant of cerebral blood flow (CBF). The zero reference point for the ICP catheter and the arterial pressure transducer should be the same. There is a small risk of catheter displacement, haematoma, and drift of the zero baseline, but this has not been found to be clinically significant; if ICP readings are incompatible with other findings, however, it is worth considering removal and reinsertion of another catheter. Other methods of measurement include ventricular catheterisation – passing a catheter into the lateral ventricle through the non-dominant frontal lobe.[58,60] There are small risks on insertion of such a catheter, and the risk of ventriculitis increases with time (particularly after 7 days), and with sampling CSF from the catheter. It can easily be checked against zero pressure, and can be used to withdraw CSF to reduce ICP. Future measurement of ICP may include a continuous estimate of intracranial compliance. Tissue perfusion is more likely to be related to compliance than pressure and critical volumetric compensatory exhaustion will be detected earlier with this measure, using, for example, the Spiegelberg device (Figure 2.2).

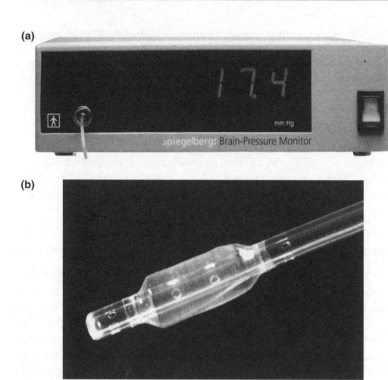

Figure 2.2 (a,b) Spiegelberg compliance monitoring device.
Future measurement of ICP may include a continuous estimate of
intracranial compliance. Tissue perfusion is more likely to be related to
compliance than pressure, and critical volumetric compensatory
exhaustion will be detected earlier with this measure. The Spiegelberg
device is such a monitor and is currently available

Cerebral metabolic monitoring

Cerebral metabolic monitoring (CMM) has a long history
and has developed as the technology has permitted. Indeed,
technology may have been the driving force for some of the
recent scientific publications. In general terms, CMM can be
divided into global and focal, and within these broad
categories bedside or remote monitors can be used.

Before describing a catalogue of the available monitors we
must ask what it is that we wish to detect. No monitor will
improve outcome itself, and this is made more likely if we
monitor intermediate physiological variables with little

relationship to consumer orientated end-points (quality of survival). There has been a tendency to "make the measurable important, rather than making the important measurable".

Ischaemia

Oxygen Secondary ischaemic damage has been shown, time and again, after TBI. Therefore a monitor that provides an early warning of impending ischaemia should offer promise. However, increasingly we believe that the pathophysiological process that leads to neuronal death is mitochondria failure. This will not be detected by any monitor of the adequacy of global oxygen delivery (jugular bulb oxygen saturation $Sjvo_2$) or regional brain tissue oxygen tension $(Ptio_2)$.[64] There are data to show a relationship between both these variables and outcome in a small number of patients but both lack sensitivity and specificity.

Cerebral blood flow Measurements of CBF, regional (PET, Xe^{133}, MRI-PWI) or global (Kety Schmidt), cannot predict what level of oxygen delivery is required to meet metabolic demand and, sadly, PET lacks the refinement of double labelling and flow and metabolism cannot be simultaneously recorded. There is increasing evidence that metabolic requirements for oxygen are extremely low after TBI and previously recognised thresholds may not equate with neuronal damage after TBI. Hyperglycolysis may be an example of mitochondria adapting to failure of oxidative metabolism.

Intermediate metabolites Intermediate metabolites of oxidative metabolism can be assessed by brain microdialysis fluid, chemical shift imaging (CSI–MRS), and sampling of the jugular venous blood. Glucose, lactate, pyruvate, their ratio, and byproducts of membrane breakdown (glycerol) have all been assessed, and phenomenology that supports current thinking has been reported.

There are few randomised trials that have compared therapy to treat therapeutic goals generated by such monitors. Robertson *et al.* conducted a pilot study in which patients were block randomised to be treated according to an $Sjvo_2$ endpoint or an ICP threshold. The result was a trend to more favourable outcomes and less intractable ICP problems in the ICP treatment cohort.[65]

Cerebral metabolic monitoring: pathobiological processes

Excitotoxicity   Brain microdialysis has been used to monitor excitatory amino acids after TBI but requires specialised equipment and does not give a continuous online measure and therefore lacks the vigilance required of a clinically useful monitor.

Inflammation   Important mediators of the inflammatory response have been measured in microdialysate and detected in jugular venous (and arterial blood giving a transcranial gradient) and in CSF after TBI. Analysis of the concentration of these mediators requires offline assay and our understanding of these processes is not yet at a level where modification of therapy (or the processes themselves) is likely to be successful.

Therefore, to date there is no CMM available with sensitivity or specificity for an intermediate physiological variable that, if modified, improves outcome. Such a device would require subsequent testing in a prospective randomised controlled trial. Current clinical management protocols aim to optimise cerebral oxygen delivery and reduce secondary insults. Therefore, we should at least monitor the endpoints of such a strategy. Currently $Sjvo_2$ recording with bad-side $Ptio_2$ monitoring is proven technology with limitations, but it is widely available and assesses the endpoint of current intensive care therapy after acute brain injury.

Brain imaging

Brain imaging is required to identify lesions that are remediable by surgery, to aid prognosis, and to facilitate/audit clinical governance. The field of imaging is advancing rapidly; blood flow and metabolism, cellular energy status, cellular repair, occult injury, and function have all been examined.

CT scanning

Marshall *et al.* described diagnostic categories by CT scanning that improve prognostic discrimination and permit more homogeneous comparisons (Table 2.3). With clinical data (Traumatic Coma Data Bank, TCDB) this scale gives better

Table 2.3 Mortality by individual categories in TCDB (Traumatic Coma Data Bank) classification of brain CT. Note that classes are not mutually exclusive

Imaging the brain – CT Scan	Mortality (%)
Diffuse injury I (no visible lesion)	9·6
Diffuse Injury II	13·5
Diffuse Injury III (swelling)	34
Diffuse Injury IV (shift)	56·2
Evacuated mass	38·8
Non-evacuated mass	52·8
Brain-stem injury	66·7

Data from Marshall et al.[78]

classification of "at risk" groups and has promoted the development of management guidelines, identifying subgroups so that new therapies can be appropriately targeted and revision of current thinking facilitated.[66] Lobato et al. attempted to identify common patterns of CT change and to validate the TCDB classification through sequential CT changes, and relating these to final outcome in severe head injury patients.[65,67,68] The final outcome was more accurately predicted using a CT scan at 48 hours than by using the initial CT scans. Because the majority of relevant CT changes developed within 48 hours after injury a pathological categorisation made by using an early elective control CT scan seems to be most useful for prognostic purposes (Figure 2.1, Table 2.3).

Magnetic resonance imaging (MRI)

Diffusion weighted imaging (DWI) is a technique that can be used to probe the microenvironment of water. Contrast in DWI is derived from the translational motion of water molecules. Quantitative assessment of the (apparent) diffusion coefficient (ADCw) is a unique method of examining tissue status.

In closed head injuries, focal lesions such as contusions resulting from mechanical distortion of tissue, and haematoma, may be detected on conventional MR and CT images. Diffuse axonal injury, including axonal shearing and hypoxic brain damage, are less identifiable using such modalities. Diffusion weighted and magnetisation transfer imaging sequences may

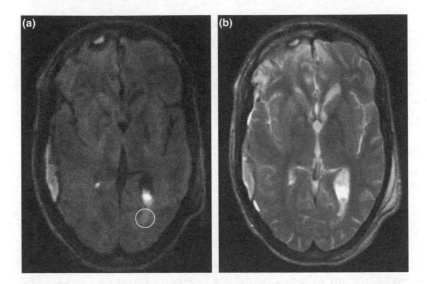

Figure 2.3 Diffusion image of patient with normal CT scan of brain but persistently abnormal neurology.

The history of the mechanism of injury suggests diffuse axonal injury and there is a history of hypoxia and hypotension. Encircled area = area with reduced ADC suggesting cellular oedema, not apparent on T2 and CT imaging

prove to be useful in highlighting axonal structural changes not obvious on T2 weighted images (Figure 2.3). With the capability of highlighting the chemical changes that accompany such diffuse head injuries, MR spectroscopy has the potential to detect such disorders in vivo.[69] Of particular interest is proton MR spectroscopy at long echo times in the metabolite N-acetyl aspartate, an amino acid found exclusively in neurons.[70] Using single slice two dimensional spectroscopic imaging, nine acute head injury patients and six controls have been successfully scanned. The problems presented by the need for ICU monitoring of these patients during MR scanning were overcome using MR compatible monitoring equipment.[71] In previous studies of head injury which used proton spectroscopy, single voxel localisation procedures have meant that the spatial extent of the spectral data has been limited, but with spectral data from a whole axial slice they have been able to identify N-acetyl aspartate abnormalities in regions remote from any T2 visible lesions. This observation suggests that spectroscopic imaging (of N-acetyl aspartate in particular) will be useful for the diagnosis of diffuse axonal injury. It may be possible to use this technique to guide therapy, monitor recovery, and aid outcome prediction.

Cerebral protection

Considerable effort[72] has gone towards the development of a neuroprotective agent, or agents, that could be given after brain trauma to reduce mortality and improve functional recovery. There have been many failed or inconclusive studies to date and the future of pharmacological neuroprotection after TBI remains in doubt. Clinicians managing patients with a head injury are therefore left with detection and prevention of secondary insults to the brain, including management of medical complications of brain injury, and non-pharmacological interventions that might beneficially modify the brain's response to trauma.

Prediction of outcome

Evaluation of effectiveness of health care delivery, stratification in clinical trials, and assessment of resource allocation requires an accurate estimator of severity of illness and probability of hospital outcome. Considerable debate exists surrounding the use of disease specific scoring systems or a one-for-all approach. The Glasgow Coma Scale (GCS) has been compared with SAPS II (Simplified Acute Physiology Score), MPM II_0, MPM II_{24} (Mortality Prediction Model), and APACHE II (Acute Physiology And Chronic Health Evaluation). The GCS was not intended to be a predictor of outcome but was described as an assessment of depression of conscious level. Although the GCS can provide a quick guide to the assessment of severity of injury, only a comprehensive system that includes the admission variables, physiological derangement, and age will provide accurate discrimination and prediction of outcome.

McQuatt *et al.* compared logistic regression with decision tree analysis of an observational, head injury dataset, including a wide range of secondary insults and 12 month outcomes.[73] Decision tree analysis highlights patient subgroups and critical values in variables assessed. Importantly, the results are visually informative and often present clear clinical interpretation about risk factors faced by patients in these subgroups. A decision tree was automatically produced from root node to target classes based on the Glasgow Outcome Scale (GOS) score (Table 2.4).[74] The most significant predictors of mortality in this patient set were duration of hypotensive, pyrexic, and hypoxaemic insults. When good and poor outcomes were compared, hypotensive insults and pupillary response on admission were significant. In certain subgroups of patients pyrexia was a predictor of good outcome. Decision tree analysis confirmed some of the results of logistic regression and challenged others and notably identified that brain stem reflexes are important predictors of outcome.[75] This was shown in the Glasgow–Liege Scale statistical analysis.[76] Additionally the decision tree analysis showed that GCS 3 patients often had a better outcome than GCS 4 patients, demonstrating that the GCS is not a linear scale, with the GCS sum score being poor at discriminating between patient outcomes.

The outcome after TBI can be subdivided grossly into hospital survival or death. There are, however, many functional outcomes among survivors. Since this population of patients is largely made up of young males, the economic costs of survival of dependent patients is great. Up to half of all head-injured patients admitted to hospital remain disabled at one year. The combination of this factor and young age makes the economic burden greater than in, for example, stroke. Future models that predict outcome must focus upon prediction of functional outcome. Factors including genetic phenotype are known to be important and will require inclusion to achieve adequate calibration and discrimination.

Rehabilitation

Brain-injured patients may benefit from advice and treatment given by a variety of experts working as a team: neurorehabilitation physician, clinical neuropsychologist, rehabilitation nurse, physiotherapist, occupational therapist,

Table 2.4 The Glasgow Outcome Scale[79-81]

Score	Outcome	Features
1	Dead	Self-explanatory
2	Persistent vegetative state	Non-sentient, no interaction with others, has sleep–wake cycles and intact brain stem reflexes
3	Severe disability	Conscious, disabled to the point of needing help from someone for basic functions for at least part of each day
4	Moderate disability	Independent in daily life, but physical or other deficits limit employability and personal development
5	Good recovery	Return to a wide range of normal activities, often employed, with a range of skills and abilities broadly similar to pre-injury, but not necessarily identical

speech and language therapist, and medical social worker/care manager. Continuity of care and information about the ability of the patient and family to cope in the community can be obtained by home visits from liaison social workers, occupational therapists, or other TBI workers. The more severe the TBI the more useful an interdisciplinary and goal orientated approach to the patient's problems is likely to be, but even moderately and mildly brain injured patients may benefit.

Conclusions

The improvement in outcome from TBI over the past 20 years has not been due to any one major breakthrough. The reduction in mortality can be attributed to improved service organisation and delivery, including the improvement in general critical care management in this patient population.

Management aspects of neuro-intensive care

- Keep sodium >140 mmol/L. A fall in serum sodium produces an osmotic gradient across the blood–brain barrier, and aggravates cerebral oedema
- Avoid hyperglycaemia (treat blood glucose >11 mmol/L). Hyperglycaemia may aggravate ischaemic brain injury by increasing cerebral lactic acidosis
- Feed via an orogastric tube. Gastric motility agents can be given as required
- Use TED stockings; avoid low dose heparin
- Apply 15–30° head up tilt with head kept in neutral position; may improve CPP
- *No parenteral non-ionic fluid must be given.*

Other guidelines available:

From Brain Trauma Foundation. Guidelines for the management of severe head injury. American Association of Neurological Surgeons. Chicago, IL, 1995. http://www.ohsu.edu/som-surgery/neurosurgery/guidelines
Recommendations for the transfer of patients with acute head injuries to neurosurgical units. The Association of Anaesthetists of Great Britain and Ireland. London, 1996. http://www.ncl.ac.uk/~nassoca

References

1 Marshall LF. Epidemiology and cost of central nervous system injury. *Clin Neurosurg* 2000;**46**:105–12.
2 Stiell IG, Lesiuk H, Wells GA, *et al*. Canadian CT head rule study for patients with minor head injury: methodology for phase II (validation and economic analysis). *Ann Emerg Med* 2001;**38**:317–22.
3 Luukinen H, Herala M, Koski K, Kivela SL, Honkanen R. Rapid increase of fall-related severe head injuries with age among older people: a population-based study. *J Am Geriatrics Soc* 1999;**47**:1451–2.
4 Richter M, Otte D, Lehmann U, *et al*. Head injury mechanisms in helmet-protected motorcyclists: prospective multicenter study. *J Trauma* 2001; **51**:949–58.
5 Pickett W, Ardern C, Brison RJ. A population-based study of potential brain injuries requiring emergency care. *Can Med Assoc J* 2001;**165**:288–92.
6 Robinson DL. Changes in head injury with the New Zealand bicycle helmet law. *Accident Analysis Prevent* 2001;**33**:687–91.
7 MacKenzie EJ. Epidemiology of injuries: current trends and future challenges. *Epidemiol Rev* 2000;**22**:112–19.
8 Klatzo I. Presidential address. Neuropathological aspects of brain edema. *J Neuropathol Exp Neurol* 1967;**26**:1–14.
9 Reulen HJ, Graham R, Spatz M, Klatzo I. Role of pressure gradients and bulk flow in dynamics of vasogenic brain edema. *J Neurosurg* 1977;**46**: 24–35.

10 Klatzo I. Aspects of the blood–brain barrier in brain edema. *Clin Neurosurg* 1969;**16**:472–3.

11 Marmarou A, Barzo P, Fatouros P, Yamamoto T, Bullock R, Young H. Traumatic brain swelling in head injured patients: brain edema or vascular engorgement? *Acta Neurochir Suppl* 1997;**70**:68–70.

12 Jafari SS, Maxwell WL, Neilson M, Graham DI. Axonal cytoskeletal changes after non-disruptive axonal injury. *J Neurocytol* 1997;**26**: 207–21.

13 Maxwell WL, Povlishock JT, Graham DL. A mechanistic analysis of nondisruptive axonal injury: a review. *J Neurotrauma* 1997;**14**:419–40.

14 Miller JD. Head injury. *J Neurol Neurosurg Psychiatry* 1993;**56**:440–7.

15 Miller JD, Sweet RC, Narayan R, Becker DP. Early insults to the injured brain. *JAMA* 1978;**240**:439–42.

16 Mascia L, Andrews PJ, McKeating EG, Souter MJ, Merrick MV, Piper IR. Cerebral blood flow and metabolism in severe brain injury: the role of pressure autoregulation during cerebral perfusion pressure management. *Intensive Care Med* 2000;**26**:202–5.

17 Mascia L, Piper IR, Andrews PJ, Souter MJ, Webb DJ. The role of endothelin-1 in pressure autoregulation of cerebral blood flow in rats. *Intensive Care Med* 1999;**25**:1282–6.

18 Beaumont A, Marmarou A, Czigner A, *et al.* The impact-acceleration model of head injury: injury severity predicts motor and cognitive performance after trauma. *Neurol Res* 1999;**21**:742–54.

19 Albrecht RF 2nd, Wass CT, Lanier WL. Occurrence of potentially detrimental temperature alterations in hospitalized patients at risk for brain injury. *Mayo Clin Proc* 1998;**73**:629–35.

20 Kilpatrick MM, Lowry DW, Firlik AD, Yonas H, Marion DW. Hyperthermia in the neurosurgical intensive care unit. *Neurosurgery* 2000;**47**:850–6.

21 Cairns CJ. Andrews PJ. Management of hyperthermia in traumatic brain injury. *Curr Opin Crit Care* 2002;**8**:106–10.

22 McQuatt A, Sleeman D, Andrews PJ, Corruble V, Jones PA. Discussing anomalous situations using decision trees: a head injury case study. *Methods Information Med* 2001;**40**:373–9.

23 Jones PA, Andrews PJ, Midgley S, *et al.* Measuring the burden of secondary insults in head-injured patients during intensive care. *J Neurosurg Anesthesiol* 1994;**6**:4–14.

24 Clifton GL, Allen S, Barrodale P, *et al.* A phase II study of moderate hypothermia in severe brain injury. *J Neurotrauma* 1993;**10**:263–71; discussion 273.

25 Clifton GL, Miller ER, Choi SC, *et al.* Lack of effect of induction of hypothermia after acute brain injury. *N Eng J Med* 2001;**344**:556–63.

26 Signorini DF, Alderson P. Therapeutic hypothermia for head injury. *Cochrane Database Systemat Rev* 2000;CD001048 [update in Cochrane Database Syst Rev. 2002;(1):CD001048;11869586].

27 Signorini DF, Alderson P. Therapeutic hypothermia for head injury. *Cochrane Database Systemat Rev* 2000;CD001048.

28 Clifton GL, Miller ER, Choi SC, Levin HS. Fluid thresholds and outcome from severe brain injury. *Crit Care Med* 2002;**30**:739–45.

29 Hutchinson PJ, Gupta AK, Fryer TF, *et al.* Correlation between cerebral blood flow, substrate delivery, and metabolism in head injury: a combined microdialysis and triple oxygen positron emission tomography study. *J Cerebral Blood Flow Metab* 2002;**22**:735–45.

30 Verweij BH, Muizelaar JP, Vinas FC, Peterson PL, Xiong Y, Lee CP. Impaired cerebral mitochondrial function after traumatic brain injury in humans. *J Neurosurg* 2000;**93**:815–20.

31 Verweij BH, Muizelaar JP, Vinas FC, Peterson PL, Xiong Y, Lee CP. Mitochondrial dysfunction after experimental and human brain injury and its possible reversal with a selective N-type calcium channel antagonist (SNX-111). *Neurol Res* 1997;**19**:334–9.

32 Clausen T, Bullock R. Medical treatment and neuroprotection in traumatic brain injury. *Curr Pharmaceut Design* 2001;**7**:1517–32.

33 McCauley SR, Levin HS, Vanier M, *et al.* The neurobehavioural rating scale-revised: sensitivity and validity in closed head injury assessment. *J Neurol Neurosurg Psychiatry* 2001;**71**:643–51.

34 McKeating EG, Andrews PJ. Cytokines and adhesion molecules in acute brain injury. *Br J Anaesth* 1998;**80**:77–84.

35 McKeating EG, Andrews PJ, Signorini DF, Mascia L. Transcranial cytokine gradients in patients requiring intensive care after acute brain injury. *Br J Anaesth* 1997;**78**:520–3.

36 McKeating EG, Andrews PJ, Mascia L. Leukocyte adhesion molecule profiles and outcome after traumatic brain injury. *Acta Neurochir Suppl* 1998;**71**:200–2.

37 McKeating EG, Andrews PJ, Mascia L. Relationship of neuron specific enolase and protein S-100 concentrations in systemic and jugular venous serum to injury severity and outcome after traumatic brain injury. *Acta Neurochir Suppl* 1998;**71**:117–19.

38 McKeating EG, Andrews PJ, Mascia L. The relationship of soluble adhesion molecule concentrations in systemic and jugular venous serum to injury severity and outcome after traumatic brain injury. *Anesth Analg* 1998;**86**:759–65.

39 Knoller N, Levi L, Shoshan I, *et al.* Dexanabinol (HU-211) in the treatment of severe closed head injury: a randomized, placebo-controlled, phase II clinical trial. *Crit Care Med* 2002;**30**:548–54.

40 Bedell EA, Prough DS. Dexanabinol as a treatment for traumatic brain injury: will another therapeutic promise be broken? *Crit Care Med* 2002;**30**:710–1.

41 Harders A, Kakarieka A, Braakman R. Traumatic subarachnoid hemorrhage and its treatment with nimodipine. German tSAH Study Group. *J Neurosurg* 1996;**85**:82–9.

42 Langham J, Goldfrad C, Teasdale G, Shaw D, Rowan K. Calcium channel blockers for acute traumatic brain injury. *Cochrane Database Systemat Rev* 2000;CD000565.

43 Anonymous. A multicenter trial of the efficacy of nimodipine on outcome after severe head injury. The European Study Group on Nimodipine in Severe Head Injury. *J Neurosurg* 1994;**80**:797–804.

44 Reinert M, Hoelper B, Doppenberg E, Zauner A, Bullock R. Substrate delivery and ionic balance disturbance after severe human head injury. *Acta Neurochir Suppl* 2000;**76**:439–44.

45 Thomas S, Prins ML, Samii M, Hovda DA. Cerebral metabolic response to traumatic brain injury sustained early in development: a 2–deoxy-D-glucose autoradiographic study. *J Neurotrauma* 2000;**17**:649–65.

46 Bergsneider M, Hovda DA, Shalmon E, *et al.* Cerebral hyperglycolysis following severe traumatic brain injury in humans: a positron emission tomography study. *J Neurosurg* 1997;**86**:241–51.

47 Yang SY, Zhang S, Wang ML. Clinical significance of admission hyperglycemia and factors related to it in patients with acute severe head injury. *Surg Neurol* 1995;**44**:373–7.

48 Walia S, Sutcliffe AJ. The relationship between blood glucose, mean arterial pressure and outcome after severe head injury: an observational study. *Injury* 2002;**33**:339–44.

49 Almkvist O, Winblad B. Early diagnosis of Alzheimer dementia based on clinical and biological factors. *Eur Arch Psychiatry Clin Neurosci* 1999;**249** (Suppl 3):3–9.

50 O'Meara ES, Kukull WA, Sheppard L, *et al.* Head injury and risk of Alzheimer's disease by apolipoprotein E genotype. *Am J Epidemiology* 1997;**146**:373–84.

51 Anonymous. The Brain Trauma Foundation. The American Association of Neurological Surgeons. The Joint Section on Neurotrauma and Critical Care. Glasgow Coma Scale score. *J Neurotrauma* 2000;**17**:563–71.

52 Stiell IG, Wells GA, Vandemheen K, *et al.* The Canadian CT Head Rule for patients with minor head injury. *Lancet* 2001;**357**:1391–6.

53 McKeating EG, Andrews PJ, Tocher JI, Menon DK. The intensive care of severe head injury: a survey of non-neurosurgical centres in the United Kingdom. *Br J Neurosurg* 1998;**12**:7–14.

54 Murray GD, Teasdale GM, Braakman R, *et al.* The European Brain Injury Consortium survey of head injuries. *Acta Neurochir* 1999;**141**:223–36.

55 Bulger EM, Nathens AB, Rivara FP, *et al.* Management of severe head injury: institutional variations in care and effect on outcome. *Crit Care Med* 2002;**30**:1870–6 [see comments].

56 Anonymous. The Brain Trauma Foundation. The American Association of Neurological Surgeons. The Joint Section on Neurotrauma and Critical Care. Methodology. *J Neurotrauma* 2000;**17**:561–2.

57 Anonymous. The Brain Trauma Foundation. The American Association of Neurological Surgeons. The Joint Section on Neurotrauma and Critical Care. Hypotension. *J Neurotrauma* 2000;**17**:591–5.

58 Anonymous. The Brain Trauma Foundation. The American Association of Neurological Surgeons. The Joint Section on Neurotrauma and Critical Care. Critical pathway for the treatment of established intracranial hypertension. *J Neurotrauma* 2000;**17**:537–8.

59 Anonymous. The Brain Trauma Foundation. The American Association of Neurological Surgeons. The Joint Section on Neurotrauma and Critical Care. Use of barbiturates in the control of intracranial hypertension. *J Neurotrauma* 2000;**17**:527–30.

60 Anonymous. The Brain Trauma Foundation. The American Association of Neurological Surgeons. The Joint Section on Neurotrauma and Critical Care. Guidelines for cerebral perfusion pressure. *J Neurotrauma* 2000;**17**: 507–11.

61 Choi SC, Clifton GL, Marmarou A, Miller ER. Misclassification and treatment effect on primary outcome measures in clinical trials of severe neurotrauma. *J Neurotrauma* 2002;**19**:17–22.

62 Dickinson K, Bunn F, Wentz R, Edwards P, Roberts I. Size and quality of randomised controlled trials in head injury: review of published studies. *Br Med J* 2000;**320**:1308–11.

63 Roberts I, Schierhout G, Alderson P. Absence of evidence for the effectiveness of five interventions routinely used in the intensive care management of severe head injury: a systematic review. *J Neurol Neurosurg Psychiatry* 1998;**65**:729–33.

64 Gupta AK, Hutchinson PJ, Fryer T, *et al.* Measurement of brain tissue oxygenation performed using positron emission tomography scanning to validate a novel monitoring method. *J Neurosurg* 2002;**96**:263–8.

65 Robertson CS, Valadka AB, Hannay HJ, *et al.* Prevention of secondary ischemic insults after severe head injury. *Crit Care Med* 1999;**27**:2086–95.

66 Vos PE, van Voskuilen AC, Beems T, Krabbe PF, Vogels OJ. Evaluation of the traumatic coma data bank computed tomography classification for severe head injury. *J Neurotrauma* 2001;**18**:649–55.

67 Lobato RD, Gamez PA, Alday R, *et al.* Sequential computerized tomography changes and related final outcome in severe head injury patients. *Acta Neurochir* 1997;**139**:385–91.

68 Anonymous. The Brain Trauma Foundation. The American Association of Neurological Surgeons. The Joint Section on Neurotrauma and Critical Care. Computed tomography scan features. *J Neurotrauma* 2000;**17**: 597–627.

69 Wild JM, Macmillan CS, Wardlaw JM, *et al.* [1]H spectroscopic imaging of acute head injury – evidence of diffuse axonal injury. *Magma* 1999;**8**: 109–15.

70 Macmillan CS, Wild JM, Wardlaw JM, Andrews PJ, Marshall I, Easton VJ. Traumatic brain injury and subarachnoid hemorrhage: in vivo occult pathology demonstrated by magnetic resonance spectroscopy may not be "ischaemic". A primary study and review of the literature. *Acta Neurochir* 2002;**144**:853–62.

71 Macmillan CS, Wild JM, Andrews PJ, *et al.* Accuracy of a miniature intracranial pressure monitor, its function during magnetic resonance scanning, and assessment of image artifact generation. *Neurosurgery* 1999;**45(1)**:188–93.

72 Narayan RK, Michel ME, Ansell B, *et al.* Clinical trials in head injury. *J Neurotrauma* 2002;**19**:503–57.

73 McQuatt A, Sleeman D, Andrews PJ, Corruble V, Jones PA. Discussing anomalous situations using decision trees: a head injury case study. *Meth Inform Med* 2001;**40**:373–9.

74 Andrews PJ, Sleeman DH, Statham PF, *et al.* Predicting recovery in patients suffering from traumatic brain injury by using admission variables and physiological data: a comparison between decision tree analysis and logistic regression. *J Neurosurg* 2002;**97**:326–36.

75 Firsching R, Woischneck D, Diedrich M, *et al.* Early magnetic resonance imaging of brainstem lesions after severe head injury. *J Neurosurg* 1998;**89**:707–12.

76 Born JD. The Glasgow–Liege Scale. Prognostic value and evolution of motor response and brain stem reflexes after severe head injury. *Acta Neurochir* 1988;**91**:1–11.

77 Teasdale G, Jennett B, Murray L, Murray G. Glasgow coma scale: to sum or not to sum? *Lancet* 1983;**2(8351)**:678.

78 Marshall LF, Marshall SB, Klauber MR, *et al.* A new classification of head injury based on computerized tomography. *J Neurosurg* 1991;**75**:S14–20.

79 Pettigrew LL, Wilson JL, Teasdale GM. Assessing disability after head injury: improved use of the Glasgow Outcome Scale. *J Neurosurg* 1998;**89**: 939–43.

80 Teasdale GM, Pettigrew LL, Lindsay WJ, *et al.* Analyzing outcome of treatment of severe head injury: a review and update on advancing the use of the Glasgow outcome scale. *J Neurotrauma* 1998;**15**:587–97.

81 Lindsay WJ, Pettigrew LL, Teasdale GM. Structured interviews for the Glasgow outcome scale and the extended Glasgow outcome scale: guidelines for their use. *J Neurotrauma* 1998;**15**:573–80.

3: Acute stroke

R DAVENPORT, M DENNIS

Introduction

In the western world, stroke is the third commonest cause of
death (after heart disease and all cancers), is probably the
commonest cause of severe disability,[1,2] and accounts for a
large proportion of healthcare resources. Its impact on
individual patients, their families, and society as a whole is
immense. About 200 people per 100 000 population will have
a first ever stroke every year.[3] Their mean age is about 72 years
and men and women are affected in roughly equal numbers.
Despite the uncertainty over whether stroke incidence is
rising, falling, or remaining static,[3,4] the absolute number of
patients is likely to increase, as incidence increases with age
and most populations are ageing.

Stroke has in the past held a low priority for many
professional groups; in 1988 the King's Fund Forum concluded
that hospital, primary care, and community services for stroke
in the United Kingdom were "haphazard, fragmented and
poorly tailored to the patients' needs".[5] However, increasing
awareness of the impact of stroke has led to it being identified
as a priority for improving services and research.[6,7] Numerous
well conducted randomised trials and systematic reviews of
medical and surgical treatments for acute stroke, as well as
primary and secondary prevention strategies, mean that we
are now considerably better equipped to know which
treatments work and which should be abandoned and what
sort of services we should be providing for our patients.

In this chapter, we will describe our approach to the
management of acute stroke, focusing mainly on the first few
days. Although the WHO definition of stroke (see below)
includes subarachnoid haemorrhage, we will not consider this

distinct syndrome further, as it is covered in detail elsewhere in this book. Our approach is based on our interpretation of the available evidence, with particular emphasis on randomised controlled trials and systematic reviews, since we believe that these provide the most reliable data on the risks and benefits of treatments. However, where such evidence is either absent or insufficient (and despite the many welcome advances, there is still much we do not know for sure), we will describe what we do in routine practice. We accept that other interpretations of the evidence are possible and are likely to be influenced by the context in which one works. For example, in the United Kingdom, unlike some other countries, our patients tend not to demand "treatment" (whether of proven benefit or not), "fee for service" is rare, and the resources available for health care are restricted so that only cost effective treatments will be advocated for widespread use. Lastly, although rehabilitation and secondary prevention are not the focus of this chapter, it is important to emphasise that for many patients, their management *after* the acute stage currently has the greater impact on their lives. With the advent of new acute strategies, this balance may change.

Is acute stroke an emergency?

Medical emergencies can be defined by certain criteria including rapidity of onset, poor prognosis, and requirement for prompt intervention. Although stroke has traditionally been treated as less of an emergency than, for instance, acute myocardial infarction or meningitis, we will illustrate that this conservative approach is no longer tenable and that stroke should now be regarded as a medical emergency.

Stroke comes on rapidly

The World Health Organization has defined stroke as a clinical syndrome characterised by rapidly developing symptoms and/or signs of focal and at times global (for patients in coma) loss of cerebral function, with symptoms lasting more than 24 hours or leading to death, with no apparent cause other than that of vascular origin.[8]

Stroke has a poor prognosis

The outcome after stroke is crucially dependent upon the extent and site of the brain damage, as well as the patient's age and prestroke health status.[9] The case fatality rates following a first ever stroke (all types combined) are 12% at seven days, 19% at 30 days, and 31% at one year;[10] haemorrhagic stroke carries a higher risk of death than ischaemic stroke.[10] Deaths occurring within the first week following stroke are mostly due to the direct effects of cerebral damage;[10-12] later on, the complications of immobility (for example, bronchopneumonia, venous thromboembolism) and cardiac events become increasingly common.[13] About 20% of those suffering a first ever stroke will be dependent on another person for everyday activities (for example, washing, dressing, mobility) at 12 months, and 50% will be independent.[14] The risk of a recurrent stroke in survivors is about 10–16% within the first year, thereafter falling to about 5% per annum.[15] The relative risk of death in stroke survivors is about twice the risk of people in the general population,[13] and this risk persists for several years; many of these deaths are due to other vascular problems (for example, ischaemic heart disease or peripheral arterial disease). This emphasises the importance of targeting these areas as well as stroke when we consider secondary prevention strategies.

Stroke patients may require immediate treatment

There are several reasons why many patients require urgent inpatient care following an acute stroke. First, stroke may lead to a variety of potentially life threatening complications such as airway obstruction and respiratory failure, swallowing problems with the risk of aspiration, dehydration, and malnutrition, venous thromboembolic complications, seizures, and infections.[16-20] These may arise within hours of stroke onset and require early assessment and intervention so that they can be anticipated, prevented, and treated. Furthermore, although stroke has represented an area of therapeutic nihilism for many years, a variety of acute and potentially effective treatments (medical and surgical) are now becoming available.

Assessment

Early assessment allows the formulation of an accurate and early diagnosis (as stroke is primarily a clinical diagnosis, the sooner a physician can elicit a history, the more likely it is to be reliable), the organisation of relevant and cost effective investigations, and the initiation of appropriate secondary prevention (which is likely to be most effective early on, when the risk of recurrence is highest). However, as with any medical emergency, the first priority in assessing a patient following a suspected stroke is to identify and treat any immediately life threatening complications. For stroke, this will usually be an obstructed airway (A), respiratory failure in a comatose patient (B), or an acute circulatory disturbance (C). Once the patient is stable, we apply a systematic, staged approach to making the diagnosis and formulating a management plan. This initial assessment should address the following questions.

Is this a vascular event?

The diagnosis depends crucially on an accurate history, taken from the patient and/or carer. We ask ourselves the following questions to help decide whether it was a vascular event.

- Are the neurological symptoms focal rather than non-focal?
- Are the focal neurological symptoms negative (that is, loss of function) rather than positive (for example, pins and needles rather than numbness)?
- Was the onset of the focal symptoms sudden?
- Were the focal symptoms maximal at onset (that is, coming on over minutes to hours) rather than progressive (that is, evolving over hours to days)?

If the answer to all these questions is yes, then a vascular cause (either cerebral ischaemia or haemorrhage) is very likely. Of course, presentations vary. Occasional patients have symptoms or signs which are not easily localised (for example, memory impairment, confusion, or a reduced conscious level), symptoms may be positive (for example, movement disorders), and many patients describe symptoms evolving over hours or even days. These exceptions simply make the clinical diagnosis less certain and should lead to early investigation to exclude alternative diagnoses which require different urgent treatment (for example, hypoglycaemia, non-convulsive seizures, cerebral infection, or subdural haematoma). When one sees a patient within the first few hours of symptom onset, it is often difficult to know whether one is witnessing a transient ischaemic attack (TIA) or stroke (or a stroke mimic), and increasingly we refer to the concept of a "brain attack" – that is, the acute onset of focal brain symptoms which are likely to be due to a vascular cause.

In addition, we consider the context in which the event has occurred. Strokes are uncommon in the young and as about 80% of stroke patients have at least one vascular risk factor at presentation,[21] the absence of risk factors should lead one to be slightly more sceptical about a diagnosis of stroke. Accurate diagnosis in the hyperacute phase (less than six hours from onset) is often difficult because symptoms and signs may be changing rapidly. The introduction of acute therapies which need to be administered within this time window suggests that early and accurate diagnoses will become increasingly important.

Which part of the brain is affected?

In reaching a diagnosis of stroke, one inevitably makes some assessment of where in the brain the lesion might be. However, it may be useful to further subclassify the stroke since this may give clues to the likely underlying cause, allow more cost effective investigations, and help in predicting both the risk of recurrence and functional outcome. Whilst there are many subclassification systems available, we use the system developed from the Oxfordshire Community Stroke Project[22] (Box 3.1), which works well at the bedside.[23–28]

Is it a haemorrhagic or ischaemic stroke?

Distinguishing between a haemorrhagic and ischaemic stroke is important in terms of acute management, prognosis, and secondary prevention. In Caucasians, about 80% of first ever strokes are ischaemic.[3,29] Although a variety of scoring systems has been devised to help differentiate between infarction and haemorrhage, none provides sufficient

Box 3.1 The Oxfordshire Community Stroke Project subclassification system[22]

Total anterior circulation syndrome (TACS); implies a large cortical stroke in middle cerebral or middle and anterior cerebral artery territories

A combination of:

— New higher cerebral dysfunction (for example dysphasia, dyscalculia, visuospatial disorder) AND
— Homonymous visual field defect AND
— An ipsilateral motor and/or sensory deficit involving at least two out of three areas of the face, arm or leg.
— **Partial anterior circulation syndrome (PACS); implies cortical stroke in middle or anterior cerebral artery territory**
— Patients with two out of the three components of the TACS OR new higher cerebral dysfunction alone OR a motor/sensory deficit more restricted than those classified as a LACS (for example isolated hand involvement).

Lacunar syndrome (LACS); implies a subcortical stroke due to small vessel disease

— Pure motor stroke
— Pure sensory stroke
— Sensorimotor stroke
— Ataxic hemiparesis

Note: evidence of higher cortical involvement or disturbance of consciousness excludes a lacunar syndrome.

Posterior circulation syndrome (POCS)

— Ipsilateral cranial nerve palsy with contralateral motor and/or sensory deficit
— Bilateral motor and/or sensory deficit
— Disorder of conjugate eye movement
— Cerebellar dysfunction without ipsilateral log-tract involvement
— Isolated homonymous visual field defect

---

accuracy to guide treatment.[30] The only reliable method of differentiating is early brain imaging. In many countries, this is best performed by computed tomography (CT). Lumbar puncture may be useful in confirming subarachnoid haemorrhage if the brain imaging is equivocal but it has no place in differentiating ischaemic and haemorrhagic stroke.

Computed tomography

Intracerebral blood immediately appears as an area of high density on CT, but thereafter decreases so that haemorrhagic lesions will eventually appear either isodense or hypodense and thus be indistinguishable from an infarct.[31] Smaller haemorrhages may become isodense within days, although usually this process takes weeks. CT in the hyperacute stage of an ischaemic stroke is often normal although there may be subtle changes which are easily overlooked by the inexperienced observer. Infarcts are most easily seen on CT after a few days or in the chronic phase, when they may become markedly hypodense and well defined, although up to 50% of patients with a clinically definite stroke never have an appropriate lesion identified on CT.[32] To help radiologists in their interpretation, we recommend that the date and time of symptom onset are always recorded on the CT request form. Although early CT will reliably identify intracerebral haemorrhage, the distinction between a primary intracerebral haemorrhage (PICH) and haemorrhagic transformation of an infarct (HTI) is unreliable and difficult. The frequency and clinical relevance of HTI is uncertain and radiologically ranges from small petechial haemorrhages to frank haematoma, which may or may not be accompanied by clinical deterioration. HTI can occur very early[33] and the only definitive way of diagnosing HTI is to have an earlier scan excluding haemorrhage, so we recommend scanning as early as possible, ideally at the time of initial assessment.

Magnetic resonance imaging

Magnetic resonance imaging (MRI) is probably more sensitive than CT for detecting stroke, particularly lacunar strokes and those occurring in the posterior fossa. However, even MRI scans can be normal in clinically definite stroke.[34] Certain MRI techniques, such as diffusion weighted imaging, are very sensitive at highlighting the "culprit" lesion, which may be useful when several areas of abnormality are shown.

The differentiation between ischaemic and haemorrhagic strokes on MRI in the first few days is less easy for the non-expert than with CT, but MRI (specifically gradient echo sequences) can help diagnose intracerebral haemorrhage months or even years after the event when CT shows only a hypodense area indistinguishable from an infarct. However, physicians in many countries do not have urgent access to MRI and it is currently a difficult technique to use safely and satisfactorily in many acutely ill patients; consequently, CT scanning is likely to remain the principal imaging technique for stroke patients for the foreseeable future.

Where available, MRI, including the use of specific sequences such as diffusion weighted imaging and MR angiography, may add significantly to the understanding of stroke mechanisms.

What caused this stroke?

The list of potential causes is long and obviously differs for ischaemic[35] and haemorrhagic stroke.[36] In individual patients, even after extensive investigation it may be difficult to establish the cause: many will have competing causes (for example, atrial fibrillation (AF) and carotid disease). Thus in practice, the precise cause of stroke is often uncertain. Accepting this, we estimate that about 50% of ischaemic strokes are due to atherothromboembolism, 25% due to intracranial small vessel disease, and 20% due to cardiac embolism, with only 5% due to rarer causes. Most haemorrhagic strokes are thought to be due to small vessel disease (often associated with hypertension), although amyloid angiopathy commonly underlies lobar haemorrhages; vascular abnormalities such as aneurysms and arteriovenous malformations may also underlie haemorrhage and the risk of haemorrhage with anticoagulants increases with the international normalised ratio (INR).

The history and examination may provide important aetiological clues (for example, the use of oral anticoagulants, the presence of an irregular pulse or heart murmur). Unusual causes are considerably more likely in younger patients (for example, evidence of drug abuse or recent cervical trauma precipitating arterial dissection). Our approach to investigation aims to be reasonably cost effective. We perform some simple investigations (full blood count, ESR, plasma glucose, urea and electrolytes, random plasma cholesterol, urinalysis, 12-lead EGG, and CT brain scan) in all patients in whom we are considering active management, even if our clinical assessment strongly suggests a common cause. These tests may identify important modifiable risk factors as well as highlighting the possibility of a rarer, unexpected cause of stroke (for example, infective endocarditis, giant cell arteritis, or thrombocythaemia) which may coexist with either cardiac or degenerative vascular disease. We reserve other more specialised tests[35] for patients in whom the cause of stroke is not clear (for example, young patients (less than 50 years) or those without risk factors), for those with clinical features of a rare cause, or where simple investigations show an abnormality (Table 3.1).

What are this particular patient's problems?

A full assessment by the various members of the multidisciplinary team should be able to identify existing problems and anticipate future ones so that a problem and goal orientated management plan can be constructed. As well as assessing individual impairments and disabilities which may lead to specific interventions (for example, positioning and physiotherapy for hemiparesis), it is important not to ignore but to treat the less specific but unpleasant symptoms such as headache, vomiting, hiccups, vertigo, constipation, and the aches and pains which so often accompany prolonged immobility. Here, we will briefly discuss some of the most common early problems which account for significant mortality and morbidity and which are most relevant to the physician. The list is not exhaustive and does not include important problems which may arise later on (for example, painful shoulders or depression).[37]

Airway and breathing

Although stroke may cause various abnormal breathing patterns[38,39] (for example, periodic respiration or hyperventilation), an intermittently obstructed airway in patients with a decreased level of consciousness may mimic this and should be excluded. The presence of significant hypoxia should stimulate a search for possible causes (for example, pulmonary oedema, pulmonary embolism, or infection). It seems reasonable to attempt to correct this with supplemental oxygen, but we do not advocate routine supplemental oxygen for all patients. We increasingly use

Table 3.1 Second-line investigations in selected stroke patients

Investigation	Indications	Disorders suggested
Liver function tests	Fever, malaise, raised ESR, malignancy	Giant cell arteritis, infective and non-bacterial thrombotic endocarditis
Calcium	Hypercalcaemia may rarely cause recurrent focal symptoms	Hypercalcaemia
Activated partial thromboplastin time, dilute Russell's viper venom time, anticardiolipin antibody, antinuclear and other antibodies	Young patient, previous or family history of venous thrombosis, recurrent miscarriages, thrombocytopenia, cardiac valve vegetations, livedo reticularis, raised ESR, malaise, positive VDRL	Antiphospholipid antibody syndrome, systemic vasculitis, SLE
Protein C and S, antithrombin III, activated protein C resistance, thrombin time	Previous or family history of thrombosis (usually venous) of young onset	Deficiency states
Serum proteins and electrophoresis, plasma viscosity	Raised ESR	Paraproteinaemias, nephrotic syndrome, cardiac myxoma
Haemoglobin electrophoresis	Afro-Caribbean patients	Sickle cell trait or disease, other haemoglobinopathies
Blood cultures	Fever, cardiac murmur, haematuria, deranged liver function tests, raised ESR, malaise	Infective endocarditis
VDRL, HIV serology	Young, unexplained, or "at risk"	Neurosyphilis, AIDS
Serum homocysteine, urinary amino acids	Marfanoid habitus, high myopia, dislocated lenses, osteoporosis, mental retardation, young	Homocystinuria

(Continued)

Table 3.1 (Continued)

Investigation	Indications	Disorders suggested
Leucocyte α-galactosidase A	Corneal opacities, cutaneous angiokeratomas, paraesthesias and pain, renal failure	Fabry's disease
Blood/CSF lactate, mitochondrial DNA analysis	Young, basal ganglia calcification, epilepsy, parietooccipital ischaemia, migraine	MELAS/mitochondrial cytopathy
Drug screen (blood or urine)	"At risk" patient, no other cause	Drug induced stroke (amphetamine, cocaine, etc.)
Chest radiograph	Hypertension, finger clubbing, cardiac murmur or abnormal ECG, young	Calcified valves, enlarged heart, pulmonary arteriovenous malformation
Carotid ultrasound/MR angiography	Carotid distribution stroke in patient suitable for surgery	Cervical internal carotid stenosis
Cerebral angiography (intraarterial digital subtraction or MR)	Young unexplained stroke, especially associated with pain or trauma, suspected arteritis, AVM, or aneurysm	Arterial dissection, vascular abnormality
Transthoracic echocardiography	Suspected cardioembolism	Cardioembolism
Transoesophageal echocardiography	Suspected cardioembolism when TTE negative (e.g. endocarditis, atrial septal aneurysm), aortic dissection or atheroma, patent foramen ovale	Cardioembolism, aortic dissection or atheroma, paradoxical embolism
24 hour ECG	Palpitations, suspicious resting ECG, clinical suspicion	Intermittent AF, heart block
Temporal artery biopsy	Older (>60), jaw claudication, headache, polymyalgia, malaise, anaemia, raised ESR	Giant cell arteritis

TTE = transthoracic echocardiography; VDRL = venereal disease reference laboratory.

pulse oximetry in the acute phase to alert us to significant oxygen desaturation.

Circulation

Hypotension is relatively uncommon in stroke patients; if it does occur, it is usually secondary to coexistent heart disease (arrhythmias, heart failure, or acute myocardial infarction), dehydration, or sepsis. As cerebral autoregulation is disturbed following stroke, with the result that cerebral blood flow becomes directly dependent upon systemic blood pressure, urgent correction is required. By contrast, hypertension is extremely common following stroke, even in patients without pre-existing hypertension.[40,41] Although some authorities recommend early pharmacological lowering of raised blood pressure, given the current absence of any convincing evidence of the effectiveness of such a policy[42-45] and the recognised potential dangers of hypotension,[46] we only give hypotensive drugs early (within the first 72 hours) to patients with features of accelerated hypertension or hypertensive encephalopathy or acute aortic dissection. We usually continue any previous antihypertensive medication a patient may have been taking, provided they are not hypotensive and can safely swallow the tablets. There is uncertainty about when hypotensive drugs should be started after the acute phase; in many cases an elevated blood pressure falls spontaneously in the days following an acute stroke. We usually delay consideration of long term drug therapy for at least a week, although we acknowledge that some physicians would start therapy earlier. Further trials assessing the effect of lowering blood pressure in acute stroke are under way (see www.nottingham.ac.uk/stroke-medicine/enostrialdb/ or www.le.ac.uk/me/shg2/COSSACShome.html).

Raised intracranial pressure

Although intracranial pressure may rise very rapidly following haemorrhagic stroke (due to the space occupying effects), it usually takes at least 48 hours, and often longer, to manifest after an ischaemic stroke (except in the unusual case of a cerebellar or brain stem infarct obliterating the cerebrospinal fluid pathways and resulting in hydrocephalus). Although treatments such as mannitol,[47] hyperventilation and

---

Box 3.2 Causes of deterioration after stroke

Neurological:

— Progression/completion of stroke
— Extension/early recurrence
— Haemorrhagic transformation of an infarct
— Developing cerebral oedema*
— Obstructive hydrocephalus*
— Epileptic seizures*
— Incorrect diagnosis*

Non-neurological:

— Infection*
— Metabolic derangement*
— Drugs*
— Hypoxia*
— Hypercapnia*

*Potentially reversible causes

---

even decompressive craniectomy[48] undoubtedly reduce intracranial pressure, it is unclear whether such aggressive interventions are associated with improved survival with acceptable quality of life. In selected patients who are deteriorating rapidly and who are judged to have some chance of a reasonable recovery, we do consider transfer to an intensive care unit for aggressive management of raised intracranial pressure. However, it is important to remember that early deteriorating conscious level is usually a very poor prognostic indicator, and such intensive treatment in an elderly patient with significant other neurological deficits is, in our view, rarely justified.

Stroke in evolution

Following the onset of symptoms, some patients continue to deteriorate over several hours or days. This is variably referred to as progressing or evolving stroke.[49,50] Such patients require prompt reassessment and investigation, as there is a wide range of potential causes of deterioration, some of which may be reversible (Box 3.2). If we suspect that the cause is progressive thromboembolism, we might use intravenous heparin despite the lack of evidence supporting its effectiveness (see below).

Swallowing, hydration, and nutrition

Dysphagia[51] and poor nutrition[52-55] are common after stroke and may lead to further complications.[56,57] All patients should have a bedside swallowing assessment[58,59] as part of their initial assessment by a suitably trained member of the multidisciplinary team. The gag reflex is an unreliable indicator of swallowing ability and should not be used for this purpose.[59] The bedside assessment should lead to a decision regarding whether or not the patient is safe to swallow and should be written down and clearly communicated to the nursing staff. For patients with an unsafe swallow, fluids should be prescribed (either intravenous or nasogastric) and arrangements made for further assessment by a speech and language therapist. The role of early enteral tube feeding, its timing, and whether this is best delivered via a nasogastric tube or percutaneous endoscopic gastrostomy remains unclear and is the subject of an ongoing multicentre trial.[60,61] Percutaneous endoscopic gastrostomy (PEG) tube feeding is clearly the best option where prolonged tube feeding is necessary. However, in the early stages, where the advantages and disadvantages of early versus delayed tube feeding and the optimal type of tube are unclear, we randomise our patients in this trial.

Glycaemic control

Hypoglycaemia, although unusual after a stroke, should always be excluded on admission, since it may mimic stroke perfectly and delay in its correction can lead to permanent disability or even death. Hyperglycaemia is much more common and has been attributed to previously recognised or occult diabetes or part of an acute stress response.[62] Hyperglycaemia is associated with poor outcomes and although work in animal models suggests that this association may be causal, it may simply reflect the severity of the stroke or underlying vascular disease. Thus, it is unclear how aggressively hyperglycaemia should be corrected and at least one randomised controlled trial is now in progress.[63] Until further evidence is available our policy is to use a glucose, potassium, and insulin infusion to correct blood sugars persistently above 11 mmol/L and to treat even at lower levels provided there are adequate facilities for close monitoring to minimise the risk of hypoglycaemia.

Pyrexia

This may be due to infection preceding the stroke (consider endocarditis and encephalitis), the stroke itself, or, most commonly, a complication such as a chest or urinary infection or venous thromboembolism. Obviously the underlying cause should be sought and treated but it is probably sensible to try to reduce the temperature using simple means (for example, antipyretic drugs) in any case since this is likely to make the patient more comfortable and there is a possibility, based on animal models and the observation that raised temperatures are associated with poor outcomes in patients,[64-67] that a raised temperature may exacerbate any ischaemic cerebral damage.[68] There are no published randomised trials of cooling therapy yet,[69] for patients with either a raised or normal temperature, but there is at least one ongoing randomised study, COOL AID 1 (see www.strokecenter.org/ trials/), and there are published small open studies.[70]

Pressure areas

Decubitus ulcers or pressure sores are an entirely avoidable complication, assuming that they did not develop before medical help was sought. When they do occur, they are painful, slow the patient's recovery, and may sometimes be fatal. Prevention relies on an early assessment of the patient's risk, expert nursing care, and the judicious use of specialised cushions and mattresses.[71]

Bladder management

Incontinence of urine is common in the first few days and a source of major distress for patients and their carers.[72] Usually it can be attributed to several factors including impaired sphincter control, immobility, communication problems, constipation, pre-existing prostatic or gynaecological problems, inadequate nursing, infection, confusion, and impaired consciousness. Obviously the cause or causes should be identified and rectified if possible. Most patients can be managed using absorbent pads, external urinary devices, and regular toileting regimes. If these are impractical and transfers very difficult and the patient's pressure areas are causing concern, we insert an indwelling catheter despite the risk of infection and trauma. Incontinence often resolves spontaneously within the first week or two, so it is wise to try removing the catheter if it seems likely that things will have improved. For patients with persisting incontinence, further investigation with bladder ultrasound or postmicturition catheterisation may be useful to assess bladder contractility and outflow. Urinary retention, particularly in men, is common and easily missed in patients with communication problems.

Venous thromboembolism prophylaxis

Studies using radiolabelled fibrinogen leg scanning suggest that deep venous thrombosis (DVT) occurs in over 50% of patients with hemiplegia.[73] However, clinically apparent DVT probably occurs in fewer than 5%.[16] Similarly, although autopsy series have identified pulmonary embolism (PE) in a large proportion,[74] clinically evident PE occurs in less than 2%,[17,19,37,75] although some PE may be unrecognised. The impact of venous thromboembolism after stroke is therefore unclear.

There are two strategies for the prevention of venous thromboembolism: physical interventions (for example, early mobilisation and compression stockings) and antithrombotic drug therapy. The evidence supporting the use of compression stockings comes from randomised controlled trials in the perioperative period[76] which may not be generalisable to stroke, because in the latter the stockings are applied *after* the onset of paralysis and immobilisation is often prolonged, and the published trials in non-surgical patients were small and inconclusive.[77] Compression stockings, apart from being uncomfortable and time consuming to apply, can occasionally cause gangrene in patients with poor peripheral circulation. It therefore seems reasonable to recommend early mobilisation wherever possible and compression stockings (usually full length, although again there is uncertainty regarding the merits of below knee versus full length stockings) for patients at high risk of DVT (those who are immobilised or who have a previous history of DVT). However, given the difficulties and risk we feel that further randomised controlled trials to evaluate their effectiveness in stroke patients are justified; CLOTS (Clots in Legs Or TEDs after Stroke) is such a trial (see www.dcn.ed.ac.uk/CLOTS).

There is reasonable evidence that aspirin reduces the risk of DVT in several clinical situations[78] and it also has a small but beneficial effect on the long term outcome of patients with ischaemic stroke (see below), so we use this routinely. Although low dose subcutaneous heparin significantly reduces the risk of DVT and PE, this effect is offset by the complications of haemorrhagic transformation and extracranial bleeding, such that at six months the average patient with ischaemic stroke has no greater chance of surviving free of dependency if treated with heparin.[79] We occasionally use heparin (standard unfractionated, at a dose of 5000 units twice daily subcutaneously) in patients we judge to be at particularly high risk of venous thromboembolism (for example those with a history of previous DVT/PE) and low risk of HTI (for example, lacunar infarction).

Epileptic seizures

Early seizures (within two weeks of stroke) occur in about 5% of patients.[80–82] They are more common in haemorrhagic stroke and large infarcts involving the cerebral cortex. Seizures should prompt a review of the diagnosis of stroke (could the focal symptoms be secondary to postictal paralysis or encephalitis?) and a search for precipitating factors (for example, alcohol withdrawal, drugs, metabolic disturbance, or infection). After treating the seizures, we would then reappraise the severity of stroke, since this is notoriously difficult in the presence of seizures. We have occasionally misdiagnosed stroke in patients with non-convulsive seizures, which requires an electroencephalogram for definitive diagnosis. The treatment of poststroke seizures is no different from other forms of secondary epilepsy.[83]

Treatment of acute ischaemic stroke

In the United Kingdom few treatments aimed specifically at the ischaemic brain lesion are routinely used. However, many treatments are used routinely in other countries and evidence is accruing that certain treatments may improve outcome in selected patients. We will therefore consider some of these further and review the available evidence to support their use. Before doing so, it may be helpful to consider briefly the main pathophysiological features of an ischaemic stroke; for a more detailed review, we refer readers elsewhere.[84,85]

Pathophysiology of ischaemic stroke

Ischaemic stroke usually occurs due to occlusion of a cerebral artery or, less often, a reduction in perfusion distal to a severe stenosis. As cerebral blood flow falls, neuronal function is affected in two stages. Initially, as blood flow falls below a critical threshold of about 20 ml of blood per 100 g of brain per minute (normal being over 50 ml/100 g/min), loss of neuronal electrical function occurs. Crucially, this is a potentially *reversible* stage. *Irreversible* damage occurs within minutes as blood flow falls below a second critical threshold of 10 ml/100 g/min; below this level, aerobic mitochondrial metabolism fails and the inefficient anaerobic metabolism of glucose takes over, rapidly leading to lactic acidosis. Consequently, the normal energy dependent cellular ion homoeostasis fails, resulting in potassium leaking out of the cell and sodium and water entering the cell, leading to cytotoxic oedema. Calcium also enters the cell, exacerbating mitochondrial failure. This loss of cellular ion homoeostasis leads to neuronal death.

The identification of these two stages of neuronal failure has led to the concept of the ischaemic penumbra; that is, an area of brain which has reached the reversible stage of electrical failure but has not yet passed onto the second irreversible stage of cellular homoeostatic failure. In theory, therefore, this tissue could be "rescued", either by early reperfusion (using agents to dissolve the acute thrombotic lesion and restore normal blood flow) or by administering agents which could protect these potentially viable neurons from further damage (neuroprotection); the combination of reperfusion and neuroprotection would seem a logical conclusion.[86] Although there is evidence that the concept of the ischaemic penumbra is valid,[87,88] it remains unclear how long ischaemic human brain might survive; in other words, the time window for intervention is unknown. It seems likely that the duration of any time window will vary between individuals and it will be increasingly important to identify the factors which influence it.

Should the mechanism of the cerebral ischaemia influence management?

Some experts believe that certain specific causes of ischaemia, such as basilar artery thrombosis or arterial dissection, warrant specific interventions, most commonly anticoagulation. There is no convincing evidence to support these views and therefore we tend to treat them in the same way as we would any other form of ischaemic stroke. A systematic review of the use of anticoagulants in cerebral venous thrombosis indicated a non-significant favourable effect.[89]

Thrombolysis

Despite having been used sporadically for over 40 years, evidence for the effectiveness of thrombolytic therapy in acute ischaemic stroke has only recently become available. A systematic review of the results of 12 of the 14 completed randomised controlled trials in the post-CT era suggests that although thrombolytic therapy (with recombinant tissue plasminogen activator, streptokinase, or urokinase) is associated with about 70 symptomatic (about 50 fatal) intracranial bleeds per 1000 patients treated, its use is associated with perhaps 65 more patients surviving free of dependency at 3–6 months post-stroke (Figure 3.1).[90] Even more compelling are the updated analyses of treatment within the first three hours.[91] These demonstrate less risk of early intracranial haemorrhage and early death and greater long term net benefit (130 extra patients alive and independent per 1000 treated).

Study	Expt n/N	Ctrl n/N	Peto OR (95%CI fixed)	Weight %	Peto OR (95%CI fixed)
Treatment within three hours					
ASK 1996	14/41	15/29		2·6	0·49 [0·19,1·28]
ECASS 1995	28/49	25/38		3·2	0·70 [0·29,1·66]
ECASS II 1998	39/81	44/77		6·2	0·70 [0·37,1·30]
MAST-E 1996	19/26	14/21		1·6	1·35 [0·39,4·68]
MAST-I 1995	46/79	69/103		6·6	0·69 [0·38,1·26]
Subtotal (95%CI)	146/276	167/268		20·3	0·70 [0·49,0·99]
Chi-square 1·61(df = 4) Z = 2·04					
Treatment between three and six hours					
ASK 1996	70/133	59/137		10·7	1·47 [0·91,2·36]
ECASS 1995	143/264	160/269		20·6	0·81 [0·57,1·13]
ECASS II 1998	148/328	167/314		25·3	0·72 [0·53,0·99]
MAST-E 1996	105/130	112/133		6·0	0·79 [0·42,1·49]
MAST-I 1995	150/234	131/223		17·1	1·25 [0·86,1·83]
Subtotal (95%CI)	616/1089	629/1076		79·7	0·93 [0·78, 1·10]
Chi-square 9·34 (df = 4) Z = 0·86					
Total (95%CI)	762/1365	796/1344		100·0	0·87[0·75, 1·02]
Chi-square 12·99 (df = 9) Z = 1·69					

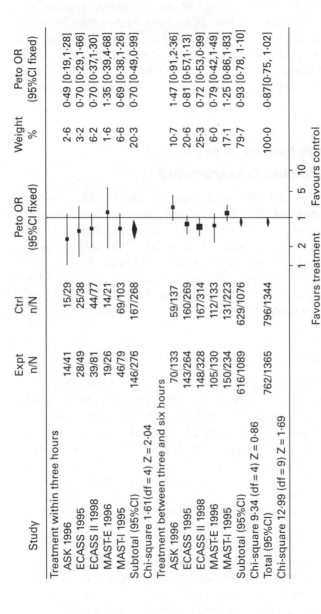

1   2   5   10

1   2

Favours treatment   Favours control

Figure 3.1 Results of a systematic review of the randomised trials of thrombolysis administered within six hours of the onset of CT proven ischaemic stroke. The estimate of treatment is expressed as an odds ratio (square, the size of the square indicating the statistical power of the estimate) and its 95% confidence intervals (horizontal bar); the diamond shapes provide estimates of the pooled trial results. An odds ratio of 1 indicates a zero treatment effect, an odds ratio less than 1 indicates treatment better than control, and an odds ratio greater than 1 indicates treatment worse than control. Treatment with thrombolysis within three hours reduced death and dependency at the end of follow up

How practicable the widespread use of thrombolysis will be (particularly for a condition which has not traditionally been thought of as an emergency) remains uncertain, although some units have published impressive figures.[92] Recombinant tissue plasminogen activator (r-TPA) is now licensed in the United States and a European licence is likely to be granted in the near future; therefore, it seems reasonable to consider using r-TPA in patients presenting within three hours, and who are similar to the patients included in the trials, provided one has a stroke service which can ensure its safe administration (Box 3.3).

Our view is that further trials are required to establish the balance of risks and benefits in a broader range of patients presenting at different stages, with differing severities and types of ischaemic stroke, different risk factors, and differing scan appearances. Many of the eligibility criteria currently in place are arbitrary and are not based on any reliable evidence. If a larger proportion of patients were eligible for treatment the potential impact on the burden of stroke would be greater and it may then be easier to justify the major changes in the delivery of acute stroke services which are required.

Anticoagulants (including standard unfractionated heparin, low molecular weight heparins, and heparinoids)

A systematic review comparing immediate anticoagulant therapy with control in acute ischaemic stroke, including over 20 000 patients, concluded that although anticoagulation started in the first day or two may reduce the risk of DVT and PE (see above), there were no short or long term benefits in terms of survival free of dependency[79] (Figure 3.2). In addition, there was no evidence to support the use of anticoagulants in any specific patient category (for example, presumed cardioembolic stroke or vertebrobasilar stroke). The only situation in which we consider starting anticoagulation (with intravenous, standard unfractionated heparin) is for patients with an evolving, CT-proven ischaemic stroke which we consider is likely to be due to progressive thromboembolism, although there is no convincing evidence to justify this policy.

Box 3.3 Suggested guidelines for the use of intravenous r-TPA in ischaemic stroke[108]

Intravenous r-TPA should be considered in all patients with a proven ischaemic stroke presenting within three hours of onset.

Recommended dose is 0·9 mg/kg, up to a maximum of 90 mg, the first 10% as a bolus, the rest as an infusion over 60 minutes.

Thrombolysis should be avoided in cases where the CT suggests early changes of major infarction (for example, sulcal effacement, mass effect, or oedema).

Thrombolytic therapy should only be administered by physicians with expertise in stroke medicine, who have access to a suitable stroke service, with facilities for identifying and managing haemorrhagic complications.

Exclusion criteria: use of oral anticoagulants or INR greater than 1·7; use of heparin in preceding 48 hours or prolonged partial thromboplastin time; platelet count less than 100 000/mm^3; stroke or serious head injury in the previous three months; major surgery within previous 14 days; pretreatment systolic BP greater than 185 mmHg or diastolic greater than 110 mmHg; rapidly improving neurological condition; mild isolated neurological deficits; previous intracranial haemorrhage; blood glucose greater than 22 mmol/L (400 mg/dl) or less than 2·8 mmol/L (50 mg/dl); seizure at stroke onset; gastrointestinal or urinary bleeding within previous 21 days; or recent myocardial infarction.

Caution is advised before giving r-TPA to patients with severe stroke (NIH Stroke Scale Score greater than 22).

It is recommended that treatment and adverse effects are discussed with patient and family prior to treatment.

The individual threshold for using early anticoagulation is very variable and some physicians use anticoagulants for specific situations such as basilar artery thrombosis or intracardiac thrombus.

Although we know that oral anticoagulation with warfarin is effective in the secondary prevention of stroke in patients with atrial fibrillation,[93,94] we have considerable difficulty deciding when to start warfarin after the primary event. We tend to delay longer (perhaps by two weeks) in patients with large ischaemic cerebral lesions, believing that they are more likely to suffer ill effects (mainly haemorrhagic transformation) from anticoagulation, although this is not evidence based. The question of whether to anticoagulate patients with other potential cardioembolic sources, such as

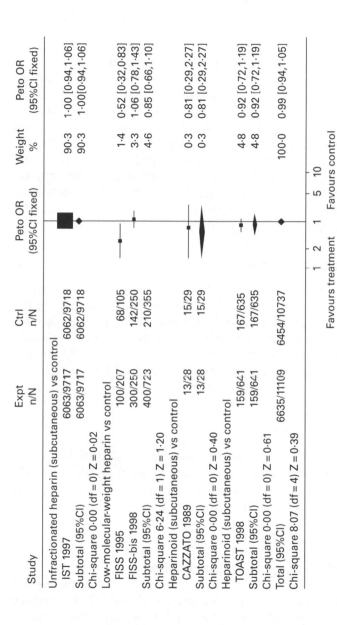

Figure 3.2 Results of a systematic review of the randomised trials of anticoagulants in acute presumed ischaemic stroke. There was no significant effect of anticoagulant treatment on death or dependency at the end of follow up (greater than one month)

mitral valve disease without AF, is very difficult, with little evidence to guide the physician.

Aspirin

The pooled results of two very large randomised controlled trials comparing aspirin with placebo concluded that medium dose aspirin (160–300 mg) started in the acute phase of an ischaemic stroke produces a small net benefit (13 fewer patients per 1000 dead or disabled).[95] Whether this benefit arose from an effect on the stroke itself or simply through earlier initiation of secondary prevention of stroke and other thrombotic complications is uncertain. We therefore start all patients on aspirin 300 mg as soon as a CT has confirmed an ischaemic stroke unless there is a specific contraindication; we later discharge patients on a maintenance dose of 75–150 mg per day.

Neuroprotective agents

To date, no neuroprotective agent has been conclusively shown to be effective and a Cochrane review summarising the current data is awaited.[96] Trials to evaluate the neuroprotective effects of magnesium (IMAGES), benzodiazepines (EGASIS), and other novel agents are in progress (see http://www. nottingham.ac. uk/stroke-medicine/enostrialdb/ and http://www. medther.gla.ac.uk/studies/images/).

Other treatments

Numerous other treatments have been used for ischaemic stroke and some have been subjected to randomised trials. However, there is currently no convincing evidence to support the routine use of any of them.

Treatment of haemorrhagic stroke

A variety of specific treatments designed to reduce intracranial pressure is often used for primary intracerebral haemorrhage, including osmotic agents such as mannitol, urea or glycerol, steroids or hyperventilation; unfortunately there is no convincing evidence that these treatments improve outcome. In view of the lack of evidence, we do not routinely use any specific medical therapy in haemorrhagic stroke, nor do we routinely use invasive devices, such as intraventricular catheters, to measure intracranial pressure directly. We would attempt to correct or reverse any clotting abnormality, including those patients on oral anticoagulant drugs, although this depends on the original indication for the anticoagulants (for example, prosthetic heart valves).

Surgery for supratentorial primary intracerebral haemorrhage

A systematic review of open surgical drainage via a craniotomy concluded that this sort of surgery was positively harmful.[97] However, safer surgical techniques are now available, in particular stereotactic aspiration, and the results of ongoing surgical trials are awaited. In a previously fit person with a large lobar intracerebral haemorrhage whose conscious level is falling, we would refer to our neurosurgeons and encourage them to drain the haematoma. In this situation, where one expects the patient to die unless action is taken, the decisions are relatively easy. More difficult are those patients with lesions deep in the hemisphere and those with severe impairments but no reduction in conscious level. These patients we usually manage conservatively or randomise into one of the ongoing trials of surgical treatment (see www.ncl.ac.uk/stich/).

Surgery for infratentorial primary intracerebral haemorrhage

Although there is general agreement that surgical intervention in this situation may be life saving (so much so that a randomised controlled trial is unlikely ever to be done), there is considerable uncertainty about which patients might benefit the most or even which procedure is optimal (haematoma evacuation versus ventricular decompression via a ventriculostomy, or both). We would always consider surgical intervention in any patient who was comatose or whose conscious level was progressively deteriorating and in whom other exacerbating causes had been excluded (Box 3.2). Once brain stem reflexes have been absent for several hours, however, death is inevitable.[98]

Organisation of stroke services

In the United Kingdom, between 40% and 70% of patients are admitted to hospital following a stroke[99–101] and mostly cared for by general internal physicians and geriatricians. In many other countries, admission rates exceed 90% and larger proportions of patients are managed by neurologists. In the United States and many European countries, professional bodies recommend hospital admission for most if not all patients following an acute stroke.[102,103] In the United Kingdom, we would recommend that most if not all patients should be referred to hospital, although not necessarily for acute admission.[104] Many patients require hospital admission on nursing grounds alone or because of diagnostic uncertainty. It is now accepted that most patients, whether admitted to hospital or not, need early access to hospital based facilities such as CT scanning.[105,106] Patients who have suffered a mild, non-disabling stroke may not require inpatient care but do need rapid assessment (within a few days), the exceptions perhaps being the very infirm or elderly and those already in institutionalised care. Widespread introduction of thrombolytic therapy for ischaemic stroke, with its narrow time window will demand much improved organisation of prehospital care and the introduction of "fast tracking" within hospitals to avoid delays.

A systematic review of all randomised controlled trials evaluating stroke unit care demonstrated that patients managed in stroke units are significantly less likely to die, have severe disability, or require long term institutional care than those managed in general medical wards.[107] Although this review is often quoted to justify the establishment of acute stroke units (that is, those which admit patients directly for just a few days to facilitate acute treatment and intensive monitoring), it did not include such units. Thus the evidence from randomised controlled trials only applies to units which can also offer at least several weeks of care coordinated by a multidisciplinary team.

Having said this, we believe that patients should have access to comprehensive and well organised services, whatever their need. An acute unit run by interested specialists is more likely to ensure high quality care and will facilitate the introduction of evidence-based protocols for investigation and treatment, as well as further research. It seems likely that the sooner acute specific treatments can be given, the more effective they will be ("time is brain"). It is likely that there will be increasing emphasis on systems of pre-hospital care which facilitate earlier transfer to an acute stroke unit. However, this must not inhibit the development of other aspects of the services (for example, rehabilitation) which have been shown to have important benefits for patients.

Therefore hospitals need to develop both inpatient and outpatient services in collaboration with primary care, which can respond rapidly. As an important adjunct to developing these services, the general public should be educated about the symptoms of stroke and the importance of early presentation to medical services.

Conclusions

Stroke causes a vast amount of death and disability throughout the world, yet for many healthcare professionals it remains an area of therapeutic nihilism and thus uninteresting. This negative perception is shared by the general public, who often have a poor understanding of the early symptoms and significance of a stroke. Yet within the last few years there have been many important developments in the approach to caring for stroke patients, for both the acute management and secondary prevention.

Following the completion of numerous clinical trials, we now have robust evidence either to support or discredit various interventions. Even more exciting is the prospect of yet more data becoming available in the near future, testing a whole array of treatments, as clinical interest in stroke expands exponentially.

Management of acute stroke

- Acute stroke is hugely important worldwide as a cause of death and serious disability.
- Acute stroke represents a medical emergency, and should be managed as such.
- Management is crucially dependent upon an early and accurate diagnosis; investigations should be aimed to help to identify the type of stroke and its possible causes. They should be performed promptly and be cost effective.
- Patients should be managed within an organised stroke unit, which is the only intervention proven to reduce death and disability for most patients.
- Intravenous thrombolysis is currently only applicable to a small proportion of patients with proven ischaemic stroke presenting within three hours.
- There is no evidence to support the use of anticoagulants in any patient category. However we consider starting intravenous standard unfractionated heparin in evolving CT-proven ischaemic stroke which is likely to be due to progressive thromboembolism.
- We start all patients on aspirin 300 mg as soon as CT has confirmed an ischaemic stroke unless there is a contraindication.
- We would refer a patient with a large lobar intracerebral haemorrhage and falling conscious level for drainage of the haematoma.
- We would consider a patient in coma or deteriorating with a cerebellar haematoma for surgical intervention.
- It is likely that new, effective strategies to treat acute stroke will become available soon.

References

1　Harris AI. *Handicapped and impaired in Great Britain*. London: HMSO, 1971.
2　Martin J, Meltzer H, Elliot D. *OPCS surveys of disability in Great Britain report 1. The prevalence of disability amongst adults*. London: HMSO, 1988.
3　Sudlow C, Warlow C. Comparing stroke incidence worldwide. What makes studies comparable? *Stroke* 1996;**27**:550–8.
4　Warlow CP, Dennis MS, van Gijn J, *et al*. The organisation of stroke services. In: *Stroke. A practical guide to management,* 2nd edn. Oxford: Blackwell Science, 2001;723–61.
5　King's Fund Forum. Treatment of stroke. *Br Med J* 1988;**297**:126–8.
6　Department of Health. National Service Framework for older people. 2001. www.doh.gov.uk/nsf/olderpeople.htm.
7　Scottish Executive. Coronary heart disease and stroke strategy for Scotland. 2002. www.show.scot.nhs.uk/sehd/stroke/.
8　Hatano S. Experience from a multicentre stroke register: a preliminary report. *Bull WHO* 1976;**54**:541–53.

9   Counsell C, Dennis M, McDowall M, Warlow C. Predicting outcome after acute stroke: development and validation of new models. *Stroke* 2002;**33**:1041–7.

10 Bamford J, Dennis M, Sandercock P, *et al*. The frequency, causes and timing of death within 30 days of a first stroke: the Oxfordshire Community Stroke Project. *J Neurol Neurosurg Psychiatry* 1990;**53**:824–9.

11 Bounds JV, Wiebers DO, Whisnant JP, *et al*. Mechanisms and timing of deaths from cerebral infarction. *Stroke* 1981;**12**:474–7.

12 Silver FL, Norris JW, Lewis AJ, *et al*. Early mortality following stroke: a prospective review. *Stroke* 1984;**15**:492–6.

13 Dennis MS, Burn JP, Sandercock PA, *et al*. Long-term survival after first-ever stroke: the Oxfordshire Community Stroke Project. *Stroke* 1993;**24**:796–800.

14 Warlow CP, Dennis MS, van Gijn J, *et al*. A practical approach to the management of stroke patients. In: *Stroke. A practical guide to management*, 2nd edn. Oxford: Blackwell Science, 2001;414–41.

15 Burn J, Dennis M, Bamford J, *et al*. Long-term risk of recurrent stroke after a first-ever stroke. The Oxfordshire Community Stroke Project. *Stroke* 1994;**25**:333–7.

16 Davenport RJ, Dennis MS, Wellwood I, *et al*. Complications after acute stroke. *Stroke* 1996;**27**:415–20.

17 Dromerick A, Reding M. Medical and neurological complications during inpatient stroke rehabilitation. *Stroke* 1994;**25**:358–61.

18 Dobkin BH. Neuromedical complications in stroke patients transferred for rehabilitation before and after diagnostic related groups. *J Neuro Rehabil* 1987;**1**:3–7.

19 Kalra L, Yu G, Wilson K, *et al*. Medical complications during stroke rehabilitation. *Stroke* 1995;**26**:990–4.

20 Langhorne P, Stott DJ, Robertson L, *et al*. Medical complications in hospitalized stroke patients: a multicentre study. *Stroke* 2000;**31**: 1223–9.

21 Sandercock PA, Warlow CP, Jones LN, *et al*. Predisposing factors for cerebral infarction: the Oxfordshire community stroke project. *Br Med J* 1989;**298**:75–80.

22 Bamford J, Sandercock P, Dennis M, *et al*. Classification and natural history of clinically identifiable subtypes of cerebral infarction. *Lancet* 1991;**337**:1521–6.

23 Anderson CS, Taylor BV, Hankey GJ, *et al*. Validation of a clinical classification for subtypes of acute cerebral infarction. *J Neurol Neurosurg Psychiatry* 1994;**57**:1173–9.

24 Lindgren A, Norvving B, Rudling O, *et al*. Comparison of clinical and neuro-radiological findings in first ever stroke: a population based study. *Stroke* 1994;**25**:1371–7.

25 Mead GE, Wardlaw JM, Dennis MS, *et al*. The validity of a simple clinical classification for acute stroke. *Age Ageing* 1998;**27**(suppl 1): 69 (abstract).

26 Al-Buhairi AR, Phillips SJ, Llewellyn G, *et al*. Prediction of infarct topography using the Oxfordshire Community Stroke Project classification of stroke subtypes. *J Stroke Cerebrovasc Dis* 1998;**7**:339–43.

27 Mead GE, Lewis SC, Wardlaw JM, Dennis MS. Warlow CP. How well does the Oxfordshire community stroke project classification predict the site and size of the infarct on brain imaging? *J Neurol Neurosurg Psychiatry* 2000;**68**:558–62.

28 Lindley RI, Warlow CP, Wardlaw JM, *et al*. Interobserver reliability of a clinical classification of acute cerebral infarction. *Stroke* 1993;**24**:1801–4.

29   Bamford J, Sandercock P, Dennis M, *et al.* A prospective study of acute cerebrovascular disease in the community: the Oxfordshire Community Stroke Project – 1981–86. 2. Incidence, case fatality rates and overall outcome at one year of cerebral infarction, primary intracerebral and subarachnoid haemorrhage. *J Neurol Neurosurg Psychiatry* 1990;**53**: 16–22.

30   Weir CJ, Murray GD, Adams FG, *et al.* Poor accuracy of scoring systems for differential clinical diagnosis of intracranial haemorrhage and infarction. *Lancet* 1994;**344**:999–1002.

31   Wardlaw JM, Keir SL, Dennis MS. The impact of delays in CT brain imaging on the accuracy of diagnosis and subsequent management in patients with minor stroke. *J Neurol Neurosurg Psychiatry* 2003 (in press).

32   Warlow CP, Dennis MS, van Gijn J, *et al.* What pathological type of stroke is it? In: *Stroke. A practical guide to management*, 2nd edn. Oxford: Blackwell Science, 2001;151–222.

33   Bogousslavsky J, Regli F, Uske A, *et al.* Early spontaneous haematoma in cerebral infarct. *Neurology* 1991;**41**:837–40.

34   Alberts MJ, Faulstich ME, Gray L. Stroke with negative brain magnetic resonance imaging. *Stroke* 1992;**23**:663–7.

35   Warlow CP, Dennis MS, van Gijn J, *et al.* What caused this transient or persisting ischaemic event? In: *Stroke. A practical guide to management*, 2nd edn. Oxford: Blackwell Science, 2001;223–300.

36   Warlow CP, Dennis MS, van Gijn J, *et al.* What caused this intracerebral haemorrhage? In: *Stroke. A practical guide to management*, 2nd edn. Oxford: Blackwell Science, 2001;339–75.

37   Warlow CP, Dennis MS, van Gijn J, *et al.* What are this person's problems? A problem-based approach to the general management of stroke. In: *Stroke. A practical guide to management*, 2nd edn. Oxford: Blackwell Science, 2001;572–652.

38   Rout MW, Lane DJ, Wollner L. Prognosis in acute cerebrovascular accidents in relation to respiratory pattern and blood gas tensions. *Br Med J* 1971;**3**:7–9.

39   Nachtmann A, Siebler M, Rose G, *et al.* Cheyne–Stokes respiration in ischemic stroke. *Neurology* 1995;**45**:820–1.

40   Carlsson A, Britton M. Blood pressure after stroke. A one-year follow-up study. *Stroke* 1993;**24**:195–9.

41   Wallace JD, Levy LL. Blood pressure after stroke. *JAMA* 1981;**246**:2177–80.

42   Blood pressure in Acute Stroke Collaboration (BASC). Interventions for deliberately altering blood pressure in acute stroke. In: Cochrane Collaboration. *Cochrane Library*. Issue 4. Oxford: Update Software, 2002.

43   Powers WJ. Acute hypertension after stroke: the scientific basis for treatment decisions. *Neurology* 1993;**43**:461–7.

44   Bath FJ, Bath PMW. What is the correct management of blood pressure in acute stroke? The Blood Pressure in Acute Stroke Collaboration. *Cerebrovasc Dis* 1997;**7**:205–13.

45   Potter JF. What should we do about blood pressure and stroke? *Q J Med* 1999;**92**:63–6.

46   Britton M, de Faire U, Helmers C. Hazards of therapy for excessive hypertension in acute stroke. *Acta Med Scand* 1980;**207**:253–7.

47   Bereczki D, Liu M, do Prado GF, Fekete I. Mannitol for acute stroke. In: Cochrane Collaboration. *Cochrane Library*. Issue 4. Oxford: Update Software, 2002.

48   Hacke W, Berge E, Dennis M, Morley N. Decompressive surgery for malignant middle cerebral artery territory infarction. *Pract Neurol* 2002;**2**:144–53.

49 Gautier JC. Stroke-in-progression. *Stroke* 1985;**16**:729–33.
50 Asplund K. Any progress on progressing stroke? *Cerebrovasc Dis* 1992;**2**:317–19.
51 Gordon C, Hewer RL, Wade DT. Dysphagia in acute stroke. *Br Med J* 1987;**295**:411–14.
52 Axelsson K, Asplund K, Norberg A, Eriksson S. Eating problems and nutritional status during hospital stay of patients with severe stroke. *J Am Dietary Assoc* 1989;**8**:1092–6.
53 Davalos A, Ricart W, Gonzalex-Huix F, *et al*. Effect of malnutrition after acute stroke on clinical outcome. *Stroke* 1996;**27**:1028–32.
54 Smithard DG, Renwick D, O'Neill PA. Change in nutritional status following acute stroke. *Age Ageing* 1993;**22** (suppl 3):11 (abstract).
55 Unosson M, Ek AC, Bjurulf P, von Schenk H, Larsson J. Feeding dependence and nutritional status after acute stroke. *Stroke* 1994;**25**: 366–71.
56 Smithard DG, O'Neill PA, Park C, *et al*. Complications and outcome after stroke. Does dysphagia matter? *Stroke* 1996;**27**:1200–4.
57 Gariballa SE, Parker SG, Taub N, Castleden CM. Influence of nutritional status on clinical outcome after acute stroke. *Am J Clin Nutr* 1998;**68**: 275–81.
58 Scottish Intercollegiate Guidelines Network. *Management of patients with stroke. III: Identification and management of dysphagia*. Edinburgh: SIGN, 1997.
59 Smithard DG, O'Neill PA, Park C, *et al*. Can bedside assessment reliably exclude aspiration following acute stroke? *Age Ageing* 1999;**27**:99–106.
60 Dennis MS. The FOOD Trial Collaboration. Performance of a statistical model to predict stroke outcome in a large simple randomized controlled trial of feeding. *Stroke* 2003 (in press).
61 Bath PMW, Bath FJ, Smithard DG. Interventions for dysphagia in acute stroke. In: Cochrane Collaboration. *Cochrane Library*. Issue 4. Oxford: Update Software, 2002.
62 Scott JF, Gray CS, O'Connell JE, *et al*. Glucose and insulin therapy in acute stroke; why delay further? *Q J Med* 1998;**91**:511–15.
63 Scott JS, Robinson GM, O'Connell JE, *et al*. Glucose potassium insulin (GKI) infusions in the treatment of acute stroke patients with mild to moderate hyperglycaemia: the glucose insulin in stroke trial. *Stroke* 1999;**30**:793–99.
64 Castillo J, Martinez F, Leira R, *et al*. Mortality and morbidity of acute cerebral infarction related to temperature and basal analytic parameters. *Cerebrovasc Dis* 1994;**4**:66–71.
65 Chen H, Chopp M, Welch KM. Effect of mild hyperthermia on the ischemic infarct volume after middle cerebral artery occlusion in the rat. *Neurology* 1991;**41**:1133–5.
66 Azzimondi G, Bassein L, Nonino F, *et al*. Fever in acute stroke worsens prognosis. A prospective study. *Stroke* 1995;**26**:2040–3.
67 Reith J, Jorgensen HS, Pedersen PM, *et al*. Body temperature in acute stroke: relation to stroke severity, infarct size, mortality, and outcome. *Lancet* 1996;**347**:422–5.
68 Ginsberg MD, Busto R. Combating hyperthermia in acute stroke. A significant clinical concern. *Stroke* 1998;**29**:529–34.
69 Correia M, Silva M, Veloso M. Cooling therapy for acute stroke. In: Cochrane Collaboration. *Cochrane Library*. Issue 4. Oxford: Update Software, 2002.
70 Schwab S, Schwarz S, Spranger M, *et al*. Moderate hypothermia in the treatment of patients with severe middle cerebral artery infarction. *Stroke* 1998;**29**:2461–6.

71 Nuffield Institute for Health. Effective health care. The prevention and treatment of pressure sores. *Effect Health Care* 1995;**2**:1–16.

72 Nakayama H, Jorgensen HS, Pedersen PM, *et al*. Prevalence and risk factors of incontinence after stroke. The Copenhagen Stroke Study. *Stroke* 1997;**28**:58–62.

73 Warlow C, Ogston D, Douglas AS. Venous thrombosis following strokes. *Lancet* 1972;**1**:1305–6.

74 Warlow C. Venous thromboembolism after stroke. *Am Heart J* 1978;**96**: 283–5.

75 McClatchie G. Survey of the rehabilitation outcomes of stroke. *Med J Aust* 1980;**1**:649–51.

76 Wells PS, Lensing AWA, Hirsch J. Graduated pressure stockings in the prevention of postoperative venous thromboembolism: a meta analysis. *Arch Intern Med* 1994;**154**:67–72.

77 Muir KW, Watt A, Baxter G, Grosset DG, Lees KR. Randomised trial of graded compression stockings for prevention of deep-vein thrombosis after acute stroke. *Q J Med* 2000;**93**:359–64.

78 Antiplatelet Trialists' Collaboration. Collaborative overview of randomised trials of antiplatelet therapy – III: Reduction in venous thrombosis and pulmonary embolism by antiplatelet prophylaxis among surgical and medical patients. *Br Med J* 1994;**308**:235–46.

79 Gubitz G, Counsell C, Sandercock P, Signorini D. Anticoagulants for acute ischaemic stroke. In: Cochrane Collaboration. *Cochrane Library*. Issue 4. Oxford: Update Software, 2002.

80 Kilpatrick CJ, Davis SM, Tress BM, *et al*. Epileptic seizures in acute stroke. *Arch Neurol* 1990;**47**:157–60.

81 So EL, Annegers JF, Hauser WA, *et al*. Population-based study of seizure disorders after cerebral infarction. *Neurology* 1996;**46**:350–5.

82 Burn J, Dennis M, Bamford J, Sandercock P, Wade D, Warlow C. Epileptic seizures after a first stroke: the Oxfordshire Community Stroke Project. *Br Med J* 1997;**315**:1582–7.

83 Scottish Intercollegiate Guidelines Network. *Diagnosis and management of epilepsy in adults*. Edinburgh: SIGN, 1997.

84 Sharp FR, Swanson RA, Honkaniemi J, Kogure K, Massa SM. Neurochemistry and molecular biology. In: Barnett HJM, Mohr JP, Stein BM, Yatsu FM, eds. *Stroke. Pathophysiology, diagnosis, and management*. Philadelphia: Churchill Livingstone, 1998.

85 Kristian T, Siesjo BK. Calcium in ischemic cell death. *Stroke* 1998;**29**: 705–18.

86 Steiner T, Hacke W. Combination therapy with neuroprotectants and thrombolytics in acute ischaemic stroke. *Eur Neurol* 1998;**40**:1–8.

87 Marchal G, Beaudouin V, Rioux P, *et al*. Prolonged persistence of substantial volumes of potentially viable brain tissue after stroke: a correlative PET–CT study with voxel-based data analysis. *Stroke* 1996; **27**:599–606.

88 Baron JC. Mapping the ischaemic penumbra with PET: implications for acute stroke treatment. *Cerebrovasc Dis* 1999;**7**:205–13.

89 Stam J, de Bruijn SFTM, DeVeber G. Anticoagulation for cerebral sinus thrombosis. In: Cochrane Collaboration. *Cochrane Library*. Issue 4. Oxford: Update Software, 2002.

90 Wardlaw JM, Warlow CP, Counsell C. Systematic review of evidence on thrombolytic therapy for acute ischaemic stroke. *Lancet* 1997;**350**: 607–14.

91   Wardlaw JM, del Zoppo G, Yamaguchi T. Thrombolysis for acute ischaemic stroke. In: Cochrane Collaboration. *Cochrane Library.* Issue 4. Oxford: Update Software, 2002.

92   Grond M, Stenzel C, Schmulling S, *et al.* Early intravenous thrombolysis for acute ischemic stroke in a community-based approach. *Stroke* 1998;**29**:1544–9.

93   Koudstaal P. Anticoagulants for preventing stroke in patients with non-rheumatic atrial fibrillation and a history of stroke or transient ischaemic attacks. In: Cochrane Collaboration. *Cochrane Library.* Issue 4. Oxford: Update Software, 2002.

94   Koudstaal P. Anticoagulants versus antiplatelet therapy for preventing stroke in patients with nonrheumatic atrial fibrillation and a history of stroke or transient ischaemic attacks. In: Cochrane Collaboration. *Cochrane Library.* Issue 4. Oxford: Update Software, 2002.

95   CAST (Chinese Acute Stroke Trial) Collaborative Group. CAST: randomised placebo-controlled trial of early aspirin use in 20000 patients with acute ischaemic stroke. *Lancet* 1997;**349**:1641–9.

96   Lees KR, Muir KW. Excitatory amino acid antagonists for acute stroke (Protocol for a Cochrane Review). In: Cochrane Collaboration. *Cochrane Library.* Issue 4. Oxford: Update Software, 2002.

97   Hankey GJ, Hon C. Surgery for primary intracerebral hemorrhage: is it safe and effective? A systematic review of case series and randomized trials. *Stroke* 1997;**28**:2126–32.

98   Gerritsen van der Hoop R, Vermeulen M, van Gijn J. Cerebellar hemorrhage: diagnosis and treatment. *Surg Neurol* 1988;**29**:6–10.

99   Bamford J, Sandercock P, Warlow C, *et al.* Why are patients with acute stroke admitted to hospital? *Br Med J* 1986;**292**:1369–72.

100 Wade DT, Hewer RL. Hospital admission for acute stroke: who, for how long, and to what effect? *J Epidemiol Community Health* 1985;**39**: 347–52.

101 Brocklehurst JC, Andrews K, Morris P, *et al.* Why admit stroke patients to hospital? *Age Ageing* 1978;**7**:100–8.

102 Lanska DJ. Review criteria for hospital utilization for patients with cerebro-vascular disease. Task Force on Hospital Utilization for Stroke of the American Academy of Neurology. *Neurology* 1994;**44**:1531–2.

103 Adams HP, Brott TG, Crowell RM, *et al.* Guidelines for the management of patients with acute ischaemic stroke. A statement for healthcare professionals from a special writing group of the Stroke Council, American Heart Association. *Stroke* 1994;**25**:1901–14.

104 Dennis M. Who to admit and when? That is the question. *Proc R Coll Physicians Edinb* 2001;**31**(suppl 8):25–28.

105 Scottish Intercollegiate Guidelines Network. *Management of patients with stroke. I: Assessment, investigation, management and secondary prevention.* Edinburgh: SIGN, 1997.

106 Royal College of Physicians of Edinburgh. Consensus conference on the medical management of stroke. *J Neurol Neurosurg Psychiatry* 1999;**66**: 128–9.

107 Stroke Unit Trialists' Collaboration. Organised inpatient (stroke unit) care for stroke. In: Cochrane Collaboration. *Cochrane Library.* Issue 4. Oxford: Update Software, 2002.

108 Adams HP, Brott TG, Furlan AJ, *et al.* Guidelines for thrombolytic therapy for acute stroke: a supplement to the guidelines for the management of patients with acute ischemic stroke. *Circulation* 1996;**94**:1167–74.

Useful websites

http://www.strokecenter.org/trials/ A useful register of completed and ongoing trials in stroke, with links to individual websites.

http://www.dcn.ed.ac.uk/CSRG The Cochrane Stroke Review Group home page, with lists of completed Cochrane reviews and protocols in stroke, and information on how to undertake a systematic review.

http://www.basp.ac.uk The home web site of the British Association of Stroke Physicians.

4: Delirium

S TURNER, S LEWIS

The concept of delirium has been with us for over 2000 years. Greek physicians, such as Hippocrates, described its essential features[1] and the Roman writer Celsus distinguished it from mania and depression.[2] Galen differentiated between primary (idiopathic) and secondary (symptomatic) forms.[3]

Delirium is common in the hospital setting.[4] It often goes undiagnosed in its early stages[5] and may present as a neurological emergency. If untreated, it is associated with a high mortality.[6]

Terminology

A general problem in psychiatry has been the complex etymology of clinical terms. This problem has been improved as a result of the move towards operational definitions in both the *International Classification of Mental and Behavioural Disorders* (ICD10; Box 4.1);[7] and the American *Diagnostic and Statistical Manual of Mental Disorders*, 4th edition (DSMIV; Box 4.2).[8]

"Delirium" is now the accepted term for acute, transient, global, organic disorders of higher nervous system function involving impaired consciousness and attention. It is synonymous with the "acute confusional state" of ICD9,[9] which has been replaced, and is also referred to as "acute organic reaction" and "acute brain syndrome". The DSMIV definition has changed markedly (Box 4.2). The aim of the change was to increase the accuracy of diagnosis.[10] The new definition emphasises those symptoms most specific to delirium in the medically ill elderly (for example, perceptual disturbances and incoherent speech) instead of those found to be less specific (for example, sleep disturbance and psychomotor change).[11]

Definitions of delirium remain problematical, particularly with respect to dementia in the elderly. The distinctions

---

Box 4.1 ICD10 diagnostic criteria for delirium

For a definite diagnosis, symptoms, mild or severe, should be present in each one of the following areas:

1. Impairment of consciousness and attention (on a continuum from clouding to coma; reduced ability to direct, focus, sustain, and shift attention).
2. Global disturbance of cognition (perceptual distortions, illusions, and hallucinations – most often visual; impairment of abstract thinking and comprehension, with or without transient delusions but typically with some degree of incoherence; impairment of immediate recall and of recent memory but with relatively intact remote memory; disorientation for time as well as, in more severe cases, for place and person).
3. Psychomotor disturbances (hypoactivity or hyperactivity and unpredictable shifts from one to the other; increased reaction time; increased or decreased flow of speech; enhanced startle reaction).
4. Disturbance of the sleep–wake cycle (insomnia or, in more severe cases, total sleep loss or reversal of the sleep–wake cycle; daytime drowsiness; nocturnal worsening of symptoms; disturbing dreams or nightmares, which may continue as hallucinations after awakening).
5. Emotional disturbances, for example, depression, anxiety, or fear, irritability, euphoria, apathy, or wondering perplexity.

The onset is usually rapid, the course diurnally fluctuating, and the total duration of the condition less than six months. The above clinical picture is so characteristic that a fairly confident diagnosis of delirium can be made even if the underlying cause is not firmly established. In addition to a history of an underlying physical or brain disease, evidence of cerebral dysfunction (such as an abnormal EEG, usually but not invariably showing a slowing of the background activity) may be required if the diagnosis is in doubt.

---

between the two have been called into question.[12] For instance, abrupt deterioration in cognitive state is typical of vascular dementia. Visual hallucinations and fluctuating cognitive states are typical of Lewy body dementia.[13] Also some studies of prognosis of delirium have shown that symptoms can be more prolonged than previously acknowledged.[14]

In this chapter, symptoms and signs will be defined with regard to their clinical utility in diagnosing delirium. It should be borne in mind, however, that many terms such as "consciousness"[15] and "memory"[16] are used slightly differently

> **Box 4.2 DSMIV diagnostic criteria for delirium**
>
> Disturbance of consciousness (that is, reduced clarity of awareness of the environment) with reduced ability to focus, sustain or shift attention.
>
> A change in cognition (such as memory deficit, disorientation, language disturbance) or the development of a perceptual disturbance that is not better accounted for by a pre-existing, established or evolving dementia.
>
> The disturbance develops over a short period of time (usually hours to days) and tends to fluctuate during the course of the day.
>
> There is evidence from the history, physical examination or laboratory findings that the disturbance is caused by the direct physiological consequences of a general medical condition.

by different groups, even within medicine. The terms "confusion", "clouding", and "sensorium" in particular should be avoided because of their lack of standard definitions.

Epidemiology

Sophisticated epidemiological data are now available for most psychiatric disorders. Accurate data on incidence, prevalence, and mortality in delirium, however, are difficult to come by. The comparison of estimates across studies is hampered by methodological differences. Methods of case finding and diagnosis will influence rates obtained, as will the patient population and the setting (community, general medical, surgical, or geriatric inpatient) in which the disorder is diagnosed.[17] Most incidence and prevalence studies of delirium have been conducted in inpatient settings. One notable exception is the Eastern Baltimore Mental Survey, a large community based survey forming part of the Epidemiologic Catchment Area (ECA) programme.[18] This study aimed to look at the prevalence of delirium in the general adult population aged between 18 and 64 years. A total of 810 individuals were subjected to psychiatric evaluation and a point prevalence rate of 0·4% was calculated, rising to 1·1% for those aged 55 years and over.

Whereas prevalence rates in the community are low, in hospital settings they are high. It has been estimated that 10% of all medical and surgical inpatients meet criteria for delirium at some point during their stay.[4] Delirium may therefore represent the mental disorder with the single highest incidence.[19]

As with community subjects, advanced age is a potent risk factor for delirium in inpatient surveys. Among elderly general medical inpatients, rates of 30%[20] or even 50%[21] have been reported, although a more conservative estimate of 17%[22] is probably more realistic. Rates of delirium in elderly surgical patients are broadly similar, although following operation for hip fracture the rate may be as high as 50%.[23]

A pre-existing dementia seems also to be a risk factor, independent of age. A large Finnish study[24] found that in 2000 patients aged 55 and over admitted to medical wards, delirium was present in over 40% of those patients with evidence for an established dementia, compared with 15% on admission for the group as a whole.

The diagnosis of delirium carries a significant mortality rate.[6] It is significantly higher than non-delirious controls during hospital admission and long term follow up. In most studies, hospital mortality in the elderly varies from 8% to 16% compared to 1–5% in controls.[25–28] A few studies have an even higher mortality, up to 65%.[29,30] One explanation for this is that they tend to include younger patients, who usually require a severe underlying illness to produce delirium. In the elderly the higher mortality persists even up to two years later with a mortality of 39% compared to 23% in controls.[31] Some studies have found delirium to be an independent predictor of both hospital[28] and long term mortality.[30] Other studies, however, have found that delirium is not associated with increased mortality when confounding factors such as severity of acute illness, cognitive impairment, and co-morbid disease were taken into account.[25,27] It is important to stress that the successful treatment of delirium eliminates much of the excess hospital mortality. This underlines the importance of early detection and urgent treatment.

The course of the symptoms has been found in some studies to be much less transient than previously acknowledged. In one study only 18% of patients had resolved all new symptoms six months after discharge.[14] Delirium has also been found to be associated with prolonged hospital stay, increased risk of hospital acquired complications, and increased risk of admission to institutional care.[27]

In the elderly, delirium is best thought of as a multifactorial condition similar to other old age conditions, such as falls or incontinence. Risk factors can be divided into vulnerability factors (present on admission) and precipitating factors (acquired during hospital stay). Most studies have examined both factors simultaneously; they are certainly highly interrelated. Those patients with a high number of vulnerability factors only require a small precipitating insult to produce delirium, whereas those with a low vulnerability require a much greater insult to produce the same effect.[32]

Despite using different populations and definitions, there is consensus between studies about three vulnerability factors: pre-existing cognitive impairment, severe chronic illnesses, and functional impairment.[33] The precipitating factors commonly mentioned in the literature include medications (particularly those with psychoactive and/or anticholinergic properties), infections, metabolic disturbances, alcohol withdrawal, dehydration, and malnutrition. Factors that reduce mobility, such as intravenous lines, indwelling catheters, and use of physical restraints (in the United States), have also been suggested as having a precipitant role.

Aetiology

Delirium is a consequence either of a primary brain lesion or of cerebral involvement secondary to systemic illness, including those cases caused by exogenous substances such as drugs and poisons. A wide variety of causes act by way of a common pathway of neurochemical disturbance to produce the clinical syndrome.[34]

It is important to stress that in the elderly, delirium may be the sole presentation of a serious acute illness, such as myocardial infarction or sepsis.[33] Almost any sufficiently severe acute medical or surgical condition may, under the right circumstances, cause the syndrome. Some of the more common causes of delirium are given in Box 4.3.

Although most cases of the clinical syndrome present little difficulty in determining a cause, a substantial minority of patients (as high as 5–20% of the elderly delirious)[35] never receive an aetiological diagnosis. In this situation it may be necessary to reconsider the diagnosis, but cases remain where

Box 4.3 Causes of delirium

Primary central nervous system causes:
  Head injury
  Cerebrovascular: stroke, subdural haematoma, transient ischaemic attack
  Raised intracranial pressure
  Intracranial infection: encephalitis, meningitis
  Epilepsy: ictal, postictal

Secondary to systemic illness:
  Infections: chest, urinary tract, septicaemia, malaria, HIV
  Cardiovascular: infarction, cardiac failure, arrhythmia
  Metabolic: hypo/hyperglycaemia, uraemia, hepatic failure, electrolyte disturbances
  Endocrine: Addisonian crisis, disturbance of thyroid, parathyroid
  Alcohol: Wernicke's encephalopathy, delirium tremens
  Prescribed drugs: psychotropic drugs, steroids, digoxin, cimetidine, anticonvulsants, anticholinergics, overdosage
  Illicit drugs

Rare causes:
  Systemic lupus erythematosus, porphyria, vitamin B_{12} or folate deficiency, pellagra, heavy metal poisoning, hypothermia, Wilson's disease, remote effect of carcinoma, hypertensive encephalopathy

the clinical diagnosis is not in doubt, yet the aetiological agent simply remains unidentified. It must also be remembered that more than one aetiological factor may be contributing to the patient's delirium, particularly in the elderly.[32]

The commonest causes of delirium include alcohol abuse and withdrawal, stroke, diabetes, ischaemic heart disease, pneumonia, and urinary tract infections.[36] Almost any medically prescribed drug can cause delirium if taken in sufficient dose, but anticholinergic, psychotropic, and hypnotic agents are especially known for their propensity to provoke the disorder, particularly in the elderly.[37]

Pathology and pathogenesis

It has been known since the nineteenth century that the brains of patients who have died from delirium show no obvious macroscopic or microscopic changes.[38] The abnormalities associated with delirium are functional rather than anatomical. There have been studies of patients with delirium resulting from localised anatomical lesions of the brain. These have highlighted certain areas as having an important role in producing the symptoms of delirium. These include the right cerebral hemisphere (particularly the parietal cortex)[39] and subcortical structures (particularly the thalamus).[40] The frontal lobes are also suspected to be involved as they are known to subserve functions of major importance in delirium, such as attention.[41]

Much of the functional research of delirium has been obtained from EEG studies. An important conclusion from the early research by Engel and Romano was that delirium was probably due to a global reduction in brain metabolic rate. This was proposed from the finding that delirium produced slowing of EEG activity.[42]

In the delirious patient, the deviation of electrical activity on the EEG from that of the normal waking state correlates well with the clinical condition:[43] in most cases, the greater the slowing of the EEG trace, the more clinically impaired the patient. Delirium associated with withdrawal states such as delirium tremens does not follow this general rule and tends to be associated with fast wave activity superimposed on generalised slowing of the trace, suggesting additional pathogenic mechanisms.[42] The rate of change of frequency is important: single EEG recordings may occasionally give a false impression in delirious patients with unusually high or low premorbid baseline frequencies,[44] implying the desirability of serial EEG recordings in the diagnosis of delirium. These changes are reversible and mirrored in the patient's recovery.[42,45]

Modern functional imaging studies, such as single photon emission computed tomography (SPECT), are small in number and inconclusive. They are often limited to small numbers of cases. A SPECT study of delirium tremens showed an association with widespread increased cerebral blood flow (CBF), suggesting increases in cerebral oxidative metabolism.[46] A review of SPECT studies of subclinical hepatic encephalopathy[47] has shown associations with decreased cortical CBF, with lateralising tendencies to the right side and frontal cortex. Some of the hepatic studies have shown a decrease in subcortical metabolism while others have shown an increase.

Many studies concerned with the neurochemical basis of delirium have indicated a major role for acetylcholine.

Acetylcholine is involved with the brain functions of memory, attention, and the sleep–wake cycle, all of which are affected in delirium.[48] Anticholinergic drugs, taken medically or recreationally, have the capacity to induce delirious states.[48] Hypoxia or hypoglycaemia, both known causes of delirium, lead to a marked decrease in cellular synthesis of acetylcholine.[49] Deterioration in cholinergic function is associated with normal ageing and is even more marked in Alzheimer's disease.[50] This fits with the known increased vulnerability of both of these groups to develop delirium. Also, Lewy body disease, a condition with symptoms which closely resemble delirium, is associated with an even greater neocortical cholinergic deficit than Alzheimer's disease.[51]

It is unlikely that acetylcholine is the only neurotransmitter associated with delirium. Other neurotransmitters implicated include dopamine, serotonin, GABA, and glutamate. Dopamine is implicated by the improvement in symptoms of delirium when treated with a dopamine blocker, such as haloperidol. It is also known that hypoxia leads to an increase in extracellular dopamine.[52] An imbalance in acetylcholine and dopamine levels may be responsible for some of the symptoms of delirium. This is suggested by the effects of giving large doses of L-dopa to patients with Parkinson's disease who have low cortical cholinergic activity. When exposed to L-dopa, these patients develop complex visual hallucinations, often combined with sleep disturbance, similar to those in delirium and Lewy body disease.[53]

Delirium is a syndrome of global cerebral dysfunction. Most cases appear to be associated with widespread reductions in cerebral metabolism, apart from the known exception of delirium tremens. The various causes of delirium appear to work by affecting neurotransmitter function, particularly the cholinergic system. Neurotransmission may be affected directly by anticholinergic drugs or indirectly by interference with brain cell metabolism.[54]

Clinical features

As noted by Lishman,[55] one of the most intriguing aspects of delirium is the constancy of the clinical picture despite the wide variety of different causes.

In the past, the central feature of delirium has been held to be a reduced level of consciousness. In an effort to identify a less complex core cognitive feature, delirium has increasingly been stressed as a disorder of *attention*. Patients have difficulties in directing, maintaining, and shifting their attention. Typically, the patient may need to have questions repeated, becomes distracted by other events on the ward, and repeats the answer to the previous question (perseveration).

A patient's level of attention can be assessed by basic bedside tasks such as serial sevens (subtraction of seven from 100, then seven from 93, and so on), and digit span (immediate verbal repeating of a string of six or seven digits). It is, however, essential to appreciate that impairment on any basic test of attention is not an absolute indication of dysfunction. Possible confounding factors include the patient's age, level of educational attainment, and coexisting anxiety. It has been claimed that serial sevens and digit span do not even allow differentiation of organic from "functional" disorders, let alone delirium from dementia.[56,57] If doubt remains about the presence of attentional deficit, one means of helping to decide the matter is to give increasingly simple tasks, such as requesting the months of the year or days of the week in reverse, serial threes or serial ones (asking the patient to subtract one from 20, then one from 19 and so on).

Alertness to environmental stimuli may be abnormally elevated or lowered. If hyperalert, the patient (within this section male) responds to stimuli without discrimination, with the clinical result that he is distracted by irrelevant events at the expense of the more relevant. It is characteristic of delirium tremens and may be accompanied by overactivity. If hypoalert, there is an overall reduction in response to environmental stimuli; for example, the patient may remain mute as the physician attempts to take a history. This is characteristically seen in metabolic encephalopathies and may be associated with underactivity. Any one individual delirious patient, however, may alternate between hyper- and hypoalertness, as well as exhibiting relatively lucid periods. Abnormalities in attention are present regardless of the level of the patient's alertness.

Attention and alertness are parts of a larger group of functions known as consciousness. Delirium was traditionally described as a disorder of consciousness. This description is currently out of favour due to difficulties in defining and rating changes of consciousness.

A number of forms of *memory impairment* may be seen in delirium. Immediate ("working") memory relates to the ability to hold information for very short periods of only a few seconds. By contrast, short term memory refers to information recalled after a delay of minutes. Long term memory refers to the recall of events that occurred days, weeks, months, or years previously.[58]

In delirium, disordered immediate memory is primary. Secondary, anterograde short term deficits result, and long term memory deficits may also be present, although generally there is relative preservation of long term memory except in the most severe cases. Thus the memory deficit, although primarily anterograde, may in severe cases be retrograde.

Short term memory deficit may be elicited by the patient's inability to recall completely after five minutes a seven-unit name and address or even three nouns (for example, dog, wall, sun) after correct registration. Registration (the immediate repetition of the units) is obviously contingent on adequate attentional processes and it therefore follows that if those processes are impaired to such an extent that the patient cannot correctly register the units, then formal testing of short term memory is not possible.

Clinical information on both short term and long term memory can sometimes be inferred from the patient's spontaneous behaviour and speech. For example, he may insist that he is seeing his wife for the first time that day even though she has been talking with him at his bedside just a few minutes earlier (impaired short term memory). He may believe, despite being in hospital, that he is living at a location he left many years earlier and he may talk of going out to work at what was his occupation there at the time (impaired short term memory with inappropriate accessing of long term memory). If severely ill, he may claim never to have met his wife and children before (impairment of long term memory). Confabulation is the term for the giving of false past personal information in the context of a short term memory deficit and is presumed to be an attempt by the patient to obscure the memory deficit.

Disorientation for time, place, and person reflects abnormalities in immediate and short term memory.

Disorientation for the exact time of day is considered a sensitive indicator of delirium. As the disorder progresses and becomes more established the patient characteristically loses the ability to identify correctly the day of the week, the month of the year, or even the year itself. In relatively mild cases the patient may be fully orientated for place and person but disorientated for time.

Disorientation for place refers to inability to identify correctly where the person is physically located at the time of interview. Some consideration must be given to the context in which the interview occurs when assessing this. For example, a patient at home may be able to identify this correctly, yet become totally disorientated for place when taken from his familiar surroundings and admitted to hospital.[59,60] Presumably in such cases a relatively unimpaired access to the long term memory store compensates for the underlying functional deficit.

Abnormalities in thought are evident through *lack of coherence of speech*. Incoherence can be mild with rambling speech, peculiar word use, and some expressions of tangentiality or circumstantiality in individuals who remain understandable. Severe incoherence presents as prominent tangential and circumstantial speech so that it is no longer possible to understand the patient.[11] Thought content in delirium has often been noted to have an oneroid (dream-like) quality.[61,62] Delusions, when they occur, are typically transitory and fragmentary and usually of a persecutory nature. Different studies put their prevalence at between 40% and 100%.[63-65]

Patients often experience *abnormal perceptions*. These have been shown to be related to impairments of perceptual processing.[66] The percept may be distorted and happens most often in the visual modality. Distortions can occur in the perceived size and shape of objects. In addition, the patient may have difficulty in distinguishing between internal mental events and external percepts. Perceptual misidentifications (illusions) are also common, as in delirium tremens where, for example, an innocuous wallpaper pattern may be perceived as a host of unpleasant scurrying animals. Misidentification of persons often occurs and usually involves mistaking unfamiliar persons for familiar. Here again context is important. For example, a patient's inability to identify his recently acquired hospital doctor would not give as much cause for concern as being unable to recognise a spouse.

Less commonly the abnormal percepts have no basis in external reality (hallucinations). They occur in between 40% and 75% of all cases of delirium[63-65,67] and are more common in younger patients. Again, they are most often visual. They vary in complexity from simple geometric shapes and colours to the highly detailed, such as people, animals, or the physical environment. They are most frequently associated with hyperalert states of delirium such as occur commonly with withdrawal states associated with alcohol, hypnotics, and anxiolytics, and intoxication states associated, for example, with anticholinergic drugs.

Mood disturbance is frequent, in particular irritability, agitation, aggression, anxiety, depression, apathy, perplexity, or suspiciousness.[64,68] Euphoria may also occur, but is less common.[34] The mood and its behavioural consequences shift frequently and rapidly from one state to another, giving a characteristic lability of mood. Anxiety or fear is often seen in hyperalert states and will be accompanied by overactivity of the autonomic nervous system. Mood disturbances can be marked and present an urgent management problem: undertreated agitation may result in injury to the patient or others.

The abnormalities in mentation present in delirium result in directly observable *abnormalities of behaviour*. The patient may be either underactive or overactive or may irregularly alternate between the two. The level of activity tends to correlate with the level of conscious alertness exhibited by the patient at the time. In general, hyperalertness is associated with general motor overactivity which is at best semipurposeful, such as repeatedly getting out of bed in an attempt to leave the hospital. On other occasions the behaviour is essentially purposeless, for example, picking at the bedclothes and purposeless tossing and turning in bed. By contrast, hypoactivity is associated with general underactivity and prolongation of the reaction time. In severe cases the patient may be stuporous and mute. It is important to emphasise that these two dimensions of the clinical syndrome are not distinct subtypes of delirium, as both may occur in irregular alternation during any one illness.[69]

It is important to bear in mind that the popular medical conception of delirium corresponds to hyperactivity; it follows that in hypoactive patients a diagnosis of delirium may be missed.[42] This important aspect of delirium has been vividly conveyed by Mulligan and Fairweather[70]:

To the experienced clinician the sight of an elderly lady immobile for no obvious cause (typically identified as a 'social admission'), untidily slouched in her chair with a bewildered expression on her face, with a slow and variable response to queries with a hint of dysarthria, a mild tremor and infrequent jerky movements, all observed while the history is being taken, shrieks delirium.

The *sleep–wake cycle* is invariably disturbed in delirium: the patient may exhibit excessive drowsiness by day with or without insomnia at night. In severe cases there may be total insomnia or reversal of the cycle. Sleep may be accompanied by nightmares which may then merge into frank hallucinations on wakening.

The *clinical course* of an episode of delirium is influenced by individual patient variables such as age and general physical condition, the cause of the disturbance, and the speed and efficacy of management interventions. Certain statements, however, apply to delirium in general. Onset is typically sudden, developing over hours or days, and often begins at night. In those cases with a relatively gradual onset, there may be a prodromal period in which the patient complains of various non-specific symptoms such as malaise, irritability, sleep disruption, nightmares, and difficulty concentrating. Once established, the clinical picture tends to fluctuate in intensity. Lucid intervals occur most commonly during the day and the usual pattern is nocturnal worsening, when levels of awareness and attention are lowered, with abnormally raised or lowered levels of alertness.

If the underlying disease is severe and progressive, the patient may lapse into an increasingly pronounced stupor, followed by coma and death. This downward spiral is sometimes marked by a period of agitated overactivity. The two most robust predictors of a fatal outcome are, unsurprisingly, advanced age and the presence of multiple physical illnesses.[6] Full recovery is the most frequent outcome, however, with a return to the patient's premorbid levels of consciousness and attention, and often occurs in less than one week. Subsequent episodes may occur in individuals at high risk such as elderly people prone to recurrent chest or urinary tract infections. In a minority of cases, resolution of the delirium leaves a chronic organic brain syndrome such as dementia following head injury, or Korsakoff's psychosis following Wernicke's encephalopathy.[71] Unipolar depressive disorder[72] and post-traumatic stress disorder[73] have been described following delirium. In all cases, following recovery there is a dense or patchy retrograde amnesia for the period of delirium which can be useful for clinching the diagnosis in hindsight.

Investigation

The list shown in Box 4.4 is a guideline of suggested first- and second-line investigations for identifying the physical agent(s) responsible for delirium in an individual patient. The choice of investigations ordered will obviously be dictated by the findings on history taking and examination. For instance, a cranial computed tomography (CT) scan or magnetic resonance imaging (MRI) is a first-line investigation if neurological signs are present or the history or examination suggests head trauma.[74] If, after initial investigation, no cause can be found for the delirium, it may then be appropriate to run a full test screen, given the serious nature of the untreated condition. In so doing one may detect uncommon presentations of relatively common diseases, such as systemic lupus erythematosus. Even after thorough investigation, some patients remain without an identified cause for their disorder. In such cases, it may be necessary to reconsider the diagnosis.

Although the process of physical investigation is successful in most cases in identifying the causes of the disorder once delirium has been diagnosed, it is of strictly limited value in confirming the diagnosis itself. Only EEG may be helpful in this respect.[75] In delirium not associated with psychoactive substance misuse, the EEG usually shows evidence of generalised slowing of background activity. In delirium associated with psychoactive substance misuse, for example alcohol or hypnotic/anxiolytic withdrawal, the EEG usually shows an excess of low amplitude fast wave activity. The limited utility of the EEG as a diagnostic aid in delirium is related to its lack of specificity, although claims have been made to the contrary.[30] The EEG often cannot enable delirium to be differentiated from dementia, as both Alzheimer's disease and multi-infarct dementia (which together account for about 90% of all dementias) are associated with a pattern of generalised slowing of the background activity similar to that seen in delirium not associated with psychoactive substance misuse.[76]

Box 4.4 Physical investigations of delirium

First line	Second line
Full blood picture	Serum folate, vitamin B_{12}
Erythrocyte sedimentation rate	Syphilis serology
Electrolytes, urea	Lumbar puncture
Liver function	Urinary illicit drug screen
Thyroid function	HIV antibodies
Blood glucose	Cardiac enzymes
Urine analysis and culture	Blood gases
EEG	Autoantibody screen
ECG	Blood cultures
Chest radiograph	Urinary porphyrins
	Calcium, phosphate
	Cranial CT scan or MRI

Differential diagnosis

In uncomplicated *dementia*, an early feature is poor short term memory in the absence of attentional deficits. This reflects the early involvement of the medial temporal lobe in the commonest form of dementia, Alzheimer's disease.[77] This contrasts with delirium where attention impairment is a cardinal feature. In Alzheimer's dementia, long term memory only becomes affected after the progression of the disease over months to years. In severe delirium both short term and long term memory become impaired within hours of the disorder developing.

Dementia is usually associated with an insidious onset over many months. In delirium onset is usually sudden.[35] In both conditions the patient's memory will be impaired. They will therefore be unable to give reliable information about onset. A reliable corroborative history from an informant, whenever possible, is invaluable. This is vital in differentiating delirium from severe dementia, due to the large overlap in symptoms between the two syndromes.

In Alzheimer's dementia, symptoms are more stable in nature than in delirium, where fluctuations in intensity are typical. Repeated bedside testing of cognitive state can reveal these fluctuations. Ward nurses, who have more prolonged contact with the patient, are a useful source of information about this feature.

The presence of dementia is a major vulnerability factor for the development of delirium. It is therefore not surprising that the two conditions can present in the same patient. This co-occurrence typically presents with a far greater deterioration in mental state over a shorter period of time than is usual for the dementia sufferer. If this is reported by an informant, the development of delirium in addition to dementia must be suspected.

The differential diagnosis of some forms of dementia can be difficult and may require expert psychiatric assessment. The *dementia from Lewy body disease* is a particular diagnostic problem with potentially fatal consequences. The symptoms of this dementia can closely resemble those of delirium. They include fluctuations in cognitive state, visual hallucinations, and paranoid delusions.[13] No causes of the delirium-like state are found on investigation. There is usually also a Parkinsonian-like syndrome present, with prominent extrapyramidal symptoms present before exposure to neuroleptics.[78] If neuroleptics have already been used there is a marked sensitivity to them. This sensitivity can be so severe at times that it can have fatal consequences.[79] Therefore if in doubt, seek expert advice from an old age psychiatrist.

Patients with *schizophrenia* can present with symptoms similar to delirium. These include incoherent speech, delusions, and hallucinations. All these symptoms are more fragmentary and fluctuant in delirium. In schizophrenia, delusions are relatively stable over time and are often part of an elaborate system of abnormal beliefs. In delirium hallucinations are usually visual. In schizophrenia auditory hallucinations are much more common.

Unlike in delirium, the attention and memory of most patients with schizophrenia is relatively unimpaired. Unfortunately, patients may be so agitated that assessment of cognition is not possible. In such situations, the importance of physical examination and investigation cannot be overstressed. In some cases, this is only possible after the patient has been sedated. Care is necessary to avoid oversedation of a possibly delirious patient, with the risk of worsening of the condition.

Variants of schizophrenia can on occasions exhibit signs of altered consciousness[80] or disorientation.[81] These disorders include acute and transient psychotic disorders (ICD10)[7] and postnatal psychosis. If there is any diagnostic uncertainty, the EEG can be particularly useful in differentiating these conditions from delirium.[33] "Functional" psychoses do not show slow wave activity typical of delirium.

In mood disorders such as *mania*, the patient may be overactive, behaviourally disturbed, and unamenable to psychiatric examination. "Confusion"[82] and transient global cognitive dysfunction[83,84] have been reported in mania. Visual hallucinations may be present in a substantial proportion of manic patients.[85] The mood state in mania, particularly in the acute stages, may be predominantly irritable as opposed to elevated or expansive, further complicating the picture.

Delirium, particularly the quieter "hypoactive form", may be mistaken for *depression*. Depression, however, tends to have a much slower onset, developing over weeks. The cognitive abnormalities associated with depressive disorder are usually more suggestive of dementia ("depressive pseudodementia").[86]

Dissociative disorders are uncommon but may be associated with impaired conscious awareness (fugue) or memory (amnesia). Mixed pictures may occur. The characteristic course of these disorders is of sudden onset, short course, and sudden termination. They may therefore be mistaken at first for delirium. In dissociative states, however, the disturbance of consciousness is often associated with a loss of sense of personal identity, which is rare in delirium. Likewise, amnesia tends to be relatively circumscribed to episodic (past personal) memory, with semantic (past impersonal) memory remaining relatively intact.[87] Such a picture is not seen in delirium. In many cases of dissociative disorder a psychosocial stressor may be identified, which may have meaningful connections with an event in the patient's distant past.

Diagnostic uncertainty can be caused by dementia, schizophrenia, and the mood disorders. More harm is possible if delirium is mistaken for another psychiatric condition than vice versa. A sensible approach in this situation is to assume a patient has delirium and manage appropriately, until it is proved otherwise.[88] Finding out that a patient has a previous psychiatric history is not sufficient information for a diagnosis of delirium to be ruled out. Patients with psychiatric conditions can neglect themselves, putting them at risk of developing conditions that can produce delirium. They also tend to be on the very medications that have the highest potential for producing delirium – psychoactive medications with anticholinergic properties.[33]

The diagnostic process in delirium is identical to that for any other medical condition. A careful history, examination, and investigation should result in the clinician identifying the syndrome and its causes. Where the diagnosis is in doubt, the responsible medical or surgical team should have access to a psychiatrist with expertise in diagnosis of the condition.[5] Referral should be made at an early stage. It is extremely helpful for the psychiatrist to have access to a nurse who has worked with the patient, an informant who can provide a reliable history, and the results of investigations. If a clinical diagnosis of delirium is made, the liaison psychiatrist should advise on investigation and management, including legal questions of consent.

Management

Delirium is managed empirically in the absence of true, formal, evidence-based guidelines.[89] As delirium is frequently undetected, the first step is identification of cases. It is often the quiet, "hypoactive" cases that are missed.[42] The cognitive screening of elderly patients on admission to medical wards is a useful aid in identification, but is often omitted.[90] An example of a simple screening instrument is the Mini Mental State Examination (MMSE) (Box 4.5).[91] It takes about 10 minutes to perform in uncomplicated cases and identifies cases of cognitive impairment. It cannot differentiate between dementia and delirium by itself. In addition, increasing age and level of educational attainment have been shown to confound its interpretation.[92] It is, however, useful in identifying a group of people who, even if they are not delirious already, are at a high risk of developing delirium during their stay. It is also helpful for identifying a later marked deterioration in cognitive state, by providing an objective baseline cognitive score. If incorrect answers are given for orientation questions the correct answers should be told to the patient. It is not only courteous to do this, it can also help orientate a delirious patient.

Some basic empirical guidelines in the management of delirium are given below. This management often requires

Box 4.5 Mini Mental State Examination

Section	Question	Max. points	Patient score
1 Orientation	a) Can you tell me today's (date)/month/(year)? Which day of the week is it today? Can you also tell me which season it is?	5	
	b) What city/town are we now in? What is the county/country? What building are we in and on what floor?	5	
2 Registration	I should like to test your memory. (Name three common objects: "ball, car, man".) Can you repeat the words I said? (*Score 1 point for each word.*) (Repeat up to six trails until all three are remembered.)	3	
3 Attention and calculation	a) From 100 keep subtracting 7 and give each answer: stop after five answers. (93_86_79_72_65_)		
	Alternatively b) Spell the word "WORLD" backwards. (D_L_R_O_W_).	5	
4 Recall	What were the three words I asked you to say earlier? (*Skip this test if all three objects were not remembered during registration test.*)	3	
5 Language Naming Repeating	Name these objects (show a watch) (show a pencil). Repeat the following: "no ifs, ands or buts".	2 1	
6 Reading	(Show card or write "CLOSE YOUR EYES".) Read this sentence and do what it says.	1	
Writing	Now can you write a short sentence for me?	1	
7 Three stage command	(Present paper.) Take this paper in your left (or right) hand, fold it in half, and put it on the floor.	3	
8 Construction	Will you copy this drawing please?	1	
Total score		30	

A score of 0–23 indicates disturbance of cognition.

considerable thought and care, tailoring the approach to each particular patient's conditions and the ward environment. The presence of behavioural problems and the pitfalls of medicating this group of patients sometimes require liaison with the psychiatric services.

The major priority is to identify and treat the underlying causes of the delirium. It is important to emphasise that general supportive and symptomatic measures should be initiated as soon as the clinical syndrome has been diagnosed, without waiting for identification of the underlying causes.

Nursing strategies should be aimed at orientating and reassuring the patient. Thought should go into making the patient's environment provide a balance between sensory overstimulation and understimulation. The patient is best placed in a side room which should be quiet and well lit by day and night. The patient's orientation may be improved by surrounding him or her with familiar objects from home. Likewise, close relatives should be encouraged to visit and should be allowed to remain outside normal visiting times. Attempts should be made to limit the number of nurses working with the patient to improve familiarity.

It is often not possible to implement all these strategies within the constraints of a working ward, but it is always possible to implement some. Certainly the practice of putting two agitated delirious patients next to each other, to give other patients a break, should be avoided. This practice is not only offensive, it is counterproductive. The last thing that is going to orientate and reassure a delirious patient is listening to another delirious patient.[88]

The patient's medication should be reviewed. Particular attention should be paid to any recent addition or withdrawal of a medication that preceded the onset of delirium. Medications are a common reversible cause of delirium.[33] If the patient is taking high risk medications (with psychoactive and/or anticholinergic properties) these should be stopped or substituted whenever possible.

The patient may be overactive and acutely disturbed in his or her behaviour. This may result in accidental or non-accidental self-injury by the patient, worsening of the patient's condition through exhaustion, or attacks on staff members. In such situations, pharmacological sedation may be necessary.

Extreme care is necessary in sedating a delirious patient in whom the cause of the delirium is unknown. Attention must also be paid to the dose of the drug prescribed. Elderly patients are sensitive to the side effects of drugs, particularly anticholinergic agents, and care is therefore necessary to prevent iatrogenic delirium or worsening of a pre-existing delirium. In fulminant hepatic encephalopathy, all forms of pharmacological sedation must be used with extreme care.

Phenothiazines, such as chlorpromazine and trifluoperazine, should be avoided in the treatment of delirium on account of their side effect profiles, especially anticholinergic effects. Their anti-adrenergic effects may lead to cardiovascular complications such as postural hypotension, tachycardia, and fatal cardiac arrhythmia. Also their antihistaminergic effects lead to excessive sedation.

The drug of choice for most delirious patients is haloperidol.[93] Haloperidol, a butyrophenone, tends to produce extrapyramidal side effects such as a Parkinsonian syndrome. However, it is less likely to cause the side effects associated with phenothiazines and is therefore preferred in the treatment of delirium. Haloperidol should be avoided in cases of benzodiazepine and alcohol withdrawal, Lewy body disease, and hepatic failure. It is highly effective in the management of agitation and has relatively low toxicity.[94] The dose regimen must always be tailored to the individual circumstances of the case in hand and only general guidelines will be given. Many elderly patients respond to the clinical effects of haloperidol at much lower doses than younger adults require. An oral dose as low as 0·5 mg twice daily can be sufficient.[95] Elderly patients are also more prone to developing extrapyramidal side effects. Severe extrapyramidal side effects require treatment with anticholinergic agents such as procyclidine, which may further exacerbate the delirium. It is not possible to predict the effective dose or the likelihood of an individual patient developing side effects. The best approach, within practical constraints, is to start low, observe, and build up gradually if necessary.

The management of agitation in Lewy body disease is very important due to the potentially fatal neuroleptic sensitivity that can occur. This can occur even with the newer atypical neuroleptics such as risperidone that are usually less prone to cause extrapyramidal side effects.[96] There has been some success with using chlormethiazole[97] and rivastigmine.[98] It is best to seek advice from an old age psychiatrist about medicating this condition.

An oral dose of haloperidol 5–10 mg twice daily has been suggested for mild to moderate agitation in young or middle aged delirious patients.[34] Oral haloperidol is detectable in the bloodstream after 60–90 minutes, and peak plasma concentrations are obtained after 4–6 hours. It is therefore not appropriate for the immediate control of severe agitation. In less severe cases, however, it should be prescribed as 1·5–15 mg per day in divided doses.[99]

Parenteral administration of haloperidol is associated with almost 100% bioavailability as opposed to approximately 66% by the oral route. Thus parenterally administered haloperidol should be given in a lower dose than the oral to achieve equivalent plasma concentrations.[100] Intravenous administration of haloperidol has a very fast onset of action (5–20 minutes). It has been reported that it causes a lower incidence of extrapyramidal side effects than oral or intramuscular administration.[101] It is not clear why this lower incidence occurs. Intravenous haloperidol should only be given in well controlled medical environments, and patients should preferably have intravenous access already in place.[94] Haloperidol can cause prolongation of the QT interval, which can lead to torsades de pointes, ventricular fibrillation, and sudden death. This complication is rare and has mainly occurred when high doses are given intravenously.[102] In this scenario, it is important to perform repeat ECGs and monitor for increases in QT interval length. If this occurs dose reduction or discontinuation should be considered.[103]

The initial oral haloperidol dose is determined by the severity of delirium, 2–5 mg for moderate and 10–20 mg for severe agitation. Intervals between repeat doses should be no less than 30 minutes. Intramuscular haloperidol reaches peak serum levels in 20–40 minutes[94] and thus may be used in the treatment of severe agitation. It is prescribed in a dose of 2–10 mg (increasing to 20 mg for emergency control), then up to 5 mg every hour if necessary (intervals of 4–8 hours may be satisfactory) to a total maximum dose of 60 mg.[99] The elderly usually require substantially lower doses.

Risperidone, an atypical neuroleptic, may have a role to play in the future management of delirium. At the moment, however, research is limited to case reports on a small number of patients.[104]

Benzodiazepines are best avoided in general cases of delirium. They are contraindicated in delirium associated with respiratory failure. They are, however, the treatment of choice in delirium associated with benzodiazepine withdrawal,[105] alcohol withdrawal,[106] and hepatic failure.[107] Delirium tremens begins about 48 hours after acute withdrawal from severe alcohol abuse. They are associated with fever, sweating, prominent visual hallucinations, tachycardia, and a marked tremor. Urgent management is necessary. Benzodiazepines should be prescribed, up to 30 mg of chlordiazepoxide per day in divided doses, gradually reducing to cessation over a 7–10 day period. Chlormethiazole is no longer recommended because of its abuse potential. Convulsions may occur, requiring specially formulated intravenous diazepam. Thiamine replacement is necessary and should be given parenterally. Acute dehydration is usual and intravenous fluids are needed once the patient is sedated.

Careful attention must be paid by medical and nursing staff to the patient's state of nutrition, fluid and electrolyte balance, and bowel and bladder function, as neglect of these will worsen the patient's condition. In patients confined to bed for long periods, expert nursing care and physiotherapy are necessary to prevent the development of pressure sores and contractures.

Delirium is underdiagnosed, underinvestigated, and undertreated: correct detection and treatment will improve outcome and reduce complications.

Management of delirium

- Delirium, otherwise known as acute confusional state, is an acute, reversible, global disorder of the higher nervous system function.
- It is common in the inpatient setting but is often undiagnosed in its early stages and may therefore present as a medical emergency.
- If not managed appropriately, it is associated with significant mortality. Early detection and treatment are therefore of paramount importance.

- Almost any acute, severe, medical or surgical condition can cause delirium. Although its pathogenesis is still poorly understood, it is generally held to represent widespread dysfunction of cerebral oxidative metabolism.
- Diagnosis of the condition involves two stages: first, the clinical syndrome itself is identified; second, the responsible aetiological agent is sought.
- Central features of the clinical syndrome (Box 4.1) are fluctuating impairments in consciousness and attention, disturbance of sleep–wake cycle with nocturnal worsening, overactivity or underactivity, disorganised thinking and speech, disorientation for time and place, and often paranoid delusions and visual hallucinations. The natural history is one of sudden onset with a fluctuating course.
- An aetiological diagnosis can be made in most patients by appropriate physical examination and investigation as suggested by the history, although a detailed test screen may be needed in a few cases. Overinvestigation is preferable to underinvestigation, given that individual cases of delirium may be caused by multiple factors.
- In those few remaining cases where the aetiological agent remains unidentified, care must be taken to exclude other psychiatric diagnoses that may occasionally mimic delirium, such as certain forms of dementia, schizophrenia, mania, depression, and dissociative disorder. Use your liaison psychiatric service.
- The proper management of delirium consists of providing general supportive measures along with treatment directed against the primary cause. Supportive measures should not be withheld until the aetiological factors have been identified, as delay may result in a deterioration in the patient's condition.
- The patient should be nursed in a well lit side room by a small group of key personnel, as overstimulation or understimulation of his or her sensory environment may exacerbate the delirium.
- Attention should be paid to nutrition, fluid, and electrolyte intake, and in those patients who are relatively immobile, physiotherapy should be instituted to avoid such potential consequences as deep venous thrombosis, pressure necrosis, and chest infection.
- Iatrogenic factors may be important in some cases and the patient's drug chart should be fully reviewed.
- Sedation should be used carefully; it may worsen the delirium if prescribed inappropriately. In those cases where sedation is necessary, such as when the patient becomes a danger to him- or herself or to others, the choice of drug is ideally informed by a knowledge of the underlying causative factors.
- Benzodiazepines are the best drugs in withdrawal states. In most other cases, butyrophenones are to be preferred. In general, mild to moderate degrees of agitation will respond to oral haloperidol whereas moderate to severe degrees require intramuscular haloperidol.

Acknowledgement

The authors thank Dr D Taylor who contributed to this chapter in earlier editions of this book.

References

1 *The medical works of Hippocrates.* Trans Chadwick J, Mann WN. Oxford: Blackwell, 1950.
2 Celsus. *De Medicina.* Trans. Spencer WG. London: Heinemann, 1938.
3 Jackson SW. Galen – on mental disorders. *J Hist Behav Sci* 1969;5:365–84.
4 Lipowski ZJ. *Delirium: acute brain failure in man.* Springfield, IL: Charles C Thomas, 1980.
5 Perez EL, Silverman M. Delirium: the often overlooked diagnosis. *Int J Psychiatry Med* 1984;14:181–9.
6 Trzepacz PT, Teague GB, Lipowski ZJ. Delirium and other organic mental disorders in a general hospital. *Gen Hosp Psychiatry* 1985;7:101–6.
7 World Health Organization. *The ICD-10 classification of mental and behavioural disorders.* Geneva: World Health Organization, 1992.
8 American Psychiatric Association. *DSM-IV: diagnostic and statistical manual of mental disorders,* 4th edn. Washington DC: American Psychiatric Association, 1994.
9 World Health Organization. *Mental disorders: glossary and guide to their classification in accordance with the ninth revision of the international classification of diseases.* Geneva: World Health Organization, 1978.
10 Tucker GJ. DSM-IV: proposals for revision of diagnostic criteria for delirium. *Int Psychogeriatr* 1991;3:197–207.
11 Gottlieb GL, Johnson J, Wanich C, *et al.* Delirium in the medically ill elderly: operationalizing the DSM-III criteria. *Int Psychogeriatr* 1991;3:181–96.
12 Macdonald AJ, Treloar A. Delirium and dementia: are they distinct? *J Am Geriatr Soc* 1996;44:1001–2.
13 McKeith IG, Perry RH, Fairbairn A, *et al.* Operational criteria for senile dementia of Lewy body type. *Psychological Med* 1992;22:911–22.
14 Levkoff SE, Evans D, Liptzin B, *et al.* Deirium, the occurrence and persistence of symptoms among elderly hospitalised patients. *Arch Intern Med* 1992;152:334–40.
15 Oakley DA. Animal awareness, consciousness and self-image. In: Oakley DA, ed. *Brain and mind.* London: Methuen, 1985:132–51.
16 Baddeley AD. Memory theory and memory therapy. In: Moffat M, ed. *Clinical management of memory problems.* London: Chapman & Hall, 1992, 4–31.
17 Levkoff S, Cleary P, Liptzin B, *et al.* Epidemiology of delirium: an overview of research issues and findings. *Int Psychogeriatr* 1991;3:149–69.
18 Folstein MF, Basset SS, Romanoski AJ, *et al.* The epidemiology of delirium in the community: the Eastern Baltimore Mental Health Survey. *Int Psychogeriatr* 1991;3:169–76.
19 Horvath TB, Siever LJ, Mohs RC, *et al.* Organic mental syndromes and disorders. In: Kaplan HI, Sadock BJ, eds. *Comprehensive textbook of psychiatry.* Baltimore: Williams and Wilkins, 1989:599–641.
20 Gillick MR, Serrell NA, Gillick LS. Adverse consequences of hospitalisation in the elderly. *Soc Sci Med* 1982;16:1033–8.

21 Warshaw GA, Moore JT, Friedman SW, *et al*. Functional disability in the hospitalised elderly. *JAMA* 1982;**248**:847–50.
22 Johnson J, Sullivan E, Gottlieb E, *et al*. Delirium in elderly patients on internal medical services. *J Am Geriatr Soc* 1987;**35**:972.
23 Williams MA, Campbell EB, Raynor WJ, *et al*. Predictors of acute confusional states in hospitalised elderly patients. *Res Nurs Health* 1985; **8**:31–40.
24 Erkinjuntti T, Wikstromm J, Palo J. Dementia among medical inpatients. *Arch Intern Med* 1986;**146**:193–6.
25 Francis J, Martin D, Kapoor WN. A prospective study of delirium in hospitalised elderly. *JAMA* 1990;**263**:1097–101.
26 Thomas RI, Cameron DJ, Fahs MC. A prospective study of delirium and prolonged hospital stay. *Arch Gen Psychiatry* 1988;**45**:937–40.
27 O'Keefe S, Lavan J. The prognostic significance of delirium in older hospital patients. *J Am Geriatr Soc* 1997;**45**:174–8.
28 Pompei P, Foreman M, Rudberg MA, *et al*. Delirium in hospitalised older persons: outcomes and predictors. *J Am Geriatr Soc* 1994;**42**:809–15.
29 Cameron DJ, Thomas RI, Mulvihill M, *et al*. Delirium: a test of the DSM III criteria on medical inpatients. *J Am Geriatr Soc* 1987;**35**:1007–10.
30 Rabins PV, Folstein MF. Delirium and dementia: diagnostic criteria and fatality rates. *Br J Psychiatry* 1982;**140**:149–53.
31 Francis J, Kapoor WN. Prognosis after hospital discharge of older medical patients with delirium. *J Am Geriatr Soc* 1992;**40**:601–6.
32 Inouye SK, Charpentier PA. Precipitating factors for delirium in hospitalised elderly persons. *JAMA* 1996;**275**:852–7.
33 Inouye SK. The dilemma of delirium: clinical and research controversies regarding diagnosis and evaluation of delirium in hospitalised elderly medical patients. *Am J Med* 1994;**97**:278–88.
34 Lipowski ZJ. *Delirium: acute confusional states*. Oxford: Oxford University Press, 1990.
35 Lipowski ZJ. Transient cognitive disorders (delirium, acute confusional states) in the elderly. *Am J Psychiatry* 1983;**140**:1426–36.
36 Sirosis F. Delirium: 100 cases. *Can J Psychiatry* 1988;**33**:375–8.
37 Blazer DG, Federspiel CF, Ray WA, *et al*. The risk of anticholinergic toxicity in the elderly: a study of prescribing practices in two populations. *J Gerontol* 1983;**38**:31–5.
38 Fordyce G. *Five dissertations on fever*. Boston: Bedlington and Ewes, 1823.
39 Mori E, Yamadori A. Acute confusional states and acute agitated delirium. *Arch Neurol* 1987;**44**:1139–43.
40 Santamaria J, Blesa R, Tolosa ES. Confusional syndrome in thalamic stroke. *Neurology* 1984;**34**:1618.
41 Ingvar DH. "Memory of the future": an essay on the temporal organisation of conscious awareness. *Hum Neurobiol* 1985;**4**:127–36.
42 Engel GL, Romano J. Delirium: a syndrome of cerebral insufficiency. *J Chronic Dis* 1959;**9**:260–77.
43 Markland ON. Electroencephalography in diffuse encephalopathies. *J Clin Neurophysiol* 1984;**1**:357–407.
44 Romano J, Engel GL. Physiologic and psychologic considerations of delirium. *Med Clin North Am* 1944;**28**:629–38.
45 Adams RD, Victor M. *Principles of neurology*. New York: McGraw-Hill, 1981:281.
46 Hemmingsen R, Vorstrup S, Clemmesen L, *et al*. Cerebral blood flow during delirium tremens and related clinical states studied with Xenon-133 inhalation tomography. *Am J Psychiatry* 1988;**145**:1384–90.
47 Trzepacz PT. The neuropathogensis of delirium: a need to focus our research. *Psychosomatics* 1994;**35**:374–91.

48 Perry EK, Perry RH. Acetylcholine and hallucinations: disease-related compared to drug-induced alterations in human consciousness. *Brain and Cognition* 1995;**28**:240–58.

49 Gibson GE, Peterson C, Sansone J. Decreases in amino acid and acetylcholine metabolism during hypoxia. *J Neurochem* 1981;**37**:192–201.

50 Perry EK, Johnson M, Kerwin JM, *et al*. Convergent cholinergic activities in aging and Alzheimer's disease. *Neurobiol Aging* 1992;**13**:393–400.

51 Perry EK, Irving D, Kerwin JM, *et al*. Cholinergic transmitter and neurotrophic activities in Lewy body dementia: similarity to Parkinson's and distribution from Alzheimer disease. *Alzheimer Dis Assoc Disord* 1993;**7**:69–79.

52 Broderick PA, Gibson GE. Dopamine and serotonin in rat striatum during in vivo hypoxic-hypoxia. *Metab Brain Dis* 1989;**4**:143–53.

53 Moskovitz C, Moses H, Klawans H. Levodopa-induced psychosis: a kindling phenomenon. *Am J Psychiatry* 1978;**135**:669.

54 Blass JP, Nolan KA, Black RS, *et al*. Delirium: phenomenology and diagnosis – a neurobiologic view. *Int Psychogeriatr* 1991;**3**:121–34.

55 Lishman WA. *Organic psychiatry*. Oxford: Blackwell Scientific, 1987.

56 Rosen AM, Fox HA. Tests of cognition and their relationship to psychiatric diagnosis and demographic variables. *J Clin Psychiatry* 1986;**47**:495–8.

57 Hinton J, Withers E. The usefulness of clinical tests of the sensorium. *Br J Psychiatry* 1971;**119**:9–18.

58 Squire LR. *Memory and brain*. Oxford: Oxford University Press, 1987.

59 Litin EM. Mental reaction to trauma and hospitalisation in the aged. *N Engl J Med* 1956;**162**:1522–4.

60 Levin M. Toxic delirium precipitated by admission to hospital. *J Nerv Ment Dis* 1952;**116**:210–14.

61 Loftus EL, Schooler JW. Information processing conceptualisations of human cognition: past, present and future. In: Rubin BD, ed. *Information and behavior*. New Brunswick, NJ: Transaction Books, 1985, 225–50.

62 Mettler CC. *History of medicine: a correlative text, arranged according to subjects*. Philadelphia, PA: Blakiston, 1947.

63 Wolff HG, Curran D. Nature of delirium and allied states. *AMA Arch Neurol Psychiatry* 1956;**75**:62–6.

64 Farber IJ. Acute brain syndrome. *Dis Nerv System* 1959;**20**:296–9.

65 Simon A, Cahan RB. The acute brain syndrome in geriatric patients. *Psychiatr Res Rep* 1963;**116**:8–21.

66 Morris GO, Singer MT. Sleep deprivation: the content of consciousness. *J Nerv Ment Dis* 1966;**143**:291–304.

67 Bleuler M, Willi J, Buhler HR. *Akute psychische Begleiter scheinungen körperlicher Krankheiten*. Stuttgart: Thieme, 1966.

68 Wolff HG, Curran D. Nature of delirium and allied states. *AMA Arch Neurol Psychiatry* 1935;**33**:1175–215.

69 Liptzin B, Levkoff SE. An empirical study of delirium subtypes. *Br J Psychiatry* 1992;**161**:843–45.

70 Mulligan I, Fairweather SA. Delirium – the geriatrician's perspective. In: Jacoby R, Oppenheimer C, eds. *Psychiatry in the elderly*. Oxford: Oxford University Press, 1997;507–26.

71 Victor M, Adams RD, Collins GH. *The Wernicke–Korsakoff syndrome*. Philadelphia, PA: FA Davis, 1971.

72 Blank K, Perry S. Relationship of psychological processes during delirium to outcome. *Am J Psychiatry* 1984;**141**:843–7.

73 MacKenzie TB, Popkin MK. Stress response syndrome occurring after delirium. *Am J Psychiatry* 1980;**137**:1433–5.

74 Francis J, Kapoor WN. Acute mental change: when are head scans needed? *Clin Res* 1991;**39**:575.

75 Brenner RP. The electroencephalogram in altered states of consciousness. *Neurol Clin* 1985;2:615–31.

76 Leuchter FA, Spar JE, Walter DO, *et al*. Electroencephalographic spectra and coherence in the diagnosis of Alzheimer-type and multi-infarct dementia. *Arch Gen Psychiatry* 1987;44:50–4.

77 Tomlinson BE. The structural and quantitative aspects of the dementias. In: Roberts PJ, ed. *Biochemistry of dementia*. Chichester: Wiley, 1980.

78 Ala TA, Yang KH, Sung JH, *et al*. Hallucinations and signs of parkinsonism help distinguish patients with dementia and cortical Lewy bodies from patients with Alzheimer's disease at presentation: a clinicopathological study. *J Neurol Neurosurg Psychiatry* 1997;62:16–21.

79 McKeith I, Fairbairn A, Perry R, *et al*. Neuroleptic sensitivity in patients with senile dementia of Lewy body type. *Br J Psychiatry* 1992;305:673–7.

80 Van Praag GE. About the impossible concept of schizophrenia. *Compr Psychiatry* 1976;17:1–97.

81 Newmark CS, Raft D, Toomet T, *et al*. Diagnosis of schizophrenia: pathognomic signs or symptom clusters. *Compr Psychiatry* 1975;16: 155–63.

82 Carlson GA, Goodwin FK. The stages of mania: a longitudinal analysis of the manic episode. *Arch Gen Psychiatry* 1973;28:221–8.

83 Van Sweden B. Disturbed vigilance in mania. *Biol Psychiatry* 1986;21: 311–13.

84 Mentzos S, Lyrakos A, Tsiolis A. Akute Virwirrtheitszustande. *Nervenarzt* 1971;42:10–17.

85 Taylor MA, Abrams R. The phenomenology of mania. *Arch Gen Psychiatry* 1973;29:520–2.

86 La Rue A, Spar J, Hill CD. Cognitive impairment in late–life depression: clinical correlates and treatment implications. *J Affect Dis* 1986;11:179–84.

87 Kopelman MD. Amnesia: organic and psychogenic. *Br J Psychiatry* 1987; 150:428–42.

88 Francis J. Delirium in older patients. *J Am Geriatr Soc* 1992;40:829–38.

89 Britton A, Russell R. Multidisciplinary team interventions for delirium in patients with chronic cognitive impairment. In: Cochrane Collaboration. *Cochrane Library*. Issue 2. Oxford: Update Software, 2002.

90 McCartney JR, Palmteer RN. Assessment of cognitive deficit in geriatric patients: a study of physician behavior. *J Am Geriatr Soc* 1985;33:467.

91 Folstein MF, Folstein SE, McHugh PR. "Mini–Mental state". *J Psychiatr Res* 1975;12:189–98.

92 Anthony JC, Le Resche L, Niaz U, *et al*. Limits of the "Mini–Mental State" as a screening test for dementia and delirium among hospital patients. *Psychol Med* 1982;12:397–408.

93 Moore DP. Rapid treatment in critically ill patients. *Am J Psychiatry* 1977;134:1431–2.

94 Settle EC, Ayd FJ. Haloperidol: a quarter century of experience. *J Clin Psychiatry* 1983;44:440–8.

95 Byrne EJ. Acute and sub–acute confusional state (delirium) in later life. In: Norman IJ, Redfern SJ, eds. *Mental health care for elderly people*. London: Churchill Livingstone, 1997;175–82.

96 Ballard C, Grace J, McKeith I, *et al*. Neuroleptic sensitivity in dementia with Lewy bodies and Alzheimer's disease. *Lancet* 1998;351:1032–3 (letter).

97 McKeith IG, Galasko D, Wilcock GK, *et al*. Lewy body dementia – diagnosis and treatment. *Br J Psychiatry* 1995;167:709–17.

98 McKeith IG, Grace JB, Walker Z, *et al*. Rivastigmine in the treatment of dementia with Lewy bodies: preliminary findings from an open trial. *Int J Geriatr Psychiatry* 2000;15:387–92.

99   *British National Formulary* (BNF 44). London: British Medical Association and the Royal Pharmaceutical Society, 2002.
100 Forsman A, Ohman R. Applied pharmacokinetics of haloperidol in man. *Curr Ther Res* 1977;**21**:396–411.
101 Menza MA, Murray GB, Holmes VF, *et al.* Decreased extrapyramidal symptoms with intravenous haloperidol. *J Clin Psychiatry* 1987;**48**: 278–80.
102 Wilt JL, Minnema AM, Johnson MD, *et al.* Torsade de pointes associated with the use of intravenous haloperidol. *Ann Intern Med* 1993;**119**: 391–4.
103 American Psychiatric Association. *Practice guideline for the treatment of patients with delirium.* Washington, DC: APA, 1999.
104 Sipahimalani A, Masand PS. Use of risperidone in delirium: case reports. *Ann Clin Psychiatry* 1997;**9**:105–7.
105 Foy A, Drinkwater V, March S, *et al.* Confusion after admission to hospital in elderly patients using benzodiazepines. *Br Med J* 1986;**293**:1072.
106 Dubin WR, Weiss KJ, Dorn JM. Pharmacotherapy of psychiatric emergencies. *J Clin Psychopharmacol* 1986;**6**:210–22.
107 Misra P. Hepatic encephalopathy. *Med Clin North Am* 1981;**65**:209–26.

5: Acute behaviour disturbances and their management

GG LLOYD, J PIMM

Psychiatric disorders are commonly encountered in neurological practice and most neurologists accept the need to assess and manage patients with behavioural problems. The more complicated cases require expert psychiatric intervention and, for optimum care, it is essential that there is close collaboration between neurologist and psychiatrist.

Many neurological conditions, particularly those with cerebral involvement, increase the risk of developing a psychiatric disorder.[1] Furthermore psychiatric disorders can be associated with symptoms such as headache, dizziness, and weakness which suggest neurological disease but for which no organic explanation can be found. This phenomenon, known as somatisation, accounts for a substantial proportion of patients who are referred to neurological departments.

Schiffer[2] evaluated a consecutive series of 241 patients attending an American neurology service and found that 101 (41·9%) had symptoms sufficient to warrant a psychiatric diagnosis according to DSM-III criteria. Of 57 inpatients, 10 were considered to have a primary psychiatric disorder and five of these had no neurological illness. Among 184 outpatients, 32 had a primary psychiatric disorder and 30 of these had no neurological illness. Kirk and Saunders[3] had previously described a retrospective survey from a neurological clinic in north east England and reported that, during a four year period, 358 (13·2%) of 2716 patients had a psychiatric disorder with no evidence of neurological illness.

If the psychiatric disorder underlying the neurological symptoms is not recognised, patients can be subjected to unnecessary and expensive investigations.[4] They may receive symptomatic treatment which fails to alleviate their condition and they will become dissatisfied with the result of their treatment and try to consult other specialists in the hope of finding a more effective remedy.

Some of the psychological symptoms and behavioural disturbances which the neurologist encounters are of sudden onset and require urgent attention. This review describes the clinical features and management of those disorders that are most likely to give rise to acute behavioural problems in neurological practice.

Affective disorders

The fundamental disturbance is a change of mood (or affect), either depression or elation. Mood disturbance is not necessarily the most prominent symptom, however, and it may be masked by a wide range of other abnormalities which at first sight suggest the presence of organic disease. Affective disorders have a tendency to recur. When the recurrences always take the same form, the condition is referred to as unipolar affective disorder; when the mood change varies between depression or elation it is described as bipolar affective disorder.

Depressive disorder

Depression not associated with organic disease usually presents to the neurologist with symptoms such as headache, dizziness, disturbance of higher mental function, and facial or bodily pain.[5] Psychological symptoms, emotional conflicts, and life stresses may not be volunteered and are only elicited by tactful, direct questioning on the part of the examining doctor. A diagnosis of depression can be made if any two of the three core symptoms and two of the other common symptoms listed in Box 5.1 have been present for a period of more than two weeks.

Box 5.1 Symptoms of depression

Core symptoms of depression
  Depressed mood
  Loss of interest and enjoyment
  Reduced energy leading to increased fatiguability and diminished activity

Common symptoms of depression
  Reduced concentration and attention
  Reduced self-esteem and self-confidence
  Ideas of guilt and unworthiness
  Bleak and pessimistic views of the future
  Ideas or acts of self-harm or suicide
  Disturbed sleep
  Diminished appetite

Fitzpatrick and Hopkins[6] assessed a series of patients referred to a neurologist with headaches not due to structural disease and found that 37% had an affective disorder of at least mild severity. The preoccupation with pain may dominate the clinical picture to such an extent that the patient does not appear depressed and does not readily admit to feeling depressed. This has been described in relation to facial pain;[7] the cognitive features of depression such as self reproach, suicidal thinking, and psychomotor retardation were uncommon but, in addition to pain, the patients complained of insomnia, fatigue, irritability, and agitation.

Depression also complicates existing neurological disease. In some cases, for example spinal cord injuries,[8] depression appears to result largely from the personal and social implications of the neurological disability. In diseases in which there is cerebral involvement, the aetiology of depression is more complex. The mood disturbance may be triggered by the emotional impact of the disease but may also result from structural pathology, possibly through interference with neurotransmitter pathways within the brain. Depressive disorders with cerebral involvement are classified as the organic mood disorders by ICD-10.[9] One of the most significant features of these disorders is that the mood disturbance, either depression or mania, may be the first manifestation of underlying neurological pathology.[10] Suspicion of unrecognised physical illness should be particularly high if there is no clear psychosocial precipitant, if the mood disorder first presents in middle or late life, and if there is no family or personal disposition to psychiatric illness.[11]

Depression has been described as a presenting feature of cerebral tumours,[12] multiple sclerosis,[13,14] Parkinson's disease,[15,16] and Huntington's disease[17,18] but most attention has been given to its association with cerebrovascular disease. Eastwood et al.[19] reported that 10% of patients in a stroke rehabilitation inpatient unit had a major depressive disorder, whereas 40% had symptoms of minor depression. Robinson et al.[20] studied patients admitted to hospital after an acute stroke and found that 27% demonstrated symptoms of major depression, whereas 20% had symptoms of minor depression. The association between mood disturbance and severity of physical impairment is not a strong one and it has been proposed that the site of the vascular lesion is an important factor in determining poststroke depression. Left-sided lesions in the frontal lobe or basal ganglia have been particularly implicated.[21] A recent systematic review offered no support for the hypothesis that the risk of depression after stroke is affected by the location of the brain lesion.[22] In addition, other reports have found a lower prevalence of depressive illness, especially when the survey has included patients not admitted to hospital.[23]

Some patients with cerebrovascular disease experience mood disturbances that are too brief to justify the diagnosis of a depressive illness.[24] This phenomenon, known as pathological emotionalism, is manifest by rapid changes of mood, sudden episodes of crying, and inappropriate and uncontrollable laughter. This type of mood change has been observed more commonly in patients with lesions in the left frontal and temporal areas.

Assessment of suicide risk

The risk of suicide is one of the reasons why depression can become an acute medical problem and it must be considered when assessing any patient who is thought to be depressed. The risk is increased in several neurological disorders,[25,26] particularly multiple sclerosis, epilepsy, head injury, and spinal cord lesions.

The most important consideration is whether the patient is expressing active suicidal intent, either spontaneously or in response to direct questioning. Box 5.2 shows the profile of demographic factors that increase the risk of suicide, which has emerged from various studies of people who have attempted suicide; a knowledge of these is important when assessing depressed patients.[27–29]

If the risk of a suicide attempt is considered to be significant, or if there is doubt about this, the neurologist should consult urgently with a psychiatrist colleague who should evaluate the patient as soon as possible. A number of management options, including outpatient or day hospital treatment, are available according to the perceived risk and availability of social support. When the risk is high and the patient has little in the way of support, admission to a psychiatric ward should be advised; in England and Wales this may have to involve applying the Mental Health Act (1983) if the patient cannot be persuaded to accept voluntary admission.

In the case of a patient already in hospital receiving any form of treatment Section 5(2) of the Act enables the patient to be detained if he or she is presenting a danger to him- or herself or others. The application must be made by the doctor in charge of the case, or the nominated deputy. The Section enables the patient to be detained for up to 72 hours during which time an assessment must be made to determine whether the patient should be detained for a further period of assessment and compulsory treatment.

Box 5.2 Risk factors for suicide attempts in depressed patients

Previous suicide attempts
Male sex
Increasing age
Living alone
Social isolation
Recent bereavement
Unemployment
Chronic physical illness
Drug and alcohol misuse
Personality disorder

Stupor

Stupor is another serious complication of depression. It is a term that leads to disagreement between neurologists and psychiatrists, who use it in different ways. It is sometimes used to describe an intermediate stage on the spectrum of impaired consciousness that eventually leads to coma. Lishman[30] argues that this is an incorrect use of the concept, which he believes is more appropriately defined as a syndrome in which the patient is conscious but makes no spontaneous movement and shows little response to external stimuli; in the most advanced form of stupor the patient is completely mute and immobile. Consciousness is inferred by the fact that there may be purposeful eye movements, following the actions of other people in the vicinity, and also by the patient's recall of events once recovery has occurred. In psychiatric practice, depression and schizophrenia are the commonest causes of stupor.[31,32] The diagnosis depends on eliciting a history of relevant symptoms during the weeks before the onset of stupor. In the case of depression there is a history of progressive psychomotor retardation in addition to the psychological symptoms of low mood, guilt, and self reproach. A full neurological evaluation, including magnetic resonance imaging (MRI) of the brain, is essential before a diagnosis can be made with confidence. Cerebral disorders that can give rise to the clinical picture of stupor include dementia, encephalitis, and cerebral tumour or cyst in the upper midbrain or posterior diencephalon causing increased intracranial pressure.

Management of depressive disorders

Depression usually responds to a combined approach of antidepressant medication and cognitive therapy. Selective serotonin re-uptake inhibitors (SSRIs: paroxetine, fluoxetine, sertraline) are replacing tricyclic antidepressants (dothiepin, amitriptyline, imipramine) as the first choice drugs in the treatment of depression. They are better tolerated, safer in overdose, and cause fewer side effects in the presence of physical illness. Other newer antidepressants, such as venlafaxine and mirtazapine, increase the availability of both serotonin and noradrenaline, and can be effective if there is an inadequate clinical response to one of the SSRI drugs.

Monoamine oxidase inhibitors (phenelzine, tranylcypromine) are also effective in depressive illness. They are used by some psychiatrists as the preferred drug when depression is accompanied by anxiety, phobic symptoms, weight gain, hypersomnia, and fatigue. For many years they have been underused because of fears of their interaction with tyramine-containing foods, potentially resulting in a catastrophic rise in blood pressure. Various foods, alcoholic drinks, and drugs have had to be avoided by patients taking monoamine oxidase inhibitors. This problem has been overcome by the introduction of reversible and selective inhibitors of monoamine oxidase subtype A, such as moclobemide.

All antidepressants take up to 2–3 weeks to produce clinical effect. In some clinical situations this delay may be unacceptable and a speedier response to treatment is required. Electroconvulsive therapy (ECT) is the preferred treatment in these situations, particularly when the risk of suicide is high, or when the patient is stuporose and is not maintaining adequate nutrition or fluid intake. ECT may have to be given under the terms of the Mental Health Act (1983) if the patient is incapable of giving informed consent to treatment; in England and Wales this involves obtaining a second opinion from a psychiatrist appointed by the Mental Health Act commission. Box 5.3 shows the main indications for ECT in depressive disorder.

There are no absolute contraindications to ECT. A decision should be taken after careful consideration of the risks of the various treatment options weighed against the risk of continuation of the depressive disorder. Box 5.4 lists the conditions in which ECT should be avoided whenever possible.

Mania

The symptoms of mania are in many ways the opposite of those of depression. There is elevation of mood accompanied by an enhanced sense of well being, physical and mental overactivity, pressure of speech, flight of ideas, increased self-confidence, and a loss of social inhibitions. Some manic patients are predominantly irritable rather than elated, particularly when other people do not share their unrealistic views of their own abilities.

> **Box 5.3 Indications for electroconvulsive therapy in depressive disorder**
>
> Severe depression with high risk of suicide
> Depressive stupor
> Depressive disorder with psychotic symptoms
> Failure to respond to an adequate course of an antidepressant
> Inability to tolerate side effects of antidepressants
> If physical illness makes antidepressants less safe than ECT

> **Box 5.4 Relative contraindications to ECT**
>
> Raised intracranial pressure
> Instability of cervical spine
> Cerebral aneurysm
> Recent history of cerebral haemorrhage
> Myocardial infarction within previous three months
> Aortic aneurysm
> Acute respiratory infection

In severe forms of mania, the inflated self-esteem may develop into delusions. Genetic and anatomical factors are important in the development of mania secondary to neurological disease.[33] A study of mania following closed head injury reported that six of 66 patients (9%) had features of mania at some stage during a 12 month follow-up period, this figure being higher than has been reported in other brain-injured people. In this study mania was associated with temporal basal polar lesions; no links were established with severity of brain-injury or previous personal or family history of psychiatric disorder.[34]

Management of acute mania

Treatment is best carried out in hospital; if the patient is already in a neurology ward, transfer to a psychiatric ward is desirable. Because of the lack of insight which is characteristic of mania, compulsory admission may have to be arranged. The two groups of drugs which are regularly used in acute mania are: (i) antipsychotics (such as chlorpromazine or haloperidol and the newer so-called atypical antipsychotics olanzapine and risperidone) and (ii) benzodiazepines (such as diazepam). Chlorpromazine can be given orally starting at a dose of 25–50 mg eight hourly, increasing to a maximum daily dose of 1500 mg according to the clinical response. When oral treatment is not accepted, an intramuscular injection of up to 150 mg can be given but this should not be repeated because of its irritant effect on muscle tissue. Haloperidol can be started at an oral dose of 5 mg eight hourly increasing to a maximum daily dose of 40 mg. When speedier control of symptoms is required, an intramuscular injection of 10–20 mg can be given.

The older antipsychotic drugs are likely to produce a variety of extrapyramidal side effects, especially in patients with existing brain damage. Akathisia, Parkinsonism, acute dystonia, and tardive dyskinesia are well established complications. Akathisia, a subjective sense of motor restlessness, leads to hyperactivity and an inability to relax. It can be wrongly attributed to a worsening of the manic condition, so an inexperienced clinician may increase the dose of antipsychotic rather than reduce it and consequently the akathisia symptoms worsen. A beta-adrenergic blocking drug such as propranolol is an effective remedy once the condition is diagnosed. Acute dystonias can also give rise to diagnostic confusion. They can present with tongue protrusion, torticollis, oculogyric crisis, or opisthotonus, and these are often wrongly diagnosed as dissociative (hysterical) reactions. Rapid relief of symptoms can be achieved by an intravenous dose of 5–10 mg of procyclidine. Sudden cardiorespiratory collapse is a potentially fatal complication of antipsychotic treatment, especially when the patient shows evidence of extreme physiological arousal and overactivity. Drug doses should be kept as low as possible and the treatment regimen monitored regularly. Pulse and blood pressure should be checked before each intramuscular injection and at regular intervals during oral treatment. In the light of these problems attention is turning to the newer antipsychotics. Olanzapine appears effective in the treatment of acute mania, with a low incidence of side effects,[35] so it may replace the more established drugs.

If manic symptoms do not respond to medication, ECT can prove to be a quick and effective treatment.

Anxiety and stress-related disorders

Patients with anxiety and allied conditions may present to neurologists if their symptoms are intermittent and of sudden onset.

Generalised anxiety disorder

There are a wide variety of physical complaints produced by:

- increased motor tension (restless fidgeting, tension headaches, trembling, and an inability to relax)
- apprehension (feeling "on edge", worries about future misfortunes, and difficulty in concentrating)
- autonomic overactivity (lightheadedness, sweating, tachycardia or tachypnoea, epigastric discomfort, dizziness, and dry mouth).

This disorder is more common in women and often related to chronic environmental stress. Its course is variable but tends to be fluctuating and chronic.

Phobic anxiety disorders

A phobia is an abnormal, disproportionate fear of an object or situation that leads to avoidance of the object or situation which precipitates it. Agoraphobia is the commonest phobia encountered clinically and symptoms attributed to neurological disease are particularly prominent; these include headache, impaired concentration, dizziness, and a fear of falling. The clue to the diagnosis comes from eliciting a link between symptoms and specific situations which invariably precipitate them. In the case of agoraphobia the commonest triggers are open spaces, crowded streets, supermarkets, and public transport.

Panic disorder

The characteristic features are recurrent episodes of overwhelming anxiety which are unpredictable and not confined to a particular situation. The somatic symptoms of anxiety, notably palpitations, chest pain, hyperventilation, and dizziness, usually dominate the picture but there is also intense psychological anxiety, often involving a fear of going mad or dying from heart attack or brain tumour. This may be accompanied by depersonalisation which patients describe as an altered sensation in their bodies which feel lifeless or unreal as if they have lost their feelings and are observing themselves from the outside. Panic attacks may be mistaken for the aura of temporal lobe epilepsy, vestibular disease, or the early manifestation of multiple sclerosis. Non-neurological conditions that need to be considered in the differential diagnoses are hyperthyroidism, phaeochromocytoma, hypoglycaemia, and supraventricular tachycardias.

A typical attack lasts only a few minutes but tends to recur. Patients become apprehensive of recurrent episodes and some learn to avoid certain places where an attack would be particularly embarrassing, such as a public place far from home from which there is no easy escape route. Thus panic attacks come to be associated with agoraphobic behaviour in some patients.

Post-traumatic stress disorder

This syndrome is a delayed response following exposure to a stressful experience of an exceptionally threatening nature which is quite outside the range of everyday experience and which is likely to cause distress to almost everyone. There is a perceived danger of death or severe physical trauma but the injuries actually sustained may be quite trivial. The experiences that evoke the response include natural disaster, road traffic accidents, military or terrorist activity, and being the victim of torture or rape. The disorder has been estimated to occur in up to one third of patients involved in road traffic accidents.[36,37]

There may be a delay between the traumatic event and the onset of symptoms which ranges from a few weeks up to six months. The typical symptoms include recurrent intrusive memories of the event ("flashbacks"), disturbed sleep, nightmares of the event, emotional blunting, avoidance of cues that evoke memories of the original trauma, depression, irritability, and autonomic arousal.

Acute stress reaction

A transient disorder which develops in response to exceptional physical and/or mental stress and which usually subsides within hours or days. The stressor may be an overwhelming traumatic experience such as a war, a natural catastrophe, rape, multiple bereavement, or fire. The symptoms show great variation but typically include an initial "daze" state with some constriction of the field of consciousness and narrowing of attention, inability to comprehend stimuli, and disorientation. Autonomic signs of panic may also be present. The symptoms usually subside within minutes, but can last hours or up to two or three days. No treatment is usually necessary.

Adjustment disorder

A varied disorder of distress and emotional disturbance usually interfering with social functioning and performance arising from a significant life change or a stressful life. The causal event does not in any way reach the level of those leading to an acute stress reaction (see above). Symptoms include depressed mood, anxiety, worry (or a mixture of these), a feeling of inability to cope and plan ahead. The individual may be prone to dramatic behaviour or outbursts of violence. The disorder is usually transient and requires no treatment.

Management of anxiety and stress-related disorders

Behaviour therapy, involving relaxation and gradual exposure to the precipitating situation, is of proven value in phobic disorders and in panic disorder when there is avoidance behaviour. A clinical psychologist should assess the patient and organise treatment if behaviour and cognitive therapy are considered appropriate. Phenelzine is a useful adjunct to psychological methods of treatment. Drug treatment is more important in spontaneous panic attacks; phenelzine, imipramine, and paroxetine have been shown to be effective.

There has been considerable interest in the psychological treatment of victims of accidents or disasters who are at risk of developing post-traumatic stress and other psychiatric disorders. Early intervention has been advocated but its efficacy has not been convincingly demonstrated. Cognitive therapy and exposure, preventing the development of avoidance therapy, are now established components of treatment.[38] If symptoms have become established, either tricyclic antidepressants or monoamine oxidase inhibitors can provide symptomatic relief.[39]

Dissociative (conversion) disorder

This group of disorders is also known as conversion hysteria. The term "hysteria" is a controversial one and is used in several different ways; as a result it has been omitted from both DSM-IV and ICD-10 but it is still widely used as a diagnostic category in clinical practice.

Dissociative disorders are characterised by symptoms that suggest lesions in the motor or sensory pathways of the voluntary nervous system. There is loss or distortion of neurological function which cannot be adequately accounted for by organic disease.[40] Psychiatrists would also want to establish positive evidence that the symptom is linked to psychological factors,[41] either previous severe stress, emotional conflict, or an associated psychiatric disorder. It is assumed that the symptoms are not intentionally produced, as in malingering, but are a result of unconscious motives. This, however, is a notoriously difficult distinction to make and it often appears that the degree of insight into the nature of the disability varies from time to time.

Dissociative disorders are thought to be declining in incidence. The commonest symptoms, which are usually of acute onset, are motor weakness, altered sensation, gait disturbance, and pseudo-seizures.[42] The neurological examination reveals characteristic abnormalities that enable the experienced neurologist to make a confident diagnosis in most cases.[43] Weakness usually involves whole movements rather than muscle groups and it affects the extremities much more often than ocular, facial, or cervical movements. Various clinical techniques can be employed to show that weakness of a limb is associated with simultaneous contraction of opposing muscle groups. There is discontinuous resistance during testing of power ("give way weakness"), muscle wasting is absent, and reflexes are normal. Sensory loss or distortion is often inconsistent when tested on more than one occasion and incompatible with peripheral nerve or root distribution. There may be discrete patches of anaesthesia or hemisensory loss which stops abruptly in the midline. Visual symptoms include monocular diplopia, triplopia, field defects, tunnel vision, and bilateral blindness associated with normal pupillary reflexes. Dissociative gait disturbance, astasia-abasia, is recognised by its bizarre character and intermittent pattern; the patient walks normally if he or she thinks that no one is observing. In some cases, when being observed, the patient actively attempts to fall and this contrasts with the patient with organic disease who tries to support him- or herself.

Pseudo-seizures are more difficult to evaluate because they are episodic and often coexist with true epilepsy. An account from a reliable observer is invaluable but it is essential for the clinician to witness an attack before making a firm diagnosis. The clinical features, which simulate epilepsy to a varying degree, have been described in detail.[44] During an attack there is marked involvement of the truncal muscles with opisthotonus and lateral rolling or jerking of the head and body. All four limbs may exhibit random thrashing movements which increase in amplitude if restraint is applied. Cyanosis is rare unless there is deliberate breath holding. Corneal and pupillary reflexes are retained although they may be difficult to elicit because the eyelids are kept firmly closed. Tongue biting and urinary incontinence are uncommon unless the patient has some degree of medical knowledge and has learned from experience that they are characteristic features of epilepsy.

In contrast to true epilepsy, pseudo-seizures usually occur in the presence of other people and not when the patient is alone or asleep. Some episodes simulate partial motor seizures or simple faints. Others occur in rapid succession without recovery of consciousness and they may be accompanied by deliberate tongue biting or incontinence so the clinical picture mimics status epilepticus. In addition to the clinical features of the attacks, certain demographic characteristics help to distinguish pseudo-seizures from true epilepsy. Patients with pseudo-seizures are more likely to have a family history of psychiatric illness, a personal history of psychiatric illness, previous suicide attempts, sexual maladjustment, and current affective disorder.[45]

Dissociative, or psychogenic, amnesia can also create diagnostic problems.[46] There is a sudden loss of memory, usually in relation to a markedly stressful event. The amnesia is selective and predominantly involves the inability to recall emotionally charged memories. The ability to learn new information is relatively preserved, as are cognitive skills such as reading and writing. A characteristic feature is a loss of personal identity; the patient is unable to recall his or her name, age, address, occupation, and family details, and may fail to recognise relatives when they visit. Recovery is usually rapid and complete. In some cases, however, dissociative amnesia lasts for several days or weeks and is accompanied by an apparently purposeful wandering away from the home or place of work. During this condition, known as a dissociative fugue, a new name and identity may be assumed. Self-care is maintained and the patient's behaviour may appear completely normal to people who do not know him or her. Recovery occurs abruptly and there is amnesia for the period of the fugue. Organic conditions that need to be considered in the differential diagnosis of dissociative amnesia include head injury, delirium, epileptic fit, Wernicke's encephalopathy, alcoholic blackout, and transient global amnesia.

Any patient suspected of having dissociative symptoms should be examined carefully by a neurologist and psychiatrist. Special investigations, such as MRI and EEG telemetry, are required in some cases before a confident diagnosis can be made and, in a few, a decision has to be deferred until the symptoms can be reviewed after a suitable time interval. The presence of organic disease does not rule out a diagnosis of dissociative disorder. Indeed it is now recognised that neurological lesions and dissociative symptoms occur together more frequently than can be explained by chance. Although the neurological lesion cannot explain the presenting symptom, coexisting disease of the nervous system may facilitate the emergence of dissociative mechanisms and provide a model for the symptom.[40] This may explain the frequent occurrence of pseudo-seizures in patients who also have genuine epilepsy.

Management of dissociative disorder

Once the diagnosis of dissociative disorder has been established, the results of the clinical examination and special investigations should be discussed with the patient together with reasons for considering the symptoms to have a psychological basis. This should not be conducted in a confrontational manner. It is best to explain that the symptoms are due to stress, that they are familiar to the clinician, that serious disease has been excluded, and that full recovery can be expected. Requests for further investigations should be resisted. A reassuring and encouraging approach is beneficial. Any associated psychiatric disorder such as depression should be treated appropriately and interpersonal conflicts discussed with the patient and key relatives. These patients are often highly suggestible so they respond well to predictions of recovery. Given that they are preoccupied with physical complaints, their recovery can be assisted by providing a physical framework for improvement. Physiotherapy is particularly effective in restoring the power to a paralysed or weakened limb. Using such an approach with patients with hysterical gait disorders, about half recover completely during a three to four day hospital stay.[47]

In resistant cases an abreaction interview under intravenous sedation is useful. Several drugs can be used to provide the required level of sedation but benzodiazepines such as diazepam are probably the safest. During the interview the patient is encouraged to explore and ventilate any emotional problems that have hitherto not been discussed. This can have a cathartic effect and is often followed by dramatic improvement, which is facilitated if the interviewer predicts recovery before and during the interview. An interview can also be useful to clarify the diagnosis and gain access to undisclosed psychopathology. It appears particularly useful for dissociative amnesia and should be used if the memory impairment does not begin to improve within a few days of its onset. Hypnosis can be employed as an alternative procedure if the clinician has sufficient experience of the technique.

Somatoform disorders and neurasthenia

These disorders tend to be chronic and are associated with repeated consultations for physical symptoms and requests for medical investigations despite previous negative findings.

They are unlikely to present as emergencies but as part of a lengthy history, at times exceeding 30 years, of chronic ill-health and contact with medical services.

Acute psychotic disorders

Psychotic symptoms are common complications of neurological and other medical illnesses. In most cases they are due to delirium and represent the acute effects on mental functioning of intracranial lesions, or metabolic or toxic disturbance elsewhere in the body. The characteristic features of delirium are alterations of consciousness, muddled thinking, mood change, psychomotor abnormalities – either retardation or excitability – and perceptual disturbances in the visual or tactile senses. In severe cases there are florid visual and tactile hallucinations. The aetiology and management of delirium have already been reviewed in this series.[48]

Psychotic symptoms arising during treatment of Parkinson's disease can often lead to diagnostic problems because psychological symptoms may be due to the disease itself or to prescribed drugs. Anticholinergic drugs such as benzhexol, procyclidine, and orphenadrine can precipitate acute delirium which resolves when the drug is withdrawn. Quicker resolution can be achieved by parenteral administration of the anticholinesterase physostigmine. Psychotic symptoms also occur during treatment with levodopa but other acute psychological reactions can develop with this drug including depression, hypomania, and hypersexuality. Antipsychotics may exacerbate the neurological symptoms of Parkinson's disease. Clozapine, which has low D_2 receptor affinity, has been recommended as an effective treatment for psychotic disorders associated with levodopa therapy.[49] The drug is currently available for the treatment of resistant schizophrenia: its use is restricted because of the appreciable risk of agranulocytosis which occurs in at least 1% of cases. Other side effects of clozapine include convulsions and hypersalivation. In the light of these complications, the more recently introduced atypical antipsychotics such as risperidone and olanzapine may be preferred to clozapine.

Psychotic symptoms without features of delirium or dementia can occur in association with a wide range of cerebral disorders, notably epileptic foci, cerebral tumour, cerebral trauma, Wilson's disease, and Huntington's disease. The psychosis can take the form of a schizophrenic or affective disorder. The site of the lesion has been considered to influence the pattern of symptoms. A schizophrenic presentation has been particularly associated with temporal lobe lesions in the dominant hemisphere, whereas affective disorders have been linked with lesions in the non-dominant hemisphere. Not all studies have demonstrated such an association with laterality.[50]

Occasionally transient psychotic disorders develop in clear consciousness in the absence of evidence of structural brain damage. The most striking clinical symptom is a well developed delusional system, nearly always of a paranoid nature. These psychotic disorders are seen most commonly in patients who have been admitted acutely to hospital and who have been treated in intensive care or coronary care units which they perceive as bewildering and threatening. The delusions typically involve members of the nursing or medical staff whom the patient may accuse of trying to poison or even kill him or her. In response to these delusions there may be sudden outbursts of aggression towards members of staff or attempts to leave hospital against medical advice. Psychoses of this nature are probably precipitated by the emotional impact of the illness and by the disruption it causes to the patient's familiar environment.

Management of acute psychoses

When the psychosis is believed to be triggered by the perceived stress of the treatment environment, it is advisable to transfer the patient as soon as possible to a less intimidating environment, for example from an intensive care unit to a general ward or from a general ward to the patient's home, if adequate care is available there. Rapid tranquillisation may be needed if there is aggressive or disruptive behaviour. Chlorpromazine or haloperidol may be given in doses similar to those used in acute mania. If very rapid control of symptoms is required, diazepam can be given intravenously in a dose of 5–10 mg as Diazemuls. Intravenous therapy ensures near immediate delivery of the drug to its site of action and effectively avoids the danger of inadvertent accumulation of slowly absorbed intramuscular doses. Note also that intravenous doses can be repeated after only 5–10 minutes if no effect is observed.[51] A recent review of rapid tranquillisation has recommended that the mainstay of pharmacological treatment should be parenteral benzodiazepines used with due care.[52] In an emergency, and if the patient is considered to lack capacity to give or withhold consent to treatment, medication can be administered under common law if it is thought to be in the person's best interest, for example to reduce the risk of violence or self-harm until a Mental Health Act assessment is arranged.[53,54] A patient's capacity to consent may be temporarily affected by many factors, including confusion, panic, shock, pain, fatigue, or drugs.

These antipsychotic drugs are well recognised as having unpleasant extrapyramidal side effects. The most dangerous of these, but fortunately the least frequent, is the neuroleptic malignant syndrome in which extrapyramidal rigidity and akathisia develop abruptly or within a few days.[55] Pyrexia is always present, together with autonomic disturbances including profuse sweating, increased salivation, hyperventilation, tachycardia, and labile blood pressure. Laboratory investigations show a leucocytosis and a raised creatinine kinase. The incidence of the condition is not known but is probably well under 1% of cases treated with antipsychotics if strict diagnostic criteria are applied. Antipsychotics should be stopped immediately once the condition is diagnosed. Rapid improvement is seen if a dopamine agonist such as bromocriptine is administered, and the mortality rate has been considerably reduced by this treatment. The newer "atypical" antipsychotics should be used in the treatment of psychotic disorders associated with organic brain lesions. If antipsychotic drugs are ineffective or contraindicated, lorazepam 2–4 mg can be given orally or intramuscularly every two hours, with a maximum daily dose of 10 mg.

Personality change due to cerebral disease

A change in personality is likely to follow diffuse, severe damage to the brain of the sort that is commonly seen after major head injury, but which can also occur in association with cerebral tumours, cerebrovascular disease, dementias, and encephalitis. The changes in behaviour are persistent and often develop gradually, but they may lead to sudden outbursts of impulsivity which create acute problems. A survey of patients who had survived a severe head injury reported that the prevalence of personality change increased with time; at five years after the injury, 74% of patients were described by their relatives as having undergone a personality change. Threats or gestures of violence had occurred in 54% while there had been an actual assault on a relative in 20% of cases. Other problems which had occurred included trouble with the law (31%), childishness (38%), and being upset by minor changes in routine (38%).[56]

Brain injury can produce an exaggeration of premorbid personality traits so that a person with an obsessional personality becomes even more meticulous and preoccupied with detail, whereas someone with an antisocial personality becomes more impulsive, irresponsible, and aggressive. Among a group of patients with Wilson's disease, psychopathic personality traits were significantly related to the severity of neurological symptoms, particularly dysarthria, bradykinesia, and rigidity.[57] If the damage is localised to particular parts of the brain, the personality changes tend to be more specific.[58,59] Frontal lobe damage is associated with apathy, lack of initiative, tactlessness, irritability, euphoria, and disinhibition. Although the patient's demeanour is predominantly listless there may be unpredictable outbursts of aggression or sexually disinhibited behaviour. Social skills tend to be lost with a failure to consider the feelings of other people and the impact of tactless remarks. The ability to plan ahead is impaired, with the result that irresponsible decisions may be taken with little concern about their outcome.

Irritability and aggressive outbursts are especially associated with temporal lobe pathology. Herpes simplex encephalitis has an affinity for the temporal lobes, so behavioural manifestations are common during the acute stages of the illness and after recovery if there is residual brain damage. Patients who survive temporal lobe damage may manifest the features of the Klüver–Bucy syndrome which include hypersexuality, aggressive outbursts, excessive oral behaviour, and visual agnosia.

Management of aggressive behaviour

Box 5.5 summarises the conditions in which unpredictable outbursts of aggression may occur.

Patients who are potentially violent should not be interviewed in an isolated room; when the risk is particularly high the doctor should not be alone with such patients. Adequate staff should be available nearby. The immediate aims are to control the risk of violence, to diagnose the underlying disorder, and to administer specific treatment. A detailed history and full physical and mental state assessment are rarely possible; immediate treatment has to be arranged until complete information is available.

Every effort should be made to calm patients by sympathetic understanding and reassurance. Violence is often a response to paranoid experiences and patients can be pacified if they believe that the doctor appreciates the reasons for their behaviour. If this can be achieved medication may be accepted voluntarily; otherwise compulsory treatment becomes unavoidable if patients are endangering themselves or others. Physical restraint should be applied with the assistance of security staff; the safety of all involved is best ensured by having more than a sufficient number of staff available. At least one person should restrain each limb while another administers medication.[60,61] Haloperidol 10–20 mg intramuscularly is the preferred drug, except for cases of alcohol or drug misuse or patients with serious physical illness. Benzodiazepines should then be given instead; for example diazepam 10 mg by slow intravenous injection or lorazepam 2 mg intramuscularly. Once the risk of aggression

---

Box 5.5 Neurological and psychiatric disorders associated with aggression

Acute delirium
Brain damage – especially to frontal and temporal lobes
Epilepsy
Functional psychoses – schizophrenia, bipolar affective disorder
Alcohol abuse – intoxication, withdrawal
Drug abuse – intoxication, withdrawal, threatening behaviour to obtain drugs
Personality disorder

has been controlled it is nearly always necessary to arrange admission to an appropriate inpatient unit to begin a diagnostic evaluation and specific treatment for the underlying condition when the diagnosis has been clarified.

Management of acute behaviour disturbances

- Acute behaviour disturbances are commonly encountered in neurological practice. Psychiatric disorders may accompany neurological disease or may present with somatic symptoms that suggest neurological lesions but for which no organic pathology can be detected.
- Evidence of intellectual impairment, particularly reduced level of consciousness, disorientation, and memory deficits, enables conditions such as delirium, which are due to overt physical disease, to be distinguished from affective, anxiety, and acute psychotic disorders. The psychotic disorders are not usually associated with overt physical disease although in a few patients they may be the presenting manifestations of an occult lesion in the central nervous system or elsewhere. The likelihood of this increases with advancing age and if there is no previous personal or family history of psychiatric illness or no apparent psychosocial precipitating factor.
- Successful management requires close collaboration between neurologists and psychiatrists. It is essential to be familiar with the psychotropic drugs that are most appropriately used for patients with neurological disorders. Tricyclic antidepressants and selective serotonin re-uptake inhibitors are both used for treating depression, but the latter group of drugs may prove more acceptable because of their lower incidence of side effects.
- Acute psychotic disorders require treatment with neuroleptic drugs, the main groups being the phenothiazines and butyrophenones. Rapid control of acute psychosis is essential when it is associated with aggressive behaviour and it is important that clinicians are familiar with regimens of parenteral neuroleptic administration and indications for compulsory treatment.

References

1 Ron MA. Psychiatric manifestations of demonstrable brain damage. In: Ron MA, David AS, eds. *Disorders of brain and mind*. Cambridge: Cambridge University Press, 1998;177–95.
2 Schiffer RB. Psychiatric aspects of clinical neurology. *Am J Psychiatry* 1983; 140:205–7.
3 Kirk C, Saunders M. Primary psychiatric illness in a neurological out-patient department in North-East England. *J Psychosom Res* 1977;21:1–5.

4   Lloyd G. Somatisation: a psychiatrist's perspective. *J Psychosom Res* 1989; **33**:665–9.

5   Kirk C, Saunders M. Primary psychiatric illness in a neurological out-patient department in North-East England: an assessment of symptomatology. *Acta Psychiatr Scand* 1977;**56**:294–302.

6   Fitzpatrick R, Hopkins A. Referrals to neurologist for headaches not due to structural disease. *J Neurol Neurosurg Psychiatry* 1981;**44**:1061–7.

7   Lascelles RG. Atypical facial pain and depression. *Br J Psychiatry* 1966;**112**: 651–7.

8   Judd FK, Stone J, Weber JE, Brown DJ, Burrows GD. Depression following spinal cord injury: a prospective in-patient study. *Br J Psychiatry* 1989; **154**:668–71.

9   World Health Organization. *The ICD-10 classification of mental and behavioural disorders: clinical descriptions and diagnostic guidelines*. Geneva: WHO, 1992.

10 Lloyd GG. Liaison Psychiatry. In: Murray R, Hill P, McGuffin P, eds. *The essentials of postgraduate psychiatry*, 3rd edn. Cambridge: Cambridge University Press, 1997;534–50.

11 Whitlock FA. *Symptomatic affective disorders*. London: Academic Press, 1982.

12 Ron MA. Psychiatric manifestations of frontal lobe tumours. *Br J Psychiatry* 1989;**155**:735–8.

13 Ron MA, Logsdail SJ. Psychiatric morbidity in multiple sclerosis: a clinical and MRI study. *Psychol Med* 1989;**19**:887–95.

14 Berrios GE, Quemada JI. Depressive illness in multiple sclerosis: clinical and theoretical aspects of the association. *Br J Psychiatry* 1990;**156**:10–16.

15 Kearney TR. Parkinson's disease presenting as a depressive illness. *J Irish Med Assoc* 1964;**54**:117–19.

16 Mindham RHS. Psychiatric symptoms in Parkinsonism. *J Neurol Neurosurg Psychiatry* 1970;**33**:188–91.

17 Lyon RL. Huntington's chorea in the Moray Firth area. *Br Med J* 1962;**1**:1301–6.

18 Folstein SE, Abbott MH, Chase GA, Jenson BA, Folstein MF. The association of affective disorder with Huntington's disease in a case series and in families. *Psychol Med* 1983;**13**:537–42.

19 Eastwood MR, Rifat SL, Nobbs H, Ruderman J. Mood disorder following cerebrovascular accident. *Br J Psychiatry* 1989;**154**:195–200.

20 Robinson RG, Starr LB, Kubos KL, *et al.* A two-year longitudinal study of post-stroke mood disorder: findings during the initial evaluation. *Stroke* 1983;**14**:736–41.

21 Starkstein SE, Robinson RG. Affective disorders and cerebrovascular disease. *Br J Psychiatry* 1989;**154**:170–82.

22 Carson AJ, MacHale S, Allen K, *et al.* Depression after stroke and lesion location: a systematic review. *Lancet* 2000;**356**:122–6.

23 House A, Dennis M, Mogridge L, Warlow C, Hawton K, Jones L. Mood disorders in the first year after stroke. *Br J Psychiatry* 1992;**158**:83–92.

24 House A, Dennis M, Molyneux A, Warlow C, Hawton K. Emotionalism after stroke. *Br Med J* 1989;**298**:991–4.

25 Stenager EN, Stenager E. Suicide and patients with neurologic diseases: methodological problems. *Arch Neurol* 1992;**49**:1296–303.

26 Stenager EN, Stenager E, Koch-Henderson N, *et al.* Suicide and multiple sclerosis: an epidemiological investigation. *J Neurol Neurosurg Psychiatry* 1992;**55**:542–5.

27 Nordentoft M, Breum L, Munck LK, Nordestgaard AG, Hunding A, Bjaeldager PAL. High mortality by natural and unnatural causes: a 10-year

follow-up study of patients admitted to a poisoning treatment centre after suicide attempts. *Br Med J* 1993;**306**:1637–41.

28 Hawton K, Fagg J, Platt S, Hawkins M. Factors associated with suicide and parasuicide in young people. *Br Med J* 1993;**306**:1641–4.

29 Appleby L. Suicide and self-harm. In: Murray R, Hill P, McGuffin P, eds. *The essentials of postgraduate psychiatry*, 3rd edn., Cambridge: Cambridge, University Press, 1997;551–62.

30 Lishman WA. Organic psychiatry: the psychological consequences of cerebral disorder, 3rd edn. Oxford: Blackwell, 1999.

31 Joyston-Bechal MP. Clinical features and outcome of stupor. *Br J Psychiatry* 1966;**112**:967–81.

32 Johnson J. Stupor: a review of 25 cases. *Acta Psychiatr Scand* 1984;**70**: 370–7.

33 Starkstein SE, Person GD, Boston J, Robinson RG. Mania after brain injury: a controlled study of causative factors. *Arch Neurol* 1988;**44**: 1069–73.

34 Jorge RE, Robinson RG, Starkstein SE, Arndt SV, Forrester AW, Geisler FH. Secondary mania following traumatic brain injury. *Am J Psychiatry* 1993;**150**:916–21.

35 Tohen M, Sanger TM, McElroy SL, *et al*. Olanzapine versus placebo in the treatment of acute mania. *Am J Psychiatry* 1999;**156**:702–9.

36 Koren D, Arnon D, Klein E. Acute stress response and post-traumatic stress disorder in traffic accident victims: a one-year prospective follow-up study. *Am J Psychiatry* 1999;**156**:367–73.

37 Ursano RJ, Fullerton CS, Epstein RS, *et al*. Acute and chronic post-traumatic stress disorder in motor vehicle accidents. *Am J Psychiatry* 1999;**156**:589–95.

38 Marks I, Lovell KI, Noshirvani H, Livanou M, Thrasher S. Treatment of post-traumatic stress disorder by exposure and/or cognitive behaviour therapy. *Arch Gen Psychiatry* 1998;**55**:317–25.

39 Davidson J. Drug therapy of post-traumatic stress disorder. *Br J Psychiatry* 1992;**160**:309–14.

40 Marsden CD. Hysteria: a neurologist's view. *Psychol Med* 1986;**16**:277–88.

41 Lloyd GG. Hysteria: a case for conservation. *Br Med J* 1986;**294**:1255–6.

42 Ljunberg L. Hysteria: a clinical prognostic and genetic study. *Acta Psychiatr Scand* 1957;**32(suppl)**:112.

43 Pincus J. Hysteria presenting to the neurologist. In: Roy A, ed. *Hysteria*, Chichester, UK: John Wiley, 1982.

44 Fenton GW. Epilepsy and hysteria. *Br J Psychiatry* 1986;**149**:28–37.

45 Roy A. Hysterical fits previously diagnosed as epilepsy. *Psychol Med* 1977; **7**:271–3.

46 Kopelman MD. Amnesia: organic and psychogenic. *Br J Psychiatry* 1987; **150**:428–42.

47 Keane JR. Hysterical gait disorders: 60 cases. *Neurology* 1989;**39**:586–9.

48 Taylor D, Lewis S. Delirium. *J Neurol Neurosurg Psychiatry* 1993;**56**: 742–51.

49 Friedman JH. The management of levodopa psychoses. *Clin Neuropharmacol* 1991;**14**:283–95.

50 Feinstein A, Ron MA. Psychosis associated with demonstrable brain diseases. *Psychol Med* 1990;**20**:793–803.

51 Taylor D, McConnell D, McConnell H, Kerwin R. *Prescribing guidelines*, 6th edn. The South London and Maudsley NHS Trust, 2001.

52 McAllister-Williams RH, Ferrier IN. Rapid tranquillisation: time for a reappraisal of options for parenteral therapy. *Br J Psychiatry* 2001;**179**: 485–9.

53 Macpherson R, Anstee B, Dix R. Guidelines for the management of acutely disturbed patients. *Adv Psychiatric Treat* 1996;2:194–201.

54 Feldman E. Use of the Mental Health Act and common law in the general hospital. In: *Liaison Psychiatry, Planning Services for Specialist Settings.* Gaskell for the Royal College of Psychiatrists, London, 2000.

55 Kellam AMP. The neuroleptic malignant syndrome, so-called: a review of the world literature. *Br J Psychiatry* 1987;**150**:752–9.

56 Brooks N, Campsie L, Symington C, Beatty A, McKinley W. The five-year outcome of severe blunt head injury: a relative's view. *J Neurol Neurosurg Psychiatry* 1986;**49**:764–70.

57 Dening TR, Berrios GE. Wilson's disease: a prospective study of psychopathology in 31 cases. *Br J Psychiatry* 1989;**155**:206–13.

58 McClelland RJ. Psychosocial sequelae of head injury: anatomy of a relationship. *Br J Psychiatry* 1988;**153**:141–6.

59 Trimble MR. Behaviour and personality disturbances. In: Bradley WG, Daroff RB, Fenichel GM, Marsden CD, eds. *Neurology in clinical practice,* vol 1. London: Butterworth-Heinemann, 1991;81–100.

60 Sheard MH. Clinical pharmacology of aggressive behaviour. *Clin Neuropharmacol* 1988;**11**:483–92.

61 Goldberg RJ, Dubin WR, Fogel BS. Behavioural emergencies: assessment and psychopharmacologic management. *Clin Neuropharmacol* 1989;**12**: 233–48.

6: Tonic-clonic status epilepticus

SIMON SHORVON, MATTHEW WALKER

Tonic-clonic status epilepticus can be defined as a condition in which prolonged or recurrent tonic-clonic seizures persist for 30 minutes or more.[1] Most tonic-clonic seizures last less than two minutes; nevertheless many seizures that continue for less than 30 minutes self-terminate.[2,3] Treatment of the premonitory stages is likely to be more successful than treatment in the later stages and so treatment should commence as soon as it is apparent that the seizure is persisting (a tonic-clonic seizure of more than five minutes duration) or there is a significant worsening of a patient's normal seizure pattern.

The annual incidence of tonic-clonic status epilepticus varies considerably from study to study depending on the population analysed; estimates have ranged from 4 to 28 cases per 100 000 persons (2000–14 000 new cases each year in the United Kingdom).[4-7] It is most frequent in the young, in whom it also tends to be longer lasting. Status epilepticus is also commoner in epileptic patients with mental handicap, or with structural cerebral pathology (especially in the frontal lobes). In established epilepsy, status epilepticus can be precipitated by drug withdrawal, intercurrent illness, or metabolic disturbance, or the progression of the underlying disease, and is more common in symptomatic than in idiopathic epilepsy. About 5% of all epileptic adult clinic patients will have at least one episode of status epilepticus in the course of their epilepsy,[1] and in children the proportion is higher (10–25%).[1,8] Most status epilepticus episodes, however, do not develop in known epileptic patients, and in such cases are almost always due to acute cerebral disturbances; common causes are cerebral infection, trauma, cerebrovascular disease, cerebral tumour, acute toxic (usually alcohol related) or metabolic disturbance, or febrile illness (in children). Studies have shown status epilepticus to account for about 4% of admissions to neurological intensive care, and 5% of all visits to a university hospital casualty department.[9] The mortality of status epilepticus is about 20%. Most patients die of the underlying condition, rather than the status epilepticus itself or its treatment.[1,5,10] Permanent neurological and mental deterioration may result from status epilepticus, particularly in young children, the risks of morbidity being greatly increased the longer the duration of the status epilepticus episode.[1] Furthermore status epilepticus can result in chronic epilepsy, and indeed 43% of those with acute symptomatic status epilepticus have a subsequent unprovoked seizure compared to 13% of those with acute symptomatic seizures. Tonic-clonic status epilepticus is only one of the forms of status epilepticus (Box 6.1), and indeed is not the most common. Nevertheless, unlike most other types, it is a medical emergency. Treatment is urgent because the longer seizures continue, the more difficult they

---

Box 6.1 Classification of status epilepticus

Confined to the neonatal period
  Neonatal status
  Status in neonatal epilepsy syndromes

Confined to infancy and childhood
  Infantile spasm (West's syndrome)
  Febrile status epilepticus
  Status in childhood myoclonic syndromes
  Status in benign childhood partial epilepsy syndromes
  Electrical status during slow wave sleep (ESES)
  Syndrome of acquired epileptic aphasia

Occurring in childhood and adult life
  Absence status
  Epilepsia partialis continua (EPC)
  Myoclonic status in coma
  Specific forms of status in mental handicap
  Myoclonic status in other epilepsy syndromes
  Non-convulsive simple partial non-convulsive status
  Complex partial status
  Boundary syndromes

Confined to adult life
  De novo absence status of late onset

Derived from Shorvon.[1]

---

become to treat, and the worse the outcome. Successful management is a balance between the often conflicting requirements of controlling seizure activity as quickly as possible, and minimising physiological changes and medical complications.

Tonic-clonic status epilepticus as a staged phenomenon

Although the original WHO definition referred to status epilepticus as an "unvarying and enduring epileptic condition", it is, on the contrary, an evolving state.[1] Indeed, it can be staged by clinical and electrographic criteria, physiological compromise, occurrence of excitotoxicity, and response to treatment.

Clinical and electrographic stages

The pattern of seizures in tonic-clonic status epilepticus evolves over time. There is often a premonitory stage of minutes or hours, during which epileptic activity increases in frequency or severity from its habitual level. This clinical deterioration is an augury, often stereotypical, of impending status epilepticus, and urgent therapy may well prevent its full development. At the onset of status epilepticus, the attacks typically take the form of discrete grand mal seizures. As time passes, however, the convulsive motor activity often evolves, first to become continuous, and then clonic jerking becomes less pronounced and less severe, and finally ceases altogether. This is the stage of "subtle status epilepticus", by which time the patient will be deeply unconscious, and the prognosis is poor. These stages are not seen in all patients; they can be modified by concomitant medication, and there is often a varying time period between each stage. In parallel to this clinical evolution, a progressive change in the EEG has also been reported in animal models.[11] The initial stage is that of discrete seizures; then there is waxing and waning of ictal discharges which progresses to continuous ictal discharges. The final stages are continuous ictal discharges punctuated by flat periods, and then periodic epileptiform discharges on a flat background. These electrographic and clinical stages importantly relate to underlying neuronal damage, and also to progressive difficulty in treating the status epilepticus (see below). The extent to which this EEG progression occurs in humans is less certain.[11-12]

Physiological stages

The physiological changes in status epilepticus are often divided into two phases, the transition from phase 1 to 2 occurring after about 30–60 minutes of continuous seizures.[1,13-15] Although this is a generally useful concept, it must be recognised that there is great variation. Both the rate and extent of physiological change are dependent on many other factors, including the anatomical site of the epileptic focus, the severity of the seizures, the underlying aetiology, and the treatment employed. Nevertheless, this staging of changes is helpful in devising a rational plan for therapy.

Phase 1

From the onset of status epilepticus, seizure activity greatly increases cerebral metabolism. Physiological mechanisms are initially sufficient largely to compensate for this perturbation. Cerebral blood flow is increased, and initially the delivery of glucose to the active cerebral tissue is maintained. Later systemic and cerebral lactate levels rise, and a profound lactic acidosis may develop.[16] There are massive cardiovascular and autonomic changes. Blood pressure rises, as does cardiac output and rate. The autonomic changes result in sweating, hyperpyrexia, bronchial secretion, salivation, vomiting, and epinephrine (adrenaline) and noradrenaline release. Endocrine and autonomic changes also cause an early rise in sugar levels.

Phase 2

As the seizure activity progresses, the compensatory physiological mechanisms begin to fail. Cerebral autoregulation breaks down progressively, and thus cerebral blood flow becomes increasingly dependent on systemic blood pressure.[13-15] Hypotension develops due to seizure-related autonomic and cardiorespiratory changes and drug treatment, and in terminal stages may be severe. The falling blood pressure results in failing cerebral blood flow and cerebral metabolism. The high metabolic demands of the epileptic cerebral tissue cannot be met and ischaemic or metabolic damage may ensue.[17,18] The tendency to hypotension can be greatly exacerbated by intravenous antiepileptic drug therapy, especially if infusion rates are too fast. Pressor agents are often necessary in prolonged therapy.

Systemic and cerebral hypoxia are common in status epilepticus, due to: central respiratory failure (greatly exacerbated by drug medication); the increased oxygen requirements of convulsions; and later pulmonary artery hypertension and pulmonary oedema.[1,14] Because of this, assisted ventilation is often required early in the course of status epilepticus.

Intracranial pressure may rise precipitously in status epilepticus. The combined effects of systemic hypotension and intracranial hypertension can result in a compromised cerebral circulation and cerebral oedema, particularly in children.[15] Intracranial pressure monitoring is advisable in prolonged severe status epilepticus, especially in children, when raised intracranial pressure is suspected; the need for active medical or surgical therapy is, however, largely determined by underlying pathology.

Cardiovascular changes in late status epilepticus can also be serious. Pulmonary hypertension and oedema are frequent, even in the presence of systemic hypotension. Pulmonary artery pressures can rise to dangerous levels, well in excess of the osmotic pressure of blood, causing oedema and stretch injuries to lung capillaries.[19] Cardiac arrhythmias in status epilepticus are the result of direct seizure-related autonomic activation, catecholamine release, hypoglycaemia, lactic acidosis, electrolyte disturbance, or cardiotoxic therapy. The autonomic effects are sometimes caused by simultaneous discharges in sympathetic and parasympathetic pathways. Intravenous sedatives depress cardiac function, and the drug effects can be potentiated by pre-existing compromise of cardiac function. In spite of the greatly increased demand, cardiac output can fall due to decreasing left ventricular contractility and stroke volume,[20] causing cardiac failure. The prodigious noradrenaline and epinephrine release also contributes to the cardiac dysfunction, arrhythmia, and tachycardia. Measures to control cardiac failure and arrhythmia are often needed.

Spectacular hyperpyrexia can also develop in status epilepticus,[16] and may also require specific treatment.

There are many metabolic and endocrine disturbances in status epilepticus, the commonest and most important being acidosis (including lactic acidosis), hypoglycaemia, hypo/hyperkalaemia, and hyponatraemia. Lactic acidosis is almost invariable in major status epilepticus, from its onset, due to neuronal and muscle activity, the acceleration of glycolysis, tissue hypoxia, impaired respiration, and catecholamine release.[16] Acute tubular necrosis due to myoglobinuria or dehydration, and occasionally fulminant renal failure, may occur. Hepatic failure is a not uncommon terminal event in status epilepticus, due to other physiological disturbances, drug treatment, or underlying disease. Rhabdomyolysis, resulting from persistent convulsive movements, can develop early in status epilepticus and precipitate renal failure if severe, and can be prevented by artificial ventilation and paralysing drugs. Disseminated intravascular coagulation is another rare but serious complication of status epilepticus, which usually requires urgent therapy. Other medical complications in status epilepticus are listed in Box 6.2, and are usually due to the autonomic activity, seizures, or drug treatment.

Excitotoxicity

The physiological compromise described above results, if unchecked, in neuronal damage. Furthermore, as shown in classic animal experiments in the 1970s and 1980s, neuronal damage can occur even without the systemic disturbance associated with status epilepticus.[21] This neuronal damage is solely dependent upon the presence of electrographic seizure activity, and is due to "excitotoxicity".[22] In both animal models and humans, the degree of excitotoxic neuronal damage relates to the duration of electrographic status epilepticus.[23-25] The occurrence of excitotoxic neuronal damage emphasises the importance of aggressively treating electrographic status epilepticus, which can occur in the absence of clinical signs of seizure activity, especially in the later stages of status epilepticus or if paralysing agents have been used.

> **Box 6.2 Medical complications in tonic-clonic status epilepticus**
>
> Cerebral
>   Hypoxic/metabolic cerebral damage
>   Seizure-induced cerebral damage
>   Cerebral oedema and raised intracranial pressure
>   Cerebral venous thrombosis
>   Cerebral haemorrhage and infarction
>
> Cardiovascular, respiratory, and autonomic
>   Hypotension
>   Hypertension
>   Cardiac failure, tachy- and bradyarrhythmia, arrest
>   Cardiogenic shock
>   Respiratory failure
>   Disturbances of respiratory rate and rhythm, apnoea
>   Pulmonary oedema, hypertension, embolism
>   Pneumonia, aspiration
>   Hyperpyrexia
>   Sweating, hypersecretion, tracheobronchial obstruction
>   Peripheral ischaemia
>
> Metabolic
>   Dehydration
>   Electrolyte disturbance (especially hyponatraemia, hyperkalaemia, hypoglycaemia)
>   Acute renal failure (especially acute tubular necrosis)
>   Acute hepatic failure
>   Acute pancreatitis
>
> Other
>   Disseminated intravascular coagulopathy/multiorgan failure
>   Rhabdomyolysis
>   Fractures
>   Infections (especially pulmonary, skin, urinary)
>   Thrombophlebitis, dermal injury

Response to treatment

As status epilepticus progresses it becomes more difficult to treat. Many of the treatments that are successful in the initial stages are ineffective later. Indeed, the potency of benzodiazepines decreases as status epilepticus progresses, although their efficacy remains;[26] the decrease in their potency is associated with a decrease in the sensitivity of

GABA receptors to benzodiazepines. Barbiturates, however, are as effective, and they appear to retain their potency throughout status epilepticus.[26]

Antiepileptic drug pharmacology in status epilepticus

As fast drug absorption is essential in status epilepticus, all drugs are ideally administered parenterally. It is desirable in status epilepticus for drugs to have a rapid onset and a prolonged duration of action. In order to accomplish this, the drugs need to cross the blood–brain barrier readily. Antiepileptic drugs achieve this either by being lipid soluble (for example, diazepam, midazolam, chlormethiazole, propofol) or by having an active transport mechanism (for example, valproate). Drugs with high lipid solubility have a biphasic concentration versus time curve. The initial phase is due to rapid redistribution from the serum to peripheral compartments (fat and muscle), and the later phase is due to elimination (usually much slower). Thus, after a single intravenous injection, there is a rapid fall in serum and consequently cerebral drug levels; the initial injection therefore can have a short-lived effect. Repeat doses, however, lead to accumulation and so a significant decrease in volume of distribution, and a decrease in the contribution of the redistribution phase to the drug's kinetics.[27] This results in greater peak concentrations and relative persistence of high serum levels. Furthermore, the cerebral drug levels following repeat dosing are maintained for longer than would be predicted from the serum data, probably due to accumulation within the brain from non-specific binding to lipid components.[27] These high, prolonged levels can precipitate hypotension, sedation, or cardiorespiratory failure – a serious risk with the repeated administration of diazepam, midazolam, chlormethiazole, clonazepam, pentobarbitone, or thiopentone. Less lipid-soluble drugs are relatively slower to act, but have a much longer lasting effect without a high risk of accumulation (for example, phenytoin, lorazepam, phenobarbitone). For lipid-soluble drugs, the rate of injection must also be carefully monitored, as too rapid administration will cause very high cerebral levels in the first pass through the cerebral circulation; this can result in sudden cardiorespiratory arrest or hypotension. For less lipid-soluble drugs (such as lorazepam), the rate of injection is not so critical.

An ideal antiepileptic drug should:

- have no active metabolites (diazepam, midazolam, lidocaine (lignocaine), and thiopentone have active metabolites)
- not interact with other medication
- not have saturable metabolism (both phenytoin and thiopentone have saturable pharmacokinetics at therapeutic levels)
- not be unduly affected by hepatic or renal blood flow or disease (chlormethiazole is an example of a drug whose metabolism is greatly affected by both hepatic disease and changes in hepatic blood flow)
- show no tendency to autoinduction (thiopentone, phenobarbitone, and phenytoin are all subject to strong autoinduction)
- have strong antiepileptic action (the non-barbiturate anaesthetics have little or no intrinsic antiepileptic action – a conundrum for their use in status epilepticus, the implications of which have not been fully considered)
- be stable in solution and unreactive with giving sets (a problem with paraldehyde, diazepam, and thiopentone).

General measures

For the new patient presenting as an emergency in status epilepticus, it is helpful to plan therapy in a series of progressive phases (Box 6.3).

First stage (0–10 minutes)

Oxygen and cardiorespiratory resuscitation

It is first essential to assess cardiorespiratory function, to secure the airway, and to resuscitate where necessary. Oxygen should always be administered, as hypoxia is often unexpectedly severe.

Box 6.3 General measures

1 (0–10 minutes)
Assess cardiorespiratory function
Secure airway and resuscitate
Administer oxygen

2 (0–60 minutes)
Institute regular monitoring (see text)
Emergency antiepileptic drug therapy (see text)
Set up intravenous lines
Emergency investigations (see text)
Administer glucose (50 ml of 50% solution) and/or intravenous thiamine (250 mg) as high potency intravenous Pabrinex where appropriate
Treat acidosis if severe

3 (0–60/90 minutes)
Establish aetiology
Identify and treat medical complications
Pressor therapy where appropriate

4 (30–90 minutes)
Transfer to intensive care
Establish intensive care and EEG monitoring (see text)
Initiate seizure and EEG monitoring
Initiate intracranial pressure monitoring where appropriate
Initiate long term, maintenance, antiepileptic therapy

These four stages should be followed chronologically; the first and second within 10 minutes, and stage 4 (transfer to intensive care unit) in most settings within 60–90 minutes of presentation.

Derived from Shorvon.[1]

Second stage (0–60 minutes)

Monitoring

Regular neurological observations and measurements of pulse, blood pressure, ECG, oxygen saturation (via a pulse oximeter), and temperature should be initiated. Metabolic abnormalities may cause status epilepticus, or develop during its course, and biochemical, blood gas, pH, clotting, and haematological measures should be monitored. The patient should continuously be attended by staff competent in resuscitation.

Emergency anticonvulsant therapy

This should be started (see below).

Intravenous lines

These should be set up for fluid replacement and drug administration (preferably with 0·9% sodium chloride (normal or physiological saline) rather than 5% glucose solutions). Drugs should not be mixed and, if two antiepileptic drugs are needed (for example, phenytoin and diazepam), two intravenous lines should be sited. The lines should be in large veins, as many antiepileptic drugs cause phlebitis and thrombosis at the site of infusion. Arterial lines must never be used for drug administration to avoid the risk of arterial necrosis.

Emergency investigations

Blood should be drawn for the emergency measurement of blood gases, sugar, renal and liver function, calcium and magnesium levels, full haematological screen (including platelets), blood clotting measures, and anticonvulsant levels. Fifty millilitres of serum should also be saved for future analysis, especially if the cause of the status epilepticus is uncertain. Other investigations depend on the clinical circumstances.

Intravenous glucose and thiamine

Fifty millilitres of a 50% glucose solution should be given immediately by intravenous injection if hypoglycaemia is suspected. If there is a history of alcoholism, or other compromised nutritional states, 250 mg of thiamine (for example, as the high potency intravenous formulation of Pabrinex, 10 ml of which contains 250 mg) should also be given intravenously. This is particularly important if glucose has been administered, as a glucose infusion increases the risk of Wernicke's encephalopathy in susceptible patients. Intravenous high dosage thiamine should be given slowly (for example, 10 ml of high potency Pabrinex over 10 minutes), with facilities for treating the anaphylaxis which is a potentially serious side effect of Pabrinex infusions. Routine glucose administration in non-hypoglycaemic patients should be avoided as there is some evidence that this can aggravate neuronal damage.

Acidosis

If acidosis is severe, the administration of bicarbonate has been advocated in the hope of preventing shock, and mitigating the effects of hypotension and low cerebral blood flow. In most cases, however, this is unnecessary and more effective is the rapid control of respiration and abolition of motor seizure activity.

Third stage (0–60/90 minutes)

Establish aetiology

The ranges of causes of status epilepticus depend primarily on age and the presence or absence of established epilepsy. The investigations required depend on clinical circumstances. CT or MRI and CSF examination are often necessary – the latter should be carried out only with facilities for resuscitation available as intracranial pressure is often elevated in status epilepticus.

If the status epilepticus has been precipitated by drug withdrawal, the immediate restitution of the withdrawn drug, even at lower doses, will usually rapidly terminate the status epilepticus.

Physiological changes and medical complications

The physiological changes of uncompensated status epilepticus, listed above, may need specific therapy. Active treatment is most commonly required for hypoxia, hypotension, raised intracranial pressure, pulmonary oedema and hypertension, cardiac arrhythmias, cardiac failure, lactic acidosis, hyperpyrexia, hypoglycaemia, electrolyte disturbance, acute hepatic or renal failure, rhabdomyolysis, and disseminated intravascular coagulation.

Pressor therapy

Dopamine is the most commonly used pressor agent, given by continuous intravenous infusion. The dose should be titrated to the desired haemodynamic and renal responses (usually initially between 2 and 5 micrograms/kg/min, but this can be increased to over 20 micrograms/kg/min in severe hypotension). Dopamine should be given into a large vein as extravasation causes tissue necrosis. ECG monitoring is required, as conduction defects may occur, and particular care is needed in dosing in the presence of cardiac failure.

Fourth stage (30–90 minutes)

Intensive care

If seizures are continuing in spite of the measures taken above, the patient must be transferred to an intensive care environment, and the usual measures instituted.

Intensive care monitoring

In severe established status epilepticus, intensive monitoring may be required, including: intra-arterial blood pressure, capnography, oximetry, central venous pressure, and pulmonary artery pressure monitoring.

Magnesium

Although effective at preventing eclampsia, there is no evidence to suggest that increasing magnesium serum concentrations to supranormal levels has any benefit in status epilepticus. Indeed, such a policy can result in motor paralysis, difficulty in detecting clinical seizure activity, and hypotension.[28] However, serum magnesium can be low in alcoholics and patients with AIDS,[29,30] and in these patients intravenous loading with 2–4 g of magnesium sulphate over 20 minutes may help with seizure control and prevention of arrhythmias.

Seizure and EEG monitoring

In prolonged status epilepticus, or in comatose ventilated patients, motor activity can be barely visible. In this situation, continuous EEG monitoring using a full EEG or a cerebral function monitor is necessary, and at the very least intermittent daily EEGs should be recorded. The latter must be calibrated individually, and then can register both burst suppression and seizure activity. Burst suppression provides an arbitrary physiological target for the titration of barbiturate or anaesthetic therapy. Drug dosing is commonly set at a level that will produce burst suppression with interburst intervals of between 2 and 30 seconds.

Intracranial pressure monitoring and cerebral oedema

Continuous intracranial pressure monitoring is advisable, especially in children in the presence of persisting, severe, or progressive elevated intracranial pressure. The need for active therapy is usually determined by the underlying cause rather than the status epilepticus. Intermittent positive pressure ventilation, high-dose corticosteroid therapy (4 mg dexamethasone every 6 hours), or mannitol infusion may be used (the latter is usually reserved for temporary respite for patients in danger of tentorial coning). Neurosurgical decompression is occasionally required.

Long term anticonvulsant therapy

Long term, maintenance, anticonvulsant therapy must be given in tandem with emergency treatment. The choice of drug depends on previous therapy, the type of epilepsy, and the clinical setting. If phenytoin or phenobarbitone has been used in emergency treatment, maintenance doses can be continued orally (through a nasogastric tube) guided by serum level monitoring. Other maintenance antiepileptic drugs can be started also, giving oral loading doses.

Drug treatment

The drug treatment of tonic-clonic status epilepticus can also be usefully divided into stages. A suggested regimen for a typical new case presenting as an emergency is given in Box 6.4.

Premonitory stage

In patients with established epilepsy, tonic-clonic status epilepticus seldom develops without warning. Usually, a prodromal phase (the premonitory stage) presages status epilepticus; during this phase seizures become increasingly frequent or severe. Urgent drug treatment will usually prevent the evolution into true status epilepticus. This stage frequently occurs prior to transfer to hospital, and indeed effective treatment may render transfer unnecessary. Thus what is needed is a drug that can be given by a route that can be used

Box 6.4 Suggested emergency antiepileptic drug regimen for status in newly presenting adult patients

Premonitory stage (pre-hospital)
Diazepam 10–20 mg given rectally, repeated once 15 minutes later if status continues to threaten
If seizures continue, treat as below

Early status
Lorazepam (IV) 0·07 mg/kg (usually a 4 mg bolus, repeated once after 10–20 minutes; rate not critical)
If seizures continue 30 minutes after first injection, treat as below

Established status
Phenytoin infusion at a dose of 15–18 mg/kg at a maximum rate of 50 mg/min or fosphenytoin infusion at a dose of 15–20 mg PE/kg at a maximum rate of 100 mg PE/minute
and/or
Phenobarbitone bolus of 10 mg/kg at a rate of 100 mg/min (usually 700 mg over seven minutes in an adult)

Refractory status
General anaesthesia, with propofol, midazolam, or thiopentone. Anaesthetic continued for 12–24 hours after the last clinical or electrographic seizure, then dose tapered

In the above scheme, the refractory stage (general anaesthesia) is reached 60/90 minutes after the initial therapy. This scheme is suitable for usual clinical hospital settings. In some situations, general anaesthesia should be initiated earlier and, occasionally, should be delayed.

outside the hospital setting, yet still has a rapid onset of action, and should not be complicated by respiratory or circulatory problems. Rectal diazepam has generally been the drug of choice. Neither suppositories nor oral diazepam have a fast enough onset of action, and intramuscular diazepam has the problem of local irritation and erratic absorption. However, 0·5–1 mg/kg rectal diazepam solution results in therapeutic serum concentrations within one hour, and has been shown to be very effective in arresting acute seizures with minimal side effects.[31]

A disadvantage of rectal diazepam is the difficulty in administration via this route, especially in children; so alternatives have been sort. Midazolam has the advantage over other benzodiazepines in that it can be administered by intranasal, buccal, and intramuscular routes. Of these, buccal midazolam (10 mg in 2 ml) seems to be the most promising.[32]

The earlier treatment is given the better. Early treatment by paramedics with intravenous diazepam or intravenous lorazepam has for instance been shown to prevent the evolution to or continuation of status epilepticus.[33] In this study, although not statistically significant, lorazepam had a more impressive effect than diazepam. Furthermore, diazepam and lorazepam resulted in less respiratory depression than placebo, suggesting that continued seizure activity carries a not insubstantial risk of respiratory depression that may offset the risk of benzodiazepine administration.[33] If the patient is at home, antiepileptic drugs should be administered before transfer to hospital, or in the casualty department before transfer to the ward. The acute administration of either diazepam or midazolam will cause drowsiness or sleep, and occasionally cardiorespiratory collapse, and should be carefully supervised.

Stage of early status epilepticus (0–30 minutes)

Once status epilepticus has developed, treatment should be carried out in hospital, under close supervision. For the first 30–60 minutes or so of continuous seizures, physiological mechanisms compensate for the greatly enhanced metabolic activity. This is the stage of early status epilepticus, and it is usual to administer a fast-acting benzodiazepine drug.

In most clinical settings, intravenous lorazepam (0·1 mg/kg) or diazepam (0·2–0·3 mg/kg) are the drugs of choice, and these doses can be repeated once if seizure activity does not stop. Diazepam has been the drug of choice, but its short distribution half-life has meant that it is usually given with a longer acting drug such as phenytoin, and is often used as repeat boluses. It is, however, very effective. Clonazepam appears to offer little advantage over diazepam. Lorazepam, however, has a longer duration of action, but a slower rate of brain penetration. Lorazepam and diazepam have been compared in a randomised study in which both were equally effective, resulting in seizure cessation in 89% and 76% of cases respectively.[34] In a recent multicentre, double-blind, randomised study of initial treatment of status epilepticus, there was no statistical difference between the efficacy of lorazepam 0·1mg/kg and the combination of diazepam 0·15 mg/kg and phenytoin 18 mg/kg.[35] Lorazepam was, however, easier to use and was faster to administer. There was no difference in side effects. Although there is little evidence supporting one benzodiazepine over another at this stage, lorazepam probably has the advantages of a longer duration of action, and ease of administration.

In patients in respiratory failure, intravenous lidocaine (lignocaine) may be preferable. In most patients, therapy will be highly effective. Continuous inpatient observation should follow. In previously non-epileptic patients, chronic antiepileptic therapy should be introduced, and in those already on maintenance antiepileptic therapy this should be reviewed.

Stage of established status epilepticus (30–60/90 minutes)

The stage of established status epilepticus can be operationally defined as status epilepticus which has continued for 30 minutes in spite of early stage treatment. The time is chosen because physiological decompensation will usually have begun. Intensive care facilities are desirable, as status epilepticus at this stage carries an appreciable morbidity. There are three alternative treatment options. These are phenobarbitone (10 mg/kg), phenytoin (15–20 mg/kg), or fosphenytoin (a phenytoin pro-drug); all are given by intravenous loading followed by repeated oral or intravenous supplementation. Diazepam is often given with phenytoin or fosphenytoin (either at this or the early stage of status epilepticus), combining the fast acting but short lasting effect of diazepam with the slow onset but long lasting effect of phenytoin.

Numerous alternative treatment options exist. Although once popular, continuous benzodiazepine and chlormethiazole infusions on the ward are hazardous and are now not recommended. Infusions of most benzodiazepines result in accumulation and so persistent action. This often results in sudden hypotension and respiratory and circulatory collapse. Unfortunately this problem is compounded by the difficulties, in most centres, of monitoring benzodiazepine plasma concentrations. Furthermore tolerance to the antiepileptic action of benzodiazepines occurs with prolonged administration, requiring higher doses that are potentially dangerous. There may also be recurrence of seizures on drug withdrawal. Chlormethiazole, which is not licensed in the United States, is an easily administered agent. Infusions, however, can be complicated by hypotension, cardiac depression, and respiratory arrest and, like benzodiazepines, this drug shows a propensity for dangerous accumulation with prolonged administration.[36,37] Of other alternatives, paraldehyde is difficult to use as an intravenous preparation, decomposes in light, and in overdose there are potentially serious toxic side effects. It may be useful in premonitory stages per rectum, but in established status epilepticus where an intravenous infusion is indicated, its use is limited.[36] There have been uncontrolled studies of the use of intravenous sodium valproate at this stage at high doses of at least 15 mg/kg followed by an infusion of 1 mg/kg/h;[38] experience of sodium valproate in status epilepticus, however, remains limited. Lorazepam and lidocaine (lignocaine) are essentially short term therapies, and so should not be employed at this stage.

Stage of refractory status epilepticus (after 60/90 minutes)

If seizures continue for 60–90 minutes after the initiation of therapy, the stage of refractory status epilepticus is reached and full anaesthesia is required.[28] In many emergency situations (for example, postoperative status epilepticus, severe or complicated convulsive status epilepticus, patients already in intensive care), anaesthesia can and should be introduced earlier. Prognosis in patients reaching this stage is poorer, and the longer the status continues the higher is the mortality and morbidity.

Anaesthesia can be induced by barbiturate or non-barbiturate drugs. A number of anaesthetics have been administered, although few have been subjected to formal evaluation and all have drawbacks. The most commonly used anaesthetics are the intravenous barbiturate thiopentone, the intravenous non-barbiturate propofol, or continuous midazolam infusion. A non-randomised comparison of propofol and thiopentone was unable to detect any clinically significant differences between the drugs.[39] Other drugs in current use include the intravenous anaesthetic pentobarbitone (not available in the United Kingdom).

Patients require the full range of intensive care facilities, including EEG monitoring, and care should be shared between anaesthetist and neurologist. Experience with long term administration (hours or days) of the newer anaesthetic drugs is very limited. The modern anaesthetics have important pharmacokinetic advantages over the more traditional barbiturates, and are thus often chosen as first–line.

Once the patient has been free of seizures for 12–24 hours and provided that there are adequate plasma levels of concomitant antiepileptic medication, then the anaesthetic should be slowly tapered. If seizures recur, anaesthesia should be reinstituted immediately and maintained for a further 24 hours. A further attempt to taper therapy can then be made. In the occasional patient, anaesthesia is needed for days or weeks, and every time withdrawal of therapy is attempted seizures recur. Although the prognosis in these cases is generally poor, there is no alternative to prolonged anaesthesia and some patients do eventually make a good recovery.

Details of recommended drugs

Diazepam

Diazepam[31,33,34,40-42] has a time honoured place as a drug of first choice in premonitory or early stages of status epilepticus. Its pharmacology and clinical effects have been extensively studied in adults, children, and the newborn, and it has been shown to be highly effective in a wide range of status epilepticus types. Diazepam can be given by intravenous bolus injections or by the rectal route in the premonitory stage, and has a rapid onset of action. Sufficient cerebral levels are reached within one minute of a standard intravenous injection, and rectal administration produces peak levels at about 20 minutes. Diazepam has a redistribution half-life of approximately 20 minutes with a large volume of distribution of 1–2 L/kg, and an elimination half-life of 20–40 hours. The drug is thus rapidly redistributed, and has a relatively short duration of action after a single intravenous injection. After repeated dosing, as drug concentrations in the peripheral compartments increase, this redistribution does not occur. Thus repeated bolus injections produce higher peak levels which persist, carrying an attendant risk of sudden and unexpected CNS depression and cardiorespiratory collapse. Diazepam is metabolised by hepatic microsomal enzymes. Respiratory depression, hypotension, and sedation are the principal side effects. Sudden apnoea can occur, especially after repeated injections or if the injection is administered at too fast a rate.

Bolus intravenous doses of diazepam should be given in an undiluted form at a rate not exceeding 2–5 mg/min, using the Diazemuls formulation. Diazepam may be given rectally, either in its intravenous preparation infused from a syringe via a plastic catheter, or as the ready made, proprietary, rectal tube preparation Stesolid, which is a convenient and easy method. Diazepam suppositories should not be used, as absorption is too slow. The adult bolus intravenous or rectal dose in status epilepticus is 10–20 mg, and additional 10 mg doses can be given at 15 minute intervals, to a maximum of 40 mg. In children, the equivalent bolus dose is 0·2–0·3 mg/kg. A continuous infusion of benzodiazepine has also been used, but there is now little place for this mode of administration. The solution should be freshly prepared, and no drugs should be admixed. The usual intravenous formulation is as an emulsion (Diazemuls) in a 1 ml ampoule containing 5 mg/ml or as a solution in 2 ml ampoules containing 5 mg/ml. Stesolid is the usual rectal formulation – a 2·5 ml rectal tube containing 5 mg or 10 mg diazepam. The intravenous solution can also be instilled rectally.

Lorazepam

Lorazepam[34,35,40–49] has a lesser volume of distribution and is less lipid soluble than diazepam. It enters the brain more slowly, taking up to 30 minutes to reach peak levels. Its distribution half-life is much longer, two to three hours, and its elimination half-life is shorter, approximately 10–12 hours. These characteristics result in a slower onset of action, but a longer duration of action. Lorazepam is indicated in the early stage of status epilepticus only, where its lack of accumulation in lipid stores, its strong cerebral binding, and long duration of action due to its distribution half-life are very significant advantages over diazepam. The pharmacology and clinical effects of lorazepam have been well characterised in adults, in children, and in the newborn, and the drug has been the subject of large scale clinical trials. Lorazepam is remarkably effective in controlling seizures in the early stage of status epilepticus. Its main disadvantage is the rapid development of tolerance. Initial injections of lorazepam are effective for about 12 hours (longer than with diazepam), but repeated doses are much less effective, and the drug has no place as long term therapy. Lorazepam has sedative effects shared by all the benzodiazepine drugs used in status epilepticus, but sudden hypotension or respiratory collapse is less likely because of its relative lipid insolubility and the lack of accumulation after single bolus injections. Lorazepam is administered by intravenous bolus injection. As distribution is slow, the rate of injection is not critical. In adults, a bolus dose of 0·07 mg/kg (to a maximum of 4 mg) is given, and this can be repeated once after 20 minutes if no effect has been observed. In children under 10 years, bolus doses of 0·1 mg/kg are recommended. Long term infusion of lorazepam should not be used. It is usually available as a 1 ml ampoule containing 4 mg of lorazepam.

Midazolam

Midazolam[43–48] has the advantage over other benzodiazepines in that it is water soluble at a suitable pH; at physiological pH it becomes highly lipophilic, permitting rapid transfer across the blood–brain barrier. This has resulted in the possibility of midazolam usage by three other routes: intranasal, buccal, and intramuscular. Recently midazolam (10 mg in 2 ml) squirted around the buccal mucosa was as effective as rectal diazepam (10 mg) in acute seizures in children, and was easier to administer. By this route, the maximum concentration is reached by 30 minutes (although the pharmacodynamic response may be quicker), and the bioavailability is 75%. Intranasal midazolam has also been used successfully; a dose of 0·2 mg/kg intranasally results in a maximum serum concentration in 12 minutes with a bioavailability of 55%. Bioavailability after intramuscular injection is about 80–100%, and peak levels are reached after about 25 minutes although there is marked individual variation.

Midazolam has a very short distribution half-life of less than 5 minutes, and a very short elimination half-life of approximately 1·5 hours. Action is short lived, and there is a strong tendency to relapse following a single bolus injection. Its kinetic characteristics and its smaller volume of distribution make it the benzodiazepine of choice for use as an infusion, as it has less propensity to accumulate. Additionally, in contrast to other benzodiazepines, it is not dissolved in propylene glycol – a vehicle that has been associated with adverse cardiac effects. It is worth noting that in the intensive care setting, midazolam can have a greater half-life and volume of distribution due to hepatic impairment. Also the lipid solubility of the drug, and hence its cerebral action, is reduced as pH falls.

Midazolam exhibits the same toxic effects as other benzodiazepines, including sedation, hypotension, and cardiorespiratory depression. Respiratory arrest may occur occasionally even after intramuscular injection so careful monitoring is imperative.

Midazolam is given in premonitory status epilepticus intramuscularly, rectally, buccally, or intranasally at a dose of 5–10 mg (in children 0·15–0·3 mg/kg), which can be repeated once after 15 minutes or so. As an intravenous infusion on the intensive care unit, it should be given as a loading dose of approximately 0·15 mg/kg followed by an infusion of 0·05–0·4 mg/kg/h. Midazolam is available in 5 ml ampoules containing 2 mg/ml or 2 ml ampoules containing 5 mg/ml.

Phenobarbitone

Phenobarbitone[50–52] is a drug of choice for the treatment of established status epilepticus. It is highly effective, has a rapid onset of action, and prolonged anticonvulsant effects. It has stable and non-reactive physical properties, and convenient pharmacokinetics. Wide experience has been gained of its use in adults and in children, and few drugs are as well tried in the newborn. It has stronger anticonvulsant properties than most other barbiturates, and may be preferentially concentrated in metabolically active epileptic foci. As well as excellent anticonvulsant properties, it may also have cerebral-protective action. Acute tolerance to the antiepileptic effect is unusual, in contrast to the benzodiazepines and, once controlled, seizures do not tend to recur. Indeed, there is evidence to suggest that given with barbiturate anaesthesia, it can reduce the relapse rate with anaesthetic withdrawal. The main disadvantages of phenobarbitone are its potential to cause sedation, respiratory depression, and hypotension, although in practice these effects seem slight except at high levels or with rapidly rising levels. Its safety at even high doses is well established. The well known chronic side effects of phenobarbitone in long term therapy are of little relevance in the emergency situation of status epilepticus. The drug is eliminated slowly and, although this is of no importance on initial phenobarbitone loading, on prolonged therapy there is a danger of accumulation and blood level monitoring is essential. In the newborn period dosing is more difficult than in adults, as the pharmacokinetics change rapidly during the first weeks and months of life. The drug has a strong tendency to autoinduction. Phenobarbitone is a stable preparation, which does not easily decompose, and the drug is not absorbed by plastic. It should not be used in a solution containing other drugs (for example, phenytoin), as this may result in precipitation.

The usual recommended adult intravenous loading dose is 10 mg/kg (doses of up to 20 mg/kg have been used and recommended), given at a rate of 100 mg/min (that is, a total of about 700 mg in seven minutes). This should be followed by daily maintenance doses of 1–4 mg/kg. In neonates, initial phenobarbitone loading doses of between 12 and 20 mg/kg have been recommended to produce therapeutic levels, with subsequent supplementation of 3–4 mg/kg per day, to a maximum dose of 40 mg/kg. In older children, loading doses of between 5 and 20 mg/kg are recommended and maintenance doses of 1–4 mg/kg, although much higher doses have been safely given. After loading, maintenance doses can be given by the oral, intravenous, or intramuscular route. Phenobarbitone is usually presented in 1 ml ampoules containing 200 mg of phenobarbitone sodium.

Phenytoin and fosphenytoin

Phenytoin[33,50,53–56] is a drug of first choice in established status epilepticus. Its pharmacology and clinical effects are well documented, and there is extensive experience in status epilepticus in adults, children, and the newborn. It is a highly effective anticonvulsant, with the particular advantage of a long duration of action. It can also be continued as chronic therapy. Phenytoin causes relatively little respiratory or cerebral depression, although hypotension is more common. The initial infusion of phenytoin takes 20–30 minutes in an adult, and the onset of action is slow. It is therefore often administered in conjunction with a short acting drug with a rapid onset of action, such as diazepam. The notorious saturable pharmacokinetics of phenytoin cause less problems in the emergency setting than in chronic therapy, but careful serum level monitoring is essential. The usual phenytoin solutions have a pH of 12, and if added to bags containing large volumes of fluid at lower than physiological pH (for example, 5% glucose) precipitation may occur in the bag or tubing; use in a solution of 0·9% sodium chloride (normal saline) (5–20 mg/ml) is safer. There is also a serious risk of precipitation if other drugs are added to the infusion solution. Administration via a side arm, or directly using an infusion pump, is preferable. Due to the high pH, phenytoin can cause thrombophlebitis (particularly with extravasation), and it is poorly and erratically absorbed after intramuscular injection. Also, its vehicle, propylene glycol, can cause hypotension.

The rate of infusion of phenytoin solution should not exceed 50 mg/min, and it is prudent to reduce this to 20–30 mg/min in the elderly. The adult dose is 15–20 mg/kg, usually about 1000 mg, therefore taking at least 20 minutes to administer. Regrettably, a lower dose is too often given, which results in suboptimal cerebral levels. This is a common and potentially serious mistake. Phenytoin therapy can be continued after intravenous loading by oral or further intravenous daily dosages of 5–6 mg/kg, guided by blood level measurements. For older children, the dose of phenytoin is as for adults. For the newborn a dose of 15–20 mg/kg, injected at a rate not exceeding 1 mg/kg/min, should be given. Phenytoin is usually available as 5 ml ampoules containing phenytoin sodium 250 mg.

In order to overcome the problems associated with phenytoin's physiochemical properties, fosphenytoin (3-phosphoryloxymethyl phenytoin disodium), a water-soluble phenytoin pro-drug, was developed.[57,58] It has a pH closer to physiological values than phenytoin and so is less irritant to the infusion site. Furthermore it is, unlike phenytoin, not prepared in propylene glycol, which may improve tolerability. Fosphenytoin is inactive, but is metabolised to phenytoin with a half-life of 8–15 minutes. It is supplied in a ready mixed solution. The equimolar equivalent of 1·5 mg of fosphenytoin is 1 mg of phenytoin, and the drug is supplied in a ready mixed solution of 50 mg phenytoin equivalents (PE) per millilitre (75 mg/ml). This is to standardise the solution to that of parenteral phenytoin. It should be given intravenously at a maximum rate of 100 mg/min in order to achieve a similar serum concentration time profile to that obtained with the present protocol of giving intravenous phenytoin in status epilepticus. Although it is more expensive than phenytoin, these costs may be balanced by less phlebitis and ease of administration. As it is water soluble, it can also be given as an intramuscular injection, although its rate of absorption by this route is too slow to be of use in status epilepticus and this route of administration is not advised. ECG monitoring is mandatory while administering intravenous phenytoin or fosphenytoin.

Propofol

In recent times, there has been a vogue for the use of non-barbiturate anaesthesia in status epilepticus; of the currently available compounds, propofol[39,59–66] is probably the drug of choice. Published experience of its use in status epilepticus is limited. Propofol is a highly effective and non-toxic anaesthetic. In experimental models, it has anticonvulsant activity at subanaesthetic doses, probably via its action in potentiating GABA receptors.[67] Propofol also has neuroexcitatory effects possibly through subcortical disinhibition resulting in muscle rigidity, opisthotonos, and abnormal movements including myoclonus; these can be and have been mistaken for seizures. Seizures have, however, been reported with propofol withdrawal, and experimental evidence suggests that this is a rebound phenomenon similar to the GABA withdrawal syndrome. Propofol has also been reported at low doses to activate the electrocorticogram, but this is a property that it shares with other anaesthetics including the barbiturates.

Propofol is extremely soluble in lipid and has a high volume of distribution. It thus acts very rapidly in status epilepticus. Its effects are maintained while the infusion is continued, and recovery following discontinuation of the drug is also very quick – in marked contrast to thiopentone. Theoretically, there is a danger of accumulation on very long term therapy, but this has not been reported in practice. Propofol administration causes profound respiratory and cerebral depression (requiring the use of assisted respiration, the full panoply of intensive care, and monitoring), but only mild hypotension, and has few cardiovascular side effects. Long term administration causes marked lipaemia and may result in acidosis and rhabdomyolysis. It also has to be noted that there is a significant mortality reported in patients treated with status, although this is usually attributed to the status itself. However, some authorities consider that prolonged therapy may carry significant risks which are currently under-recognised. This is especially so in young children in whom it should not generally be recommended. The use of propofol in refractory status epilepticus is based upon several case reports and one comparative study. This study was non-randomised and compared propofol against pentobarbital anaesthesia in 16 patients. There was no significant difference detected between the two therapies in efficacy, time on ICU, or outcome. Neither therapy was universally effective, although a greater proportion had their seizures controlled with high dose barbiturate therapy. The dose of propofol necessary to control status epilepticus is greater than that when it is used as a sedative, but less than the dose required when it is used alone for total anaesthesia.

In status epilepticus, the following regimen can be used: an initial 1–2 mg/kg bolus dose is given, which can be repeated if seizures continue, succeeded by an infusion of 1–15 mg/kg/h guided by EEG. The dose should be gradually reduced, and the infusion tapered 12 hours after seizure activity is halted. Due to the risk of rebound seizures, the dose should be tapered at a rate of 5% of the maintenance infusion per hour (that is, over approximately 24 hours). In the elderly, doses should be lower. It is available as 20 ml ampoules containing 10 mg/ml as an emulsion.

Thiopentone

Thiopentone[52,68–71] is the compound traditionally used for barbiturate anaesthesia in status epilepticus, at least in Europe. It is an effective antiepileptic drug, and may have additional cerebral-protective effects. In the doses used in status epilepticus it has an anaesthetic action, and all patients require intubation and most artificial ventilation. The most troublesome side effect is persisting hypotension and many patients require pressor therapy. Thiopentone has saturable pharmacokinetics, and a strong tendency to accumulate. Thus if large doses are given, blood levels may remain very high for protracted periods, and days may pass before consciousness is recovered after drug administration is discontinued. Blood level monitoring, both of the thiopentone and its active metabolite pentobarbitone, is therefore essential on prolonged therapy. Other toxic effects on prolonged therapy include pancreatitis and hepatic disturbance, and thiopentone may cause acute hypersensitivity. It should be administered cautiously in the elderly, and in those with cardiac, hepatic, or renal disease. Although it has been in use since the 1960s in status epilepticus, formal clinical trials of its safety and effectiveness in both adults and children are few. A full range of intensive care facilities is required during thiopentone infusions. Central venous pressure should be monitored, and blood pressure monitored via an arterial line. Pulmonary artery pressure monitoring is sometimes advisable, and EEG or cerebral function monitoring is essential if thiopentone infusions are prolonged. A concomitant dopamine infusion is frequently needed to maintain blood pressure. Thiopentone can react with polyvinyl infusion bags or giving sets. The continuous infusion should be made up in 0·9% sodium chloride (normal saline). The intravenous solution has a pH of 10·2–11·2, is incompatible with a large number of acidic or oxidising substances, and no drugs should be added. The aqueous solution is unstable if exposed to air.

The regimen commonly used is as follows: thiopentone is given as a 100–250 mg bolus over 20 seconds, with further 50 mg boluses every two to three minutes until seizures are controlled, with intubation and artificial ventilation. The intravenous infusion is then continued at the minimum dose

---

Box 6.5 Common reasons for the failure of emergency drug therapy to control seizures in status epilepticus

Inadequate emergency antiepileptic drug therapy (especially the administration of drugs at too low a dose)

Failure to initiate maintenance antiepileptic drug therapy (seizures will recur as the effect of emergency drug treatment wears off)

Hypoxia, hypotension, cardiorespiratory failure, metabolic disturbance

Failure to identify the underlying cause

Failure to identify other medical complications (including hyperthermia, disseminated intravascular coagulation, hepatic failure)

Misdiagnosis (pseudostatus epilepticus is a common differential diagnosis that is often missed)

---

required to control clinical and electrographic seizure activity, usually between 3 and 5 mg/kg/h, and at thiopentone blood levels of about 40 mg/L. After 24 hours, the dose should be controlled by blood level monitoring. At this point, metabolism may be near saturation, and daily or twice daily blood level estimations should be made to ensure that levels do not rise excessively. The dose should be lowered if systolic blood pressure falls below 90 mm/Hg, or if vital functions are impaired. There is some evidence to suggest that barbiturate anaesthesia is more successful in those who have been loaded with phenobarbitone. Thiopentone should be continued for no less than 12 hours after seizure activity has ceased, and then slowly discontinued. The usual preparation is as a 2·5 g vial with 100 ml of diluent to produce a 2·5% solution.

Failure of antiepileptic treatment

The antiepileptic drugs used in status epilepticus are highly effective. If seizures continue despite emergency therapy, it is important to reassess the clinical circumstances, as there are often complicating remediable factors influencing the response to treatment.[72] The most common of these are listed in Box 6.5.

Management of tonic-clonic status epilepticus

- The annual incidence of tonic-clonic status is about 18–28 cases per 100 000 persons. It occurs most frequently in children, the mentally handicapped, and in those with structural cerebral disorders. It can develop de novo usually due to an acute cerebral insult, or in patients with established epilepsy where drug withdrawal is often the immediate cause. The mortality rate is about 20% with most patients dying of the underlying condition rather than the status itself.

- Experimental work suggests that compensatory physiological mechanisms protect homoeostasis for the first 30–60 minutes of continuing seizures. If seizures persist for longer periods, however, a series of physiological changes occur, resulting in the breakdown of cerebral autoregulation and a fall in cerebral blood flow. The failure to meet the high metabolic demands of cerebral tissue can result in permanent cerebral damage.

- Other complications include hyperpyrexia, massive autonomic activation, pulmonary hypertension and oedema, intracranial hypertension, cardiac arrhythmia and failure, hypoglycaemia, acidosis, rhabdomyolysis, disseminated intravascular coagulation, and cardiac, respiratory, renal, or hepatic failure.

- General treatment measures should proceed in stages: (1) cardiorespiratory function should be secured; (2) regular monitoring and emergency drug therapy should be commenced, and investigations initiated; (3) aetiology should be established, and hypotension and medical complications treated. If seizures are continuing, the patient should be transferred to intensive care, and seizure, EEG, and sometimes intracranial pressure monitoring applied.

- A suggested regimen for emergency antiepileptic drug therapy is as follows: (1) *Premonitory stage (pre hospital)*: diazepam 0·2–0·3 mg/kg (usual adult dose 10–20 mg) can be given by rectal or intravenous administration, or midazolam by buccal (10 mg) or intranasal (0·2 mg/kg) administration. (2) *Early status*: lorazepam 0·07 mg/kg (usual adult dose 4 mg), which can be repeated after 10 minutes. (3) *Established status*: phenobarbitone 10 mg/kg given intravenously at an infusion rate of 100 mg/min (usual adult dose is 700 mg given over seven minutes), or phenytoin at a dose of 15–18 mg/kg at a rate of 50 mg/min (usual adult dose is 1000 mg given over 20 min) or fosphenytoin at a dose of 15–20 mg phenytoin equivalents/kg at a rate of 150 mg phenytoin equivalents/min. (4) *Refractory status*: general anaesthesia with either thiopentone initially with a 100–250 mg bolus injection, followed by further 50 mg boluses, and then a continuous infusion (usual dose 3–5 mg/kg/h), or propofol initially with a 2 mg/kg bolus dose, repeated if necessary, and then a continuous infusion of up to 15 mg/kg/h or midazolam initially with a 0·15 mg/kg bolus followed by an infusion of 0·05–0·4 mg/kg/h. Maintenance antiepileptic drug therapy should be given concurrently.

References

1 Shorvon SD. *Status epilepticus: its clinical features and treatment in children and adults*. Cambridge: Cambridge University Press, 1994.
2 DeLorenzo RJ, Garnett LK, Towne AR, *et al*. Comparison of status epilepticus with prolonged seizure episodes lasting from 10 to 29 minutes. *Epilepsia* 1999;**40**:164–9.
3 Lowenstein DH, Bleck T, Macdonald RL. It's time to revise the definition of status epilepticus. *Epilepsia* 1999;**40**:120–2.
4 Coeytaux A, Jallon P, Galobardes B, Morabia A. Incidence of status epilepticus in French-speaking Switzerland: (EPISTAR). *Neurology* 2000;**55**:693–7.
5 DeLorenzo RJ, Hauser WA, Towne AR, *et al*. A prospective, population-based epidemiologic study of status epilepticus in Richmond, Virginia. *Neurology* 1996;**46**:1029–35.
6 Hesdorffer DC, Logroscino G, Cascino G, Annegers JF, Hauser WA. Incidence of status epilepticus in Rochester, Minnesota, 1965–1984. *Neurology* 1998;**50**:735–41.
7 Knake S, Rosenow F, Vescovi M *et al*. Incidence of status epilepticus in adults in Germany: a prospective, population-based study. *Epilepsia* 2001;**42**:714–18.
8 Aicardi J, Chevrie JJ. Convulsive status epilepticus in infants and children. A study of 239 cases. *Epilepsia* 1970;**11**:187–97.
9 Pilke A, Partinen M, Kovanen J. Status epilepticus and alcohol abuse: an analysis of 82 status epilepticus admissions. *Acta Neurol Scand* 1984; **70**:443–50.
10 Logroscino G, Hesdorffer DC, Cascino G, Annegers JF, Hauser WA. Short-term mortality after a first episode of status epilepticus. *Epilepsia* 1997; **38**:1344–9.
11 Treiman DM, Walton NY, Kendrick C. A progressive sequence of electroencephalographic changes during generalized convulsive status epilepticus. *Epilepsy Res* 1990;**5**:49–60.
12 Garzon E, Fernandes RMF, Sakamoto AC. Serial EEG during human status epilepticus. Evidence for PLED as an ictal pattern. *Neurology* 2001;**57**: 1175–83.
13 Lothman E. The biochemical basis and pathophysiology of status epilepticus. *Neurology* 1990;**40**:13–23.
14 Simon RP. Physiologic consequences of status epilepticus. *Epilepsia* 1985;**26**(suppl 1):S58–66.
15 Brown JK, Hussain IH. Status epilepticus. I: Pathogenesis. *Dev Med Child Neurol* 1991;**33**:3–17.
16 Aminoff MJ, Simon RP. Status epilepticus. Causes, clinical features and consequences in 98 patients. *Am J Med* 1980;**69**:657–66.
17 Meldrum BS. Metabolic factors during prolonged seizures and their relation to nerve cell death. *Adv Neurol* 1983;**34**:261–75.
18 Siesjo BK, Ingvar M, Folbergrova J, Chapman AG. Local cerebral circulation and metabolism in bicuculline-induced status epilepticus: relevance for development of cell damage. *Adv Neurol* 1983;**34**: 217–30.
19 Benowitz NL, Simon RP, Copeland JR. Status epilepticus: divergence of sympathetic activity and cardiovascular response. *Ann Neurol* 1986;**19**: 197–9.
20 Young RS, Fripp RR, Yagel SK, Werner JC, McGrath G, Schuler HG. Cardiac dysfunction during status epilepticus in the neonatal pig. *Ann Neurol* 1985;**18**:291–7.

21 Meldrum B. Excitotoxicity and epileptic brain damage. *Epilepsy Res* 1991;**10**:55–61.
22 Olney JW, Collins RC, Sloviter RS. Excitotoxic mechanisms of epileptic brain damage. *Adv Neurol* 1986;**44**:857–77.
23 Sloviter RS. "Epileptic" brain damage in rats induced by sustained electrical stimulation of the perforant path, I. Acute electrophysiological and light microscopic studies. *Brain Res Bull* 1983;**10**:675–97.
24 Meldrum BS, Brierley JB. Prolonged epileptic seizures in primates. Ischaemic cell change and its relation to ictal physiological events. *Arch Neurol* 1973;**28**:10–17.
25 Nevander G, Ingvar M, Auer R, Siesjo BK. Status epilepticus in well-oxygenated rats causes neuronal necrosis. *Ann Neurol* 1985;**18**:281–90.
26 Kapur J, Macdonald RL. Rapid seizure-induced reduction of benzodiazepine and Zn^{2+} sensitivity of hippocampal dentate granule cell GABAA receptors. *J Neurosci* 1997;**17**:7532–40.
27 Walker MC, Tong X, Brown S, Shorvon SD, Patsalos PN. Comparison of single- and repeated-dose pharmacokinetics of diazepam. *Epilepsia* 1998;**39**:283–9.
28 Walker MC, Smith SJ, Shorvon SD. The intensive care treatment of convulsive status epilepticus in the UK. Results of a national survey and recommendations. *Anaesthesia* 1995;**50**:130–5.
29 Alldredge BK, Lowenstein DH. Status epilepticus related to alcohol abuse. *Epilepsia* 1993;**34**:1033–7.
30 van-Paesschen W, Bodian C, Maker H. Metabolic abnormalities and new-onset seizures in human immunodeficiency virus-seropositive patients. *Epilepsia* 1995;**36**:146–50.
31 Dreifuss FE, Rosman NP, Cloyd JC, *et al*. A comparison of rectal diazepam gel and placebo for acute repetitive seizures. *N Engl J Med* 1998;**338**: 1869–75.
32 Scott RC, Besag FM, Neville BG. Buccal midazolam and rectal diazepam for treatment of prolonged seizures in childhood and adolescence: a randomised trial. *Lancet* 1999;**353**:623–6.
33 Alldredge BK, Gelb AM, Isaacs SM, *et al*. A comparison of lorazepam, diazepam, and placebo for the treatment of out-of-hospital status epilepticus. *N Engl J Med* 2001;**345**:631–7.
34 Leppik IE, Derivan AT, Homan RW, Walker J, Ramsay RE, Patrick B. Double-blind study of lorazepam and diazepam in status epilepticus. *JAMA* 1983;**249**:1452–4.
35 Treiman DM, Meyers PD, Walton NY, *et al*. A comparison of four treatments for generalized convulsive status epilepticus. Veterans Affairs Status Epilepticus Cooperative Study Group. *N Engl J Med* 1998;**339**: 792–8.
36 Browne TR. Paraldehyde, chlormethiazole, and lidocaine for treatment of status epilepticus. *Adv Neurol* 1983;**34**:509–17.
37 Robson DJ, Blow C, Gaines P, Flanagan RJ, Henry JA. Accumulation of chlormethiazole during intravenous infusion. *Intensive Care Med* 1984;**10**: 315–16.
38 Giroud M, Gras D, Escousse A, Dumas R, Venaud G. Use of injectable valproic acid in status epilepticus – a pilot study. *Drug Invest* 1993;**5**: 154–9.
39 Stecker MM, Kramer TH, Raps EC, O'Meeghan R, Dulaney E, Skaar DJ. Treatment of refractory status epilepticus with propofol: clinical and pharmacokinetic findings. *Epilepsia* 1998;**39**:18–26.
40 Treiman DM. Pharmacokinetics and clinical use of benzodiazepines in the management of status epilepticus. *Epilepsia* 1989;**30**(suppl 2):S4–10.

41 Schmidt D. Diazepam. In: Levy RH, Mattson RH, Meldrum BS, eds. *Antiepileptic drugs.* New York: Raven Press, 1995;705–24.

42 Remy C, Jourdil N, Villemain D, Favel P, Genton P. Intrarectal diazepam in epileptic adults. *Epilepsia* 1992;**33**:353–8.

43 Bell DM, Richards G, Dhillon S, *et al.* A comparative pharmacokinetic study of intravenous and intramuscular midazolam in patients with epilepsy. *Epilepsy Res* 1991;**10**:183–90.

44 Kumar A, Bleck TP. Intravenous midazolam for the treatment of refractory status epilepticus. *Crit Care Med* 1992;**20**:483–8.

45 Rivera R, Segnini M, Baltodano A, Perez V. Midazolam in the treatment of status epilepticus in children. *Crit Care Med* 1993;**21**:991–4.

46 Parent JM, Lowenstein DH. Treatment of refractory generalized status epilepticus with continuous infusion of midazolam. *Neurology* 1994;**44**:1837–40.

47 Scott RC, Besag FM, Boyd SG, Berry D, Neville BG. Buccal absorption of midazolam: pharmacokinetics and EEG pharmacodynamics. *Epilepsia* 1998;**39**:290–4.

48 Rey E, Delaunay L, Pons G, *et al.* Pharmacokinetics of midazolam in children: comparative study of intranasal and intravenous administration. *Eur J Clin Pharmacol* 1991;**41**:355–7.

49 Crawford TO, Mitchell WG, Snodgrass SR. Lorazepam in childhood status epilepticus and serial seizures: effectiveness and tachyphylaxis. *Neurology* 1987;**37**:190–5.

50 Shaner DM, McCurdy SA, Herring MO, Gabor AJ. Treatment of status epilepticus: a prospective comparison of diazepam and phenytoin versus phenobarbital and optional phenytoin. *Neurology* 1988;**38**:202–7.

51 Crawford TO, Mitchell WG, Fishman LS, Snodgrass SR. Very-high-dose phenobarbital for refractory status epilepticus in children. *Neurology* 1988;**38**:1035–40.

52 Krishnamurthy KB, Drislane FW. Relapse and survival after barbiturate anesthetic treatment of refractory status epilepticus. *Epilepsia* 1996;**37**:863–7.

53 Wilder BJ, Ramsay RE, Willmore LJ, Feussner GF, Perchalski RJ, Shumate JBJ. Efficacy of intravenous phenytoin in the treatment of status epilepticus: kinetics of central nervous system penetration. *Ann Neurol* 1977;**1**:511–18.

54 Cranford RE, Leppik IE, Patrick B, Anderson CB, Kostick B. Intravenous phenytoin in acute treatment of seizures. *Neurology* 1979;**29**:1474–9.

55 Cloyd JC, Gumnit RJ, McLain-LWJ. Status epilepticus. The role of intravenous phenytoin. *JAMA* 1980;**244**:1479–81.

56 Leppik IE, Patrick BK, Cranford RE. Treatment of acute seizures and status epilepticus with intravenous phenytoin. *Adv Neurol* 1983;**34**:447–51.

57 Ramsay RE, DeToledo J. Intravenous administration of fosphenytoin: options for the management of seizures. *Neurology* 1996;**46**:S17–19.

58 Browne TR. Fosphenytoin (Cerebyx). *Clin Neuropharmacol* 1997;**20**:1–12.

59 Wood PR, Browne GP, Pugh S. Propofol infusion for the treatment of status epilepticus. *Lancet* 1988;**i**:480–1.

60 Mackenzie SJ, Kapadia F, Grant IS. Propofol infusion for control of status epilepticus. *Anaesthesia* 1990;**45**:1043–5.

61 De-Riu PL, Petruzzi V, Testa C, *et al.* Propofol anticonvulsant activity in experimental epileptic status. *Br J Anaesth* 1992;**69**:177–81.

62 Rasmussen PA, Yang Y, Rutecki PA. Propofol inhibits epileptiform activity in rat hippocampal slices. *Epilepsy Res* 1996;**25**:169–75.

63 Brown LA, Levin GM. Role of propofol in refractory status epilepticus. *Ann Pharmacother* 1998;**32**:1053–9.

64   Hewitt PB, Chu DLK, Polkey CE, Binnie CD. Effect of propofol on the electrocorticogram in epileptic patients undergoing cortical resection. *Br J Anaesth* 1999;**82**:199–202.
65   Sneyd JR. Propofol and epilepsy. *Br J Anaesth* 1999;**82**:168–9.
66   Hanna JP, Ramundo ML. Rhabdomyolysis and hypoxia associated with prolonged propofol infusion in children. *Neurology* 1998;**50**:301–3.
67   Holtkamp M, Tong X, Walker MC. Propofol in subanesthetic doses terminates status epilepticus in a rodent model. *Ann Neurol* 2001;**49**: 260–3.
68   Young GB, Blume WT, Bolton CF, Warren KG. Anesthetic barbiturates in refractory status epilepticus. *Can J Neurol Sci* 1980;**7**:291–2.
69   Partinen M, Kovanen J, Nilsson E. Status epilepticus treated by barbiturate anaesthesia with continuous monitoring of cerebral function. *Br Med J Clin Res Ed* 1981;**282**:520–1.
70   Orlowski JP, Erenberg G, Lueders H, Cruse RP. Hypothermia and barbiturate coma for refractory status epilepticus. *Crit Care Med* 1984; **12**:367–72.
71   Lowenstein DH, Aminoff MJ, Simon RP. Barbiturate anesthesia in the treatment of status epilepticus: clinical experience with 14 patients. *Neurology* 1988;**38**:395–400.
72   Walker MC, Howard RS, Smith SJ, Miller DH, Shorvon SD, Hirsch NP. Diagnosis and treatment of status epilepticus on a neurological intensive care unit. *Q J Med* 1996;**89**:913–20.

7: Raised intracranial pressure

JD PICKARD, M CZOSNYKA, LA STEINER

Epidemiology

Raised intracranial pressure is the final common pathway for many intracranial problems (Box 7.1) and has a profound influence on outcome. For example, of the 300 000–500 000 patients with head injury seen in United Kingdom accident and emergency departments per annum, 20% are admitted, of whom 10% are in coma (2% of all attenders). Over 50% of these have an intracranial pressure greater than 20 mmHg.[1,2] A total of 80% of patients with fatal head injuries (4% of all patients with head injuries admitted) show evidence of a significant increase in intracranial pressure at necropsy. Some 35% of those with severe head injuries die and 18% are left severely disabled at enormous financial and emotional cost to the family and community. Similarly, 20 per 100 000 per year are admitted with intracerebral haematoma and 10–12 per 100 000 per annum with subarachnoid haemorrhage. The average regional neurosurgical unit serving a population of two million will manage 200 patients per annum with brain tumours, some 15 patients with a cerebral abscess, and 100 patients with hydrocephalus.[3] In comatose children the incidence of raised intracranial pressure was 53% of those with head injuries, 23% with anoxic-ischaemic damage, 66% with meningitis, 57% with encephalitis, 100% with mass lesions, and 80% with hydrocephalus.[4] There is a considerable risk in all such patients of secondary brain damage with long term severe disability if raised intracranial pressure is not recognised and managed appropriately.

Box 7.1 Some common causes of raised intracranial pressure

Head injury
  Intracranial haematoma (extradural, subdural, and intracerebral)
  Diffuse brain swelling
  Contusion

Cerebrovascular
  Subarachnoid haemorrhage
  Intracerebral haematoma
  Cerebral venous thrombosis
  Major cerebral infarct
  Hypertensive encephalopathy (malignant hypertension, eclampsia)

Hydrocephalus
  Congenital or acquired
  Obstructive or communicating

Craniocerebral disproportion
  Brain "tumour" (cysts; benign or malignant tumours)
  Secondary hydrocephalus
  Mass effect
  Oedema

"Benign" intracranial hypertension (pseudotumor cerebri; idiopathic intracranial hypertension)

CNS infection
  Meningitis
  Encephalitis
  Abscess
  Cerebral malaria
  Secondary hydrocephalus

Metabolic encephalopathy
  Hypoxic-ischaemic
  Reye's syndrome, etc.
  Lead encephalopathy
  Hepatic coma
  Renal failure
  Diabetic ketoacidosis
  Burns
  Near drowning
  Hyponatraemia

Status epilepticus

Adapted from Minns,[4] Marmarou et al.,[5] Langfitt,[7] and Czosnyka et al.[10]

Pathophysiology

Resting intracranial pressure represents that equilibrium pressure at which cerebrospinal fluid (CSF) production and absorption are in balance and is associated with an equivalent equilibrium volume of CSF. CSF is actively secreted by the choroid plexus at about 0·35 ml/min and production remains constant provided cerebral perfusion pressure is adequate. CSF absorption is a passive process through the arachnoid granulations and increases with rising CSF pressure:

CSF pressure = Resistance to CSF outflow × CSF outflow rate + sagittal sinus pressure

According to the above formula (known as the Davson's equation), the mean intracranial pressure (ICP) explained solely by CSF circulation, is proportional to the resistance to CSF outflow, CSF production rate, and sagittal sinus pressure. Marmarou et al.[5] proposed a modification to this formula, stating that average ICP can be expressed by two components: CSF circulatory and vasogenic. Thus, the Davson formula can be rewritten as:

$$ICP = ICP_{CSF\ circulation} + ICP_{Vasogenic} = R_{CSF} \times I_{formation} + P_{SS} + ICP_{vasogenic}$$

where R_{CSF} is the resistance to CSF outflow and P_{ss} is the sagittal sinus pressure.

It is difficult to understand why, under steady conditions, a vascular bed which is anatomically separated from the CSF compartment may modify mean intracranial pressure. The hypothesis has been proposed recently[6] that continuous pulsation of arterial blood is transformed by both non-linear components of CSF pressure–volume compensation (exponential pressure–volume curve) and regulation of CBF (autoregulation) to appear as the additional term "$ICP_{vasogenic}$" to complete Davson's formula. Its contribution to total ICP can be as large as 60% in pathological circumstances.

The "four-lump" concept describes most simply the causes of raised intracranial pressure: the mass, CSF accumulation, vascular congestion, and cerebral oedema (Box 7.2).[7–9]

Box 7.2 Mechanisms of raised intracranial pressure

A: Mass lesions
   Haematoma, abscess, tumour

B: CSF accumulation
   Hydrocephalus (obstructive and communicating), including contralateral ventricular dilatation from supratentorial brain shift

C: Cerebral oedema
   Increase in brain volume as a result of increased water content.

   1. Vasogenic – vessel damage (tumour, abscess, contusion)
   2. Cytotoxic – cell membrane pump failure (hypoxaemia, ischaemia, toxins)
   3. Hydrostatic – high vascular transmural pressure (loss of autoregulation; post intracranial decompression)
   4. Hypoosmolar – hyponatremia
   5. Interstitial – high CSF pressure (hydrocephalus)

D: Vascular (congestive) brain swelling
   Increased cerebral blood volume
   Arterial vasodilatation (active, passive)
   Venous congestion/obstruction

The description of a patient with raised ICP as having cerebral congestion, vasogenic oedema, etc. can only be a working approximation, albeit useful, until our rather crude methods of assessment are refined. In adults the normal ICP under resting conditions is between 0 and 10 mmHg, with 15 mmHg being the upper limit of normal. Active treatment is normally instituted if ICP exceeds 25 mmHg for more than five minutes, although a treatment threshold of 15–20 mmHg has been suggested to improve outcome.[10] In the very young, the upper limit of normal ICP is up to 5 mmHg.[4,11] Small increases in mass may be compensated for by reduction in CSF volume and cerebral blood volume but, once such mechanisms are exhausted, ICP rises with increasing pulse pressure and with the appearance of spontaneous waves (plateau and B waves).[12] There is an exponential relationship between increase in volume of an intracranial mass and the increase in ICP, at least within the clinically significant range. This relationship is also helpful in understanding the most specific fluctuating component of ICP: the pulse amplitude (Figure 7.1a). It is derived from pulsation of arterial blood pressure but the change of its shape can be considerable. Classically, the pulse waveform of ICP can be depicted using the pressure–volume curve with the pulsating changes in cerebral blood volume drawn along the x (volume) axis[13] (Figure 7.1b). The curve has three major zones:[14] in the initial range ICP changes proportionally to the change of intracerebral volume. This is a zone of good compensatory reserve. Then, ICP starts to increase exponentially when intracerebral volume expands further. This is a zone of poor compensatory reserve and can be seen in clinical practice most often whenever there is any difficulty in managing a cerebrospinal volume-evolving process (head injury, poor grade subarachnoid haemorrhage, acute hydrocephalus, etc.). Finally, at very high ICP, when a decrease in cerebral perfusion pressure is too deep to secure any further arterial dilatation (that is, vessels are maximally dilated), the pressure–volume curve bends to the right (Figure 7.1b). Entering this zone represents the transition of the cerebrovascular bed from the state of active dilatation to passive collapse. When the transmural pressure further decreases, the additional compensatory reserve is gained at the expense of reduction of arterial blood volume and derangement of the autoregulatory cerebrovascular response.

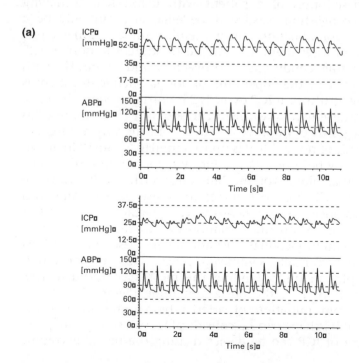

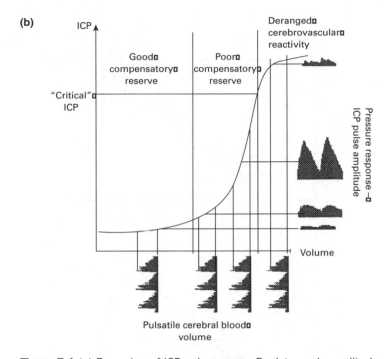

Figure 7.1 (a) Examples of ICP pulse waves. Peak-to-peak amplitude increases with increasing mean ICP (upper panel). Three distinctive "peaks" can be sometimes recorded (lower panel). (b) In a simple model, pulse amplitude of ICP (expressed along the y-axis on the right side of the panel) results from pulsatile changes in cerebral blood volume (expressed along the x-axis) transformed by the pressure–volume curve. This curve has three zones: a flat zone, expressing good compensatory reserve, an exponential zone, depicting poor compensatory reserve, and a flat zone again, seen at very high ICP (above the "critical" ICP) depicting derangement of normal cerebrovascular responses. The pulse amplitude of ICP is low and does not depend on mean ICP in the first zone. The pulse amplitude increases linearly with mean ICP in the zone of poor compensatory reserve. In the third zone, the pulse amplitude starts to decrease with rising ICP.

Adapted from Miller et al.[2] and Bingham et al.[21]; based on data from Lofgren et al.[14] and Avezaat et al.[30]

Pulse amplitude of ICP does not change with ICP in the first zone, then grows linearly with ICP in the second zone. In the third zone it starts to decrease with a further increase in ICP (Figure 7.2).

When monitored continuously, mean ICP presents a number of stereotypic patterns (Figure 7.3). The first eight

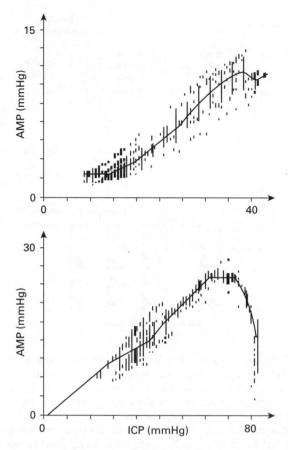

Figure 7.2 Relationship between mean intracranial pressure and amplitude of the intracranial pressure waveform in two patients. In the lower trace, there is an upper breakpoint in this relationship when cerebral perfusion pressure (mean arterial pressure – intracranial pressure) is less than 30 mmHg

panels (a–h) are representative for acute cases, such as head injury. Long term monitoring in other, non-acute cases, such as chronic hydrocephalus, produces specific but usually different patterns (Figure 7.3i,j):

1. Low and stable ICP (below 20 mmHg) – this pattern is specific for uncomplicated patients following head injury or during the first hours after trauma before ICP increases further (Figure 7.3a).

2. High and stable ICP (above 20 mmHg) – the most common picture following head injury (Figure 7.3b).
3. Vasogenic waves — B waves (Figure 7.3c), plateau waves (Figure 7.3d), or waves related to changes in arterial pressure and hyperaemic events (Figure 7.3e–g).
4. Refractory intracranial hypertension (Figure 7.3h) which usually leads to the death of the patient unless radical measures are taken (for example, surgical decompression).
5. Overnight recording of ICP in patients suffering from hydrocephalus with cyclically increased activity of B waves (Figure 7.3i) and benign intracranial hypertension (Figure 7.3j).

Spontaneous waves of intracranial pressure are usually associated with cerebrovascular dilatation. Cerebral blood volume increases during plateau waves (intracranial pressure > 50 mmHg for more than five minutes) and may be the result in some cases of inappropriate autoregulatory vasodilatation, described by Rosner and Becker[15] as the so-called vasodilatatory cascade. An increase in cerebral blood volume causes an increase in ICP, a decrease in cerebral perfusion pressure, leading to vasodilatation, and a further increase in cerebral blood volume, etc., until the system reaches the state of maximal vasodilatation. Plateau waves are observed in patients with preserved cerebral autoregulation but reduced pressure volume compensatory reserve. Very high increases in ICP when associated with a reduction in cerebral perfusion pressure may dramatically decrease cerebral blood flow (Figure 7.4, p 200).[16]

Transcranial Doppler examinations reveal that middle cerebral artery flow velocity increases at the same rate as B waves (0·5–2/min) of intracranial pressure (Figure 7.5, p 201).[17]

Gradients of intracranial pressure may develop when herniation occurs – transtentorial, subfalcine, and foramen magnum. Blockage to the free flow of CSF between intracranial compartments leads to a much greater and more rapid rise in intracranial pressure in the compartment harbouring the primary pathology and hence to the final common sequence of transtentorial and foramen magnum coning. When intracranial pressure equals arterial blood pressure, angiographic pseudo-occlusion occurs and reverberation, systolic spikes, or no flow may be seen on transcranial Doppler sonography (Figure 7.6, p 201). Patients will often satisfy the formal clinical criteria for

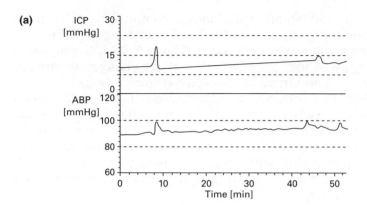

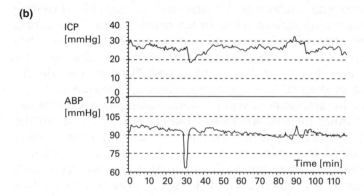

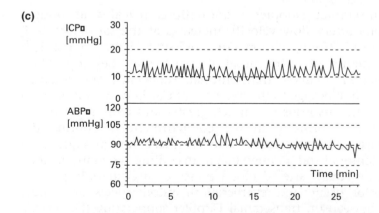

(d)

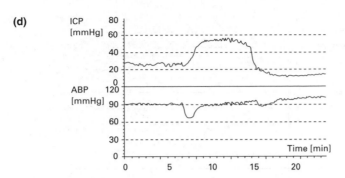

(e)

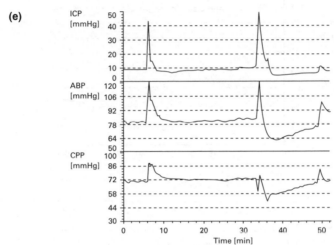

(f)

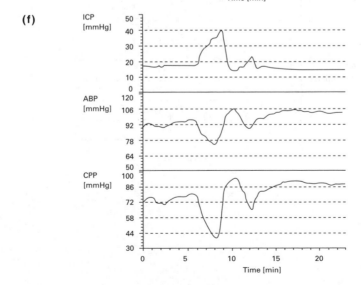

(g)

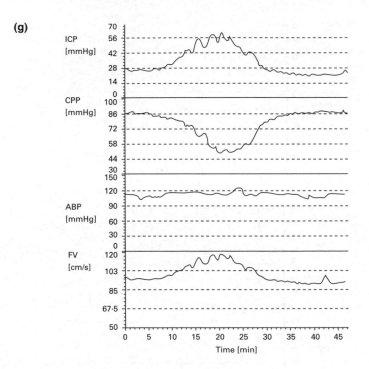

(h)

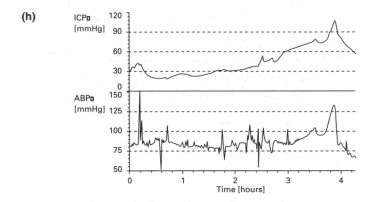

(i)

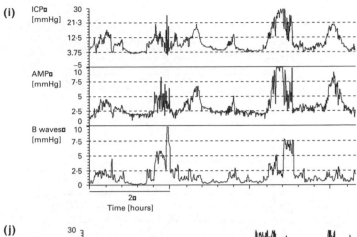

(j)

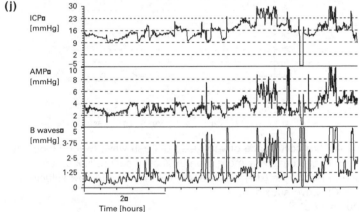

Figure 7.3 Typical recordings of intracranial pressure.

(a) Low and stable ICP.

(b) Increased and stable ICP after head injury.

(c) B waves (after head trauma).

(d) Plateau wave after head injury.

(e–g) Waves of ICP different from plateau commonly recorded after head injury:

(e) increases in ICP due to rapid increases in arterial blood pressure;

(f) changes in ICP caused by constriction/dilatation of vascular bed, due to variation in arterial pressure;

(g) longer increase in ICP associated with an increase in blood flow (monitored using TCD- FV).

(h) Intracranial hypertension – refractory (after head injury).

(i) Overnight recording in normal pressure hydrocephalus. Baseline pressure is specifically low with increased vasogenic dynamics observed as periods of increasing pulse amplitude (AMP) and magnitude of B waves.

(j) Overnight monitoring in benign intracranial hypertension. Baseline pressure is elevated with moderate dynamics and gradually increasing magnitude of B waves

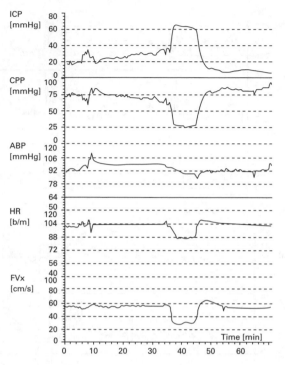

Figure 7.4 Rare occurrence of very deep plateau wave, when blood flow velocity (FVx) decreased by more than 60% of baseline. Notice the decrease in heart rate (HR) and hyperaemic increase in flow velocity after the ICP wave subsided.
From Obrist *et al.*[20]

brain stem death, for which transcranial Doppler examination is not a substitute.[18,19] When ICP rises uncontrollably, it is often called "refractory intracranial hypertension". Mean ICP may increase to well above 80 mmHg, probably due to rapid brain swelling over a period of a few hours. Pulse amplitude of ICP is commonly secondarily reduced with activation of a Cushing response and a gradual rise of mean arterial pressure. The moment of brain stem herniation is commonly marked by a rapid decrease in mean arterial pressure, a rise in a heart rate, and a terminal decrease in cerebral perfusion pressure to negative values (Figure 7.7).

Cerebral perfusion pressure (CPP) is commonly defined as mean arterial blood pressure minus mean intracranial

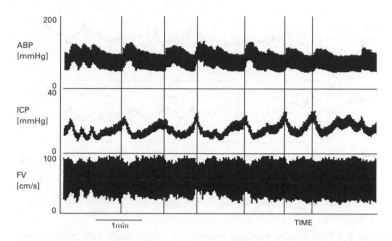

Figure 7.5 B waves of intracranial pressure in a head-injured patient and their relationship to similar variations in middle cerebral artery flow velocity compared with fluctuations in arterial blood pressure (ABP)

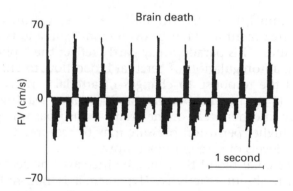

Figure 7.6 Reversal of middle cerebral artery flow velocity (FV) in a patient who fulfils the criteria for brain stem death

pressure. Mean intracranial pressure closely approximates to mean cerebral venous pressure. The lower limit of CPP which will permit autoregulation, when intracranial pressure is raised, is about 40 mmHg. There is a paradox, however: the level of cerebral perfusion pressure below which outcome after severe head injury and associated parameters deteriorate is of the order of 60–65 mmHg (mean arterial pressure < 80 mmHg;

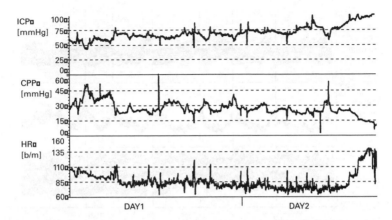

Figure 7.7 Example of two-day monitoring of a patient who died in the course of refractory intracranial hypertension on day 2. This was marked by a final decrease in CPP below 30 mmHg and an increase in heart rate (HR)

ICP >20 mmHg). Conventionally any elevation of ICP requires treatment if CPP is below 60 mmHg in adults for over five minutes. This paradox may partly reflect the "split brain" problem: autoregulation of cerebral blood flow to changes in CPP and the response to changes in arterial carbon dioxide tension ($Pa\text{CO}_2$) may be impaired focally, leaving intact reactivity in other areas of the brain. If vasospasm is present, an even higher perfusion pressure may be required to provide adequate levels of cerebral blood flow.

Total cerebral blood flow may be increased or decreased in areas with absent reactivity. Hyperaemia is non-nutritional "luxury perfusion" where cerebral blood flow is in excess of the brain's metabolic requirements[20] and accompanied by early filling of veins on angiography and "red veins" at operation. Cerebral vasodilators such as carbon dioxide will dilate "normal" arterioles, increase intracranial pressure, and may run the risk of reducing flow to damaged areas of brain (intracerebral "steal"). Inverse "steal" is one reason for the treatment of raised intracranial pressure by hyperventilation: an acute reduction of $Pa\text{CO}_2$ vasoconstricts normal cerebral arterioles, thereby directing blood to focally abnormal areas.

Normally, cerebral blood flow is coupled to cerebral oxidative metabolism via multiple mechanisms involving local concentrations of hydrogen ions, potassium, and adenosine, for example. Status epilepticus leads to gross cerebral vasodilatation and intracranial hypertension as a result of greatly increased cerebral metabolism and local release of endogenous vasodilator agents. Depression of cerebral energy metabolism by anaesthesia and hypothermia may reduce cerebral blood flow and intracranial pressure where there is a large area of the brain with reasonable electrical activity[21] and where normal flow–metabolism coupling mechanisms are intact as indicated by a reasonable cerebral blood flow carbon dioxide reactivity.[22]

There is a complex interaction between the properties of the CSF and the cerebral circulations that may be modelled (Figure 7.8).[23–25] The relative contributions of abnormalities of CSF absorption and cerebral blood volume may be approximated by calculating the proportion of CSF pressure attributable to CSF outflow resistance and venous pressure from Davson's equation. Phenomena such as the interaction of autoregulation to changing CPP with Pa_{CO_2} may be quantified.[26]

Monitoring techniques

Clinical features

In the non-trauma patient, there may or may not be a clear history of novel headache, vomiting, and visual disturbance suggestive of papilloedema (blurring of vision, obscuration) or a sixth cranial nerve palsy (lateral diplopia). The absence of papilloedema does not exclude raised ICP in patients with acute or chronic problems: disc swelling was found in only 4% of head-injured patients, 50% of whom had raised ICP on monitoring.[8] Even in the twenty-first century, it is regrettable that a clear history of raised ICP may be misinterpreted until the final denouement of disturbance of consciousness and pupillary abnormality or apnoea presents. Some patients have learnt to control their intracranial hypertension by hyperventilating, only to be dismissed as hysterics. Only slowly has the danger of lumbar puncture in the differential diagnosis of neurological patients been appreciated by the non-expert. Many of the later signs of raised ICP are the result of herniation: monitoring should detect raised ICP at an earlier stage and hence treatment should be started before irreversible damage occurs.

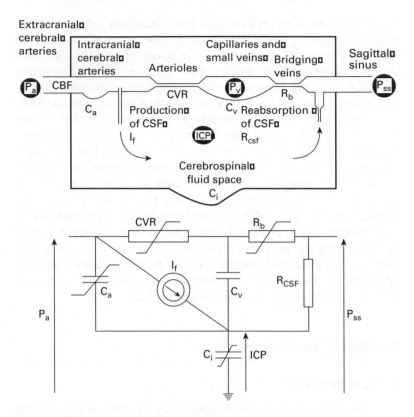

Figure 7.8 Hydrodynamic model of cerebral blood flow (CBF) and CSF circulation with the electrically equivalent circuit (for details, see Ursino[25]).

P_a = internal carotid artery blood pressure; P_v = cerebral venous pressure; P_{ss} = sagittal sinus blood pressure; ICP = intracranial pressure; I_f = CSF formation rate; CVR = resistance of cerebral arterial bed; R_b = resistance of bridging veins; R_{CSF} = resistance to CSF reabsorption; C_a = compliance of cerebral arterial bed; C_v = compliance of cerebral venous bed; C_i = compliance of lumbar CSF compartment

CT scanning

CT scanning may reveal not only a mass, hydrocephalus, or cerebral oedema, but also evidence of diffuse brain swelling such as absent perimesencephalic cisterns, compressed third ventricle, and midline shift.

Invasive methods of intracranial pressure monitoring including infusion tests

The gold standard of ICP monitoring, which was first introduced before 1951,[12,27] still remains the measurement of intraventricular fluid pressure either directly or via a CSF reservoir, with the opportunity to exclude zero drift. Subdural fluid filled catheters are reasonably accurate below 30 mmHg. Risk of infection, epilepsy, and haemorrhage is less with subdural than with intraventricular catheters, but even the latter should be less than 5% overall. Catheter tip transducers are useful particularly for waveform analysis, whether placed intraventricularly, subdurally, or intracerebrally. Ventricular catheters permit the therapeutic drainage of CSF in cases of ventricular dilatation.

In more chronic conditions of ventricular dilatation, where ICP is not greatly raised, obstruction to CSF absorption may be confirmed by CSF infusion tests (ventricular or lumbar) taking care to adapt the technique to the site of any obstruction.[28–30]

The infusion study can be performed via the lumbar CSF space or via a pre-implanted ventricular access device. In both cases two needles are inserted (22G spinal needles for lumbar tests; 25G butterfly needles for ventricular studies). One needle is connected to a pressure transducer via a stiff saline-filled tube and the other to an infusion pump mounted on a purpose-built trolley containing a pressure amplifier and an IBM-compatible personal computer running software written in house. After 10 minutes of baseline measurement, the infusion of normal saline at a rate of 1·5 ml/min or 1 ml/min (if the baseline pressure was higher than 15 mmHg) starts and continues until a steady state ICP plateau is achieved (Figure 7.9). If the ICP increases to 40 mmHg, the infusion is interrupted. Following cessation of the saline infusion, ICP is recorded until it decreases to steady baseline levels. All compensatory parameters are calculated using computer-supported methods based on physiological models of the CSF circulation.[30–33] Baseline ICP and R_{CSF} characterise static conditions of CSF circulation. R_{CSF} is calculated as the pressure increase during the infusion, divided by the infusion rate. A value below 13 mmHg/(ml/min) characterises normal CSF circulation.[28] Above 18 mmHg/(ml/min) the CSF circulation is clearly disturbed.[34] Between 13 and 18 mmHg/(ml/min) there is a grey zone, when other

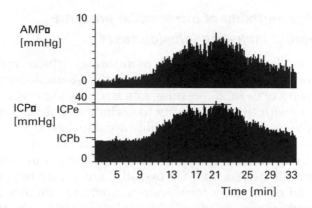

Figure 7.9 Recording of ICP and pulse amplitude (AMP) during infusion study.
Constant rate infusion (1 ml/min) started 9 minutes after insertion of needles into Ommaya reservoir and finished 13 minutes later. ICP increased from 11 to 32 mmHg, indicating resistance to CSF outflow of 21 mmHg/(m/min)

compensatory parameters and clinical investigation should be considered to make a decision about shunting.[33]

The cerebrospinal elasticity coefficient (E_1) and pulse amplitude of ICP waveform (AMP) express the dynamic components of CSF pressure volume compensation.

E_1 describes the compliance of the CSF compartment according to the formula:

$$\text{Compliance of CSF space} = Ci = 1/ \{E_1 \times (ICP-p_0)\},$$

where p_0 is the unknown reference pressure level, representing hydrostatic difference between the site of ICP measurement and pressure indifferent point of cerebrospinal axis.[35,36] Cerebrospinal compliance is inversely proportional to ICP, therefore comparison between different subjects can be made only at the same level of the difference: $ICP - p_0$. The elastance coefficient E_1 is independent of ICP, thus this coefficient is a much more convenient parameter when comparing individual patients. A low value of E_1 (less 0·2 L/ml) is specific for a compliant system, whilst a high value indicates decreased pressure–volume compensatory reserve.

The pulse amplitude of ICP (AMP) increases proportionally when the mean ICP rises. The proportionality ratio (the AMP/P index) characterises both elastance of the cerebrospinal space and the transmission of arterial pulsations to the CSF compartment.[30]

Finally, the production of CSF fluid can be estimated using Davson's equation. However, the sagittal sinus pressure is unknown and cannot be easily measured without increasing the invasiveness of the whole procedure. Consequently, the P_{ss} and CSF formation are estimated jointly using a non-linear model utilising the least square distance method during the computerised infusion test.[33] It is important to mention that such an "estimate" of CSF production rate approximates CSF absorption, rather than the actual production rate. It is based upon the assumption that all circulating CSF is reabsorbed via the arachnoid granulations. In cases where significant CSF leakage into brain parenchyma occurs, CSF production may be grossly underestimated.

Twenty-four hour intracranial pressure monitoring in patients with so-called normal pressure hydrocephalus may reveal a high incidence of B waves during sleep which is a very helpful prognostic sign for the outcome following shunting (see also Figure 7.3i).[29,36–38] Benign intracranial hypertension seldom requires more than CSF pressure monitoring through a lumbar catheter or needle for an hour.

Considerable effort continues into the detailed analysis of the ICP trace to determine whether it is possible to reveal the mechanism of raised ICP and whether autoregulatory reserve remains intact. The pulsatile waveform of ICP hypothetically includes information about both transmission of the arterial pulse pressure through the arterial walls and the compliance of the brain. This information is not always clear and demands specific computer analysis and critical interpretation, thereby restricting its use to only a few centres.

It has been proposed[9] that congestion or vascular brain swelling may be present when the ratio of the amplitudes of the pulse and respiratory components of the ICP trace exceeds two, when there is an increase in the high frequency centroid,[39] or when there is a high amplitude transfer function for the harmonics from arterial pressure to ICP. Such a transfer function is calculated from the Fourier transform of the digitised signal.[40] Continuous multimodality monitoring is required to draw any

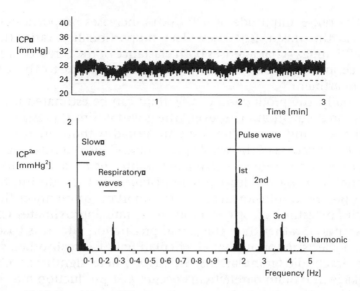

Figure 7.10 Example of ICP recording showing pulse, respiratory, and "slow waves" overlapped in time-domain (upper panel) and separated in frequency domain (lower panel)

safe conclusions, however, and should include some measure of cerebral blood flow (for example, transcranial Doppler sonography) and indirect measures of cerebral metabolism (for example, EEG, jugular venous oxygen saturation). Indices of imminent decompensation would be very helpful but volume pressure responses,[41] pressure volume indices, or definition of the contribution of CSF outflow resistance to intracranial pressure[5] are not suitable for routine clinical use.

Using computer analysis the ICP waveform can be interpreted far more precisely. Basic breakdown to pulse wave, respiratory wave, and slow waves (of a period from 20 seconds to 3 minutes) can be done using frequency analysis (Figure 7.10).

A few complex indices describing cerebrospinal dynamics have been introduced. Although they are not in standard use, more advanced readers may benefit from this methodology.

Pressure–volume compensatory reserve index (RAP)

The RAP index (correlation coefficient [R] between AMP amplitude [A] and mean pressure [P]) was derived by linear correlation between 40 consecutive, time-averaged data points of AMP and ICP acquired over 6.4 seconds. This index indicates the degree of correlation between AMP and mean ICP over short periods of time (~ 4 minutes). Its clinical significance has been discussed before.[9] Theoretically, the RAP coefficient indicates the relationship between ICP and changes in volume of the intracerebral space, known as the "pressure–volume curve".[2,20,30] An RAP coefficient close to 0 indicates lack of synchronisation between changes in AMP and mean ICP. This denotes a good pressure–volume compensatory reserve at low ICP (Figure 7.1b). When RAP rises to +1, AMP varies directly with ICP and this indicates that the "working point" of the intracranial space shifts to the right towards the steep part of the pressure–volume curve. Here compensatory reserve is low, therefore any further rise in volume may produce a rapid increase in ICP. Following head injury and subsequent brain swelling RAP is usually close to +1. With further increase in ICP, AMP decreases and RAP values fall below zero. This occurs when the cerebral autoregulatory capacity is exhausted and the pressure–volume curve bends to the right as the capacity of cerebral arterioles to dilate in response to a cerebral perfusion pressure decrement is exhausted, and they tend to passively collapse. This indicates terminal cerebrovascular derangement with a decrease in pulse pressure transmission from the arterial bed to the intracranial compartment (Figure 7.11).

Cerebrovascular pressure–reactivity index (PRx)

A second ICP-derived index is the pressure–reactivity index (PRx), which incorporates the philosophy of assessing cerebrovascular pressure reactivity by observing the response of ICP to spontaneous changes in arterial blood pressure (ABP).[10] Using computational methods similar to calculation of the RAP index, PRx is determined by calculating the correlation coefficient between 40 consecutive, time-averaged data points of ICP and ABP. A positive PRx signifies a positive gradient of the regression line between the slow components of ABP and ICP, which we hypothesise to be associated with a passive behaviour of a non-reactive vascular bed. A negative value of PRx reflects a normally reactive vascular bed, as ABP waves provoke inversely correlated waves in ICP (Figure 7.12). This index correlates well with indices of autoregulation based on transcranial Doppler ultrasonography.[42,43] Furthermore,

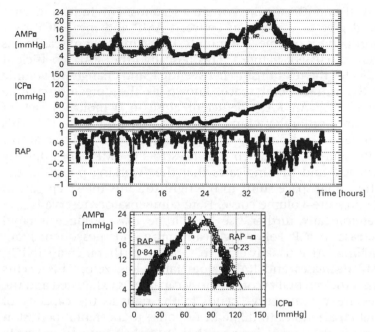

Figure 7.11 Example of the relationship between pulse wave amplitude (AMP) and mean intracranial pressure (ICP) recorded during a 46 hour period, during which terminal intracranial hypertension developed.

Pulse amplitude increased first proportionally to the change in ICP but started to decrease when ICP increased above 80 mmHg. The regression plot between AMP and ICP (bottom panel) indicated a biphasic relationship of positive and negative slopes. The correlation coefficient between AMP and ICP (RAP) was positive before 32 hours but negative after that, indicating terminal cerebrovascular deterioration

abnormal values of both PRx and RAP, respectively indicative of poor autoregulation or deranged cerebrospinal compensatory reserve, have been demonstrated to be predictive of a poor outcome following head injury (Figure 7.13).[44,45]

Non-invasive intracranial pressure measurement

It would be very helpful to measure ICP or cerebral perfusion pressure without invasive catheters. Transcranial Doppler examination, tympanic membrane displacement,

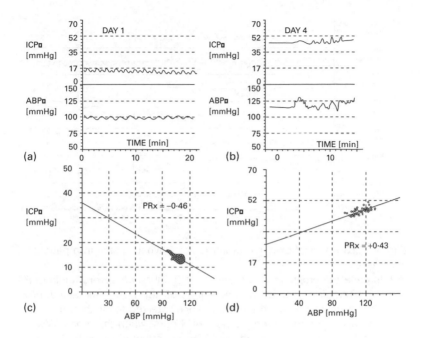

Figure 7.12 Relationship between slow waves of arterial pressure (ABP) and intracranial pressure (ICP).
This patient had low ICP on the first day after admission (a,c). Coherent waves both in ABP and ICP (a) produced negative correlation coefficient, when plotted on the regression graph (c), giving values of PRx clearly negative. On day 4 patient developed secondary intracranial hypertension. The nature of slow waves in ICP and ABP has changed (b) and correlation became obviously positive (d), giving a positive value of PRx. This indicated loss of cerebrovascular pressure reactivity

and even skull compliance studies have been advocated. Also it would be very helpful to have answers to the following questions: what is the cerebral perfusion pressure at any given time? What is the relative contribution of each possible mechanism to raised ICP? What features may predict decompensation? Is it possible to have an online assessment of cerebrovascular reactivity either to changes in cerebral perfusion pressure (autoregulation) or to carbon dioxide? Which therapy or cocktail is best suited to the sum of that individual's "split brain" problems?

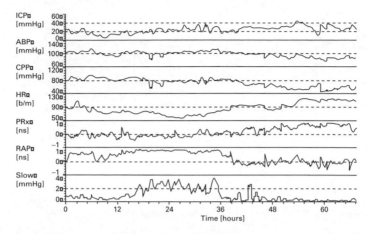

Figure 7.13 A typical example of intracranial hypertension in a patient who died.

In this case the progressive increase in ICP caused a severe fall in CPP (time = 48 hours), although normal values of ABP were maintained. PRx was at first slightly above the normal range, started to climb in the second part of the monitoring (time > 40 hours) when the progressive increase in ICP was associated with CPP reduction; similarly RAP, initially above 0·6, started to fall, suggesting a loss in vasomotor reserve (time > 40 hours). Slow waves were low at the beginning

A non-invasive method which monitored continuously both cerebral perfusion pressure and cerebral blood flow autoregulatory reserve would be very helpful in refining management of the swollen brain.

Transcranial Doppler

Aaslid's description of transcranial Doppler sonography in 1982 permitted bedside monitoring of one index of cerebral blood flow, non-invasively, repeatedly, and even continuously.[46,47] The problem has been that it is a "big tube technique", which measures flow velocity in branches of the circle of Willis, most commonly the middle cerebral artery. Changes in velocity may reflect changes in either blood flow or diameter of the insonated artery. Unfortunately, diameter and flow may not change in the same direction and great care must be taken with the interpretation.[48] Low velocity may indicate low flow or arterial dilatation at constant flow. High velocity may indicate high flow or arterial constriction/ vasospasm at constant flow.

Compliant branches of the middle cerebral artery can be compared approximately to two physiological pressure transducers. Pattern of blood flow inside these tubes is certainly modulated by transmural pressure (that is, cerebral perfusion pressure) and the proximal vascular resistance (also modulated by cerebral perfusion pressure). But what is the calibration factor and how should we compensate for unknown non-linear distortion?

There is a reasonable correlation between the pulsatility index of middle cerebral artery velocity and cerebral perfusion pressure after head injury but absolute measurements of cerebral perfusion pressure cannot be extrapolated.[49]

Others have suggested that "critical closing pressure" derived from flow velocity and arterial pressure waveform approximates the ICP.[50] The accuracy of this method has, however, never been satisfactory.[51]

Aaslid suggested[52] that an index of cerebral perfusion pressure could be derived from the ratio of the amplitudes of the first harmonics of the arterial blood pressure and the middle cerebral artery velocity (detected by transcranial Doppler sonography) multiplied by mean flow velocity.

Recently a new method for the non-invasive assessment of cerebral perfusion pressure has been reported, derived from mean arterial pressure multiplied by the ratio of diastolic to mean middle cerebral artery flow velocity.[53,54] This estimator can predict real cerebral perfusion pressure with an error of less than 10 mmHg for more than 70% of the time. This is of potential benefit for continuous monitoring of changes in real cerebral perfusion pressure over time in situations where the direct measurement of cerebral perfusion pressure is not readily available (Figure 7.14).

A more complex method aimed at the non-invasive assessment of ICP has been introduced and tested by Schmidt et al.[55] The method is based on the presumed linear transformation between arterial pressure and ICP waveforms. Coefficients of this transformation are derived from the database of real ABP and ICP recordings. Similar linear transformation is built, using the same database between flow velocity and arterial pressure. Then, the model assumes linear relationship between arterial pressure and flow velocity and

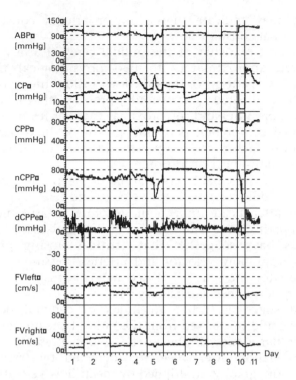

Figure 7.14 Daily recordings of mean ICP, arterial pressure (ABP), cerebral perfusion pressure (CPP = ABP – ICP), left and right mean flow velocity (FVleft and FVright), non-invasive CPP (nCPP), and left-to-right difference in nCPP (dCPPe) in a patient following head injury. Signals were recorded for at least half an hour each day

arterial pressure to ICP transformations. Multiple regression coefficients are calculated. Finally for each prospective study, ICP is calculated using ABP to ICP transformation, formed from ABP to flow velocity transformation transposed using precalculated regression coefficients. Simple? Not at all, but the method gives amazingly promising results (Figure 7.15).

Recent studies[56] have reported a good relationship between the flow velocity of venous blood in the straight sinus and ICP. Increasing ICP is supposed to squeeze the sinus and produce a proportional rise in blood flow velocity. The calibration coefficient was reported to be convergent in a group of patients, making this method possibly quantitative.

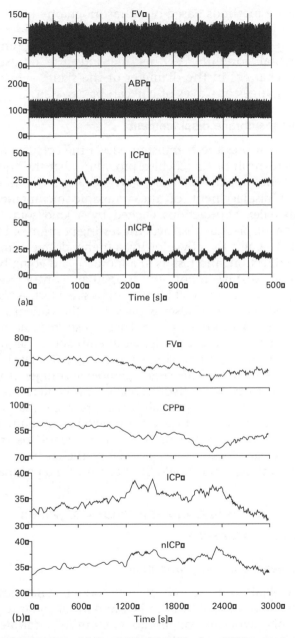

Figure 7.15 Examples of "simulation" (nICP) of real ICP recorded during B waves (a) and during intermittent elevation of ICP (5 minutes long), probably due to unstable arterial pressure (b)

There are methods based on ultrasonography but not using the Doppler principle. Time of flight of ultrasound through the skull is theoretically dependent on the tension of intracerebral contents.[57] Other methods use ultrasound to measure changes in the diameter of the skull[58] – in this way relative changes or waves of ICP can be assessed.

Tympanic membrane displacement

Intracranial pressure is transmitted via the cochlear aqueduct to the perilymph of the cochlea providing that the aqueduct is patent. Perilymphatic pressure may be assessed indirectly by recording displacement of the tympanic membrane during stapedial reflex contractions elicited by a loud sound.[59] High perilymphatic pressure displaces the resting position of the stapes footplate laterally, thereby allowing a higher degree of motion in a medial direction, and results in a more inward going tympanic membrane displacement on stapedial contraction. Low perilymphatic pressure will have an opposite effect. A transducer probe attached to a headset is placed in the patient's external auditory meatus and computer based instrumentation allows small movements of the tympanic membrane to be measured when 1000 Hz of increasing sound pressure level induces stapedial contraction. This very ingenious technique is useful in younger patients with hydrocephalus or benign intracranial hypertension on a sequential basis, provided that a skilled audiologist is available. It does not provide an absolute measure of ICP. It is of no value in patients on ventilators receiving neuromuscular blockers. The patency of the cochlear aqueduct decreases with age and should be checked with a postural test.

Indirect monitoring: consequences of raised intracranial pressure

Cerebral venous oxygen saturation

The cerebral arteriovenous oxygen content difference should normally be 5–7 ml/dl. Values below 4 ml/dl indicate cerebral hyperaemia, whereas values above 9 ml/dl indicate global cerebral ischaemia. Jugular bulb oxygen saturation may be monitored, preferably continuously, with an indwelling catheter. Single measurements of jugular venous oxygen are of little value given the many fluctuations during the day. Overenthusiastic treatment, which on occasion may induce cerebral ischaemia, may be monitored with this technique. Hyperventilation and barbiturate induced falls in cerebral perfusion pressure have been shown in individual patients to be counterproductive. An index of regional oxygen metabolism is required. Transcutaneous, transcranial near infrared spectroscopy is completely non-invasive.[60] This is a promising technique, however the scope for technological refinement is still huge.

Intraparenchymal probes

The oxygen content of cerebral tissue is reactive to high ICP.[61] However low oxygen tension may be provoked by other factors such as hyperventilation, low arterial blood pressure, microvascular problems, mitochondrial dysfunction, etc. Therefore, specificity of the method is low. Moreover, the measurement covers only a very small area of the brain.

Similar criticism can be raised in case of microdialysis. The lactate/pyruvate ratio is an accepted marker of brain ischaemia. Similarly, glutamate is supposed to be a marker of neuronal disintegration. Both markers have, however, non-established relationship to ICP. Recently, concerns were raised that ICP may modulate microdialysis recovery rate, as it acts as enviromental pressure.

Recent studies have explored other tracers of intracranial hypertension such as potassium ions.[62,63]

Cerebral electrical activity

The compressed EEG (cerebral function monitoring) is helpful in deciding whether cerebral metabolic depressants may be indicated in the treatment of intracranial hypertension.[21] Such drugs will obviously not be helpful if the EEG is flat or greatly reduced in amplitude.

Management strategies

Emergency resuscitation and diagnosis

Patients who are rapidly deteriorating or already are unconscious require immediate resuscitation followed by a diagnostic CT scan. In head-injured patients it is recommended to keep systolic blood pressure higher than 90 mmHg and arterial partial pressure of oxygen (Pao_2) higher than 8 kPa or arterial oxygen saturation greater than 90%. Patients with a Glasgow Coma Score (GCS) of 8 or less need to be intubated and ventilated to protect their airways *prior* to scanning. An intravenous bolus of mannitol 20% (2 ml/kg over 15 minutes) may be required if there is evidence of coning such as pupillary dilatation. Acute ventricular dilatation demands immediate ventricular drainage – bilateral if the lesion is midline. Hyperacute ventricular dilatation following subarachnoid haemorrhage or in association with a third ventricular lesion need not be gross to cause death. Significant space occupying lesions require surgical intervention, and abscesses require tapping. If an intracranial tumour or abscess is identified as the cause of intracranial hypertension, dexamethasone (initial dose 10–20 mg IV bolus) can be given.

Management of raised intracranial pressure

Based on data from head-injured patients showing worse outcome in patients with ICP greater than 20–25 mmHg,[66,67] raised ICP should be treated above this threshold. However, ICP therapy has side effects and needs to be selectively targeted if it is not to be counterproductive. As clinical signs, particularly in unconscious patients on a ventilator, are not reliable, ICP should be monitored when it is expected to be high or when active treatment is instigated in unconscious patients. For head-injured patients there are guidelines when monitoring of ICP is appropriate.[68] For all other patients the decision to insert monitors must be based on the CT scan and the clinical presentation. Possible indications for ICP monitoring are listed in Box 7.3. Raised ICP has been predominantly studied in head-injured patients and most treatment algorithms are designed for this group of patients. However, depending on the dominant mechanism leading to intracranial hypertension, these algorithms can easily be adapted to suit the needs of patients with other forms of brain injury. Based on an algorithm that has been successfully used in a wide range of brain-injured patients over recent years (Figure 7.16), the therapeutic options to lower ICP are discussed in the following section.

Addenbrooke's NCCU: ICP/CPP management algorithm

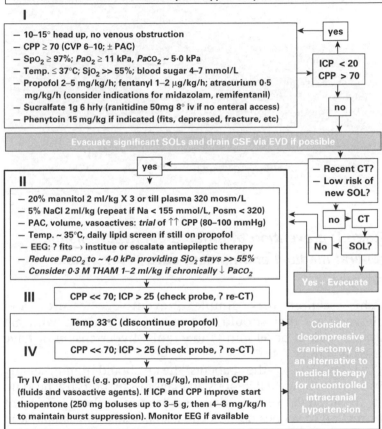

All patients with or at risk or intracranial hypertension *must* have invasive arterial monitoring, CVP line, ICP monitor, and RT $SjvO_2$ catheter at admission to NCCU.
— Aim to establish multimodality monitoring within the first six hours of NCCU stay.
— Interventions in stage II targeted to clinical picture.
— CPP 70 mmHg set as a target, although CPP > 60 mmHg is often acceptable.
— Check recruitment to research protocols.
Evacuate significant SOLs and consider CSF drainage before escalating medical Rx. Rx in italics and Grades III and IV only after approval by NCCU consultant

I

— 10–15° head up, no venous obstruction
— CPP ≥ 70 (CVP 6–10; ± PAC)
— SpO_2 ≥ 97%; PaO_2 ≥ 11 kPa, $PaCO_2$ ~ 5·0 kPa
— Temp. ≤ 37°C; SjO_2 >> 55%; blood sugar 4–7 mmol/L
— Propofol 2–5 mg/kg/h; fentanyl 1–2 µg/kg/h; atracurium 0·5 mg/kg/h (consider indications for midazolam, remifentanil)
— Sucralfate 1g 6 hrly (ranitidine 50mg 8° iv if no enteral access)
— Phenytoin 15 mg/kg if indicated (fits, depressed, fracture, etc)

yes

ICP < 20
CPP > 70

no

Evacuate significant SOLs and drain CSF via EVD if possible

— Recent CT?
— Low risk of new SOL?

yes

II

— 20% mannitol 2 ml/kg X 3 or till plasma 320 mosm/L
— 5% NaCl 2ml/kg (repeat if Na < 155 mmol/L, Posm < 320)
— PAC, volume, vasoactives: *trial* of ↑↑ CPP (80–100 mmHg)
— Temp. ~ 35°C; daily lipid screen if still on propofol
— EEG: ? fits → institue or escalate antiepileptic therapy
— *Reduce $PaCO_2$ to ~ 4·0 kPa providing SjO_2 stays >> 55%*
— *Consider 0·3 M THAM 1–2 ml/kg if chronically ↓ $PaCO_2$*

no — CT

No — SOL?

Yes → Evacuate

III   CPP << 70; ICP > 25 (check probe, ? re-CT)

Temp 33°C (discontinue propofol)

IV   CPP << 70; ICP > 25 (check probe, ? re-CT)

Try IV anaesthetic (e.g. propofol 1 mg/kg), maintain CPP (fluids and vasoactive agents). If ICP and CPP improve start thiopentone (250 mg boluses up to 3–5 g, then 4–8 mg/kg/h to maintain burst suppression). Monitor EEG if available

Consider decompressive craniectomy as an alternative to medical therapy for uncontrolled intracranial hypertension

Figure 7.16 Addenbrooke's Hospital Neurosciences Critical Care Unit algorithm for treatment of raised ICP.
Abbreviations: ICP = intracranial pressure; CPP = cerebral perfusion pressure (cerebral perfusion pressure = mean arterial blood pressure – ICP); CVP = central venous pressure; $SjvO_2$ = jugular venous oxygen saturation; SOL = space occupying lesion, Rx = therapy; PAC = pulmonary artery catheter; SpO_2 = oxygen saturation (pulse-oximeter); PaO_2 and $PaCO_2$ = arterial partial pressure of O_2 and CO_2; EVD = external ventricular drainage. Reproduced with permission of DK Menon

Box 7.3 Indications for intracranial pressure monitoring

Head injury (based on guidelines of the Brain Trauma Foundation[64])
Severe head injury (GCS 3–8) with abnormal admission CT scan
Severe head injury (GCS 3–8) with normal admission CT scan and
two of the following criteria:
Age > 40 years
Systolic blood pressure < 90 mmHg
Unilateral or bilateral motor posturing

Intracerebral and subarachnoid haemorrhage
GCS < 9
Postoperatively following intraoperative complications
Hydrocephalus

Various aetiologies with GCS < 9 and CT evidence of brain oedema
Metabolic (e.g. hepatic failure)
Hypoxia/ischaemia (e.g. large stroke, post cardiac arrest)
CNS infections (see Box 7.1)

Hydrocephalus and benign intracranial hypertension

Adapted from Minns,[4] Miller and Dearden,[9] and Campkin and
Turner.[65]

Stage I: prevention of intracranial hypertension: general medical and nursing care — avoidable factors

This section lists simple preventive measures and interventions that should be used in all patients who are either at risk of developing intracranial hypertension or have raised ICP (Box 7.4).[9,65]

The position of the patients' head should minimise any obstruction to cerebral venous drainage. Many units use head up tilt to improve venous drainage from the head. Relevant obstruction to venous outflow can also be caused by lateral head tilt, neck collars used for stabilisation of the cervical spine, tight bands used for the fixation of endotracheal tubes, or inappropriate amounts of positive end expiratory pressure (PEEP). There is a certain reluctance to use a PEEP greater than 5 cm H_2O in head-injured patients, but PEEP needs to be selected based on individual patient characteristics and by optimising the effects on intracranial pressure *and* arterial partial pressure of oxygen. When patients are nursed in a head up position, care must be taken that

---

Box 7.4 Potential problems exacerbating raised intracranial pressure

Incorrect calibration of intracranial pressure and arterial blood pressure transducers and monitors

- check calibration and proper position of arterial transducer reference point

Obstruction of venous drainage from the head

- inappropriate position of head and neck
- avoid constricting tape/tube fixations around neck

Cardiovascular problems

- inadequate cerebral perfusion pressure (too low (hypovolaemia?) or too high)
- cerebral vasodilating drugs

Respiratory problems

- hypercapnia/hypoxia
- inappropriate positive end expiratory pressure
- secretions, bronchospasm, etc.

Metabolism: fever, hyperglycaemia, infusion of hypo-osmotic fluids

Insufficient analgesia, insufficient sedation

- consider using muscle relaxants if analgesia and sedation are adequate

Seizures

Developing or new space occupying lesions

---

cerebral perfusion pressure is maintained. Direct measurement of global cerebral blood flow and cerebral perfusion pressure suggests that a head up tilt of up to 30 degrees is safe but cerebral perfusion pressure needs to be monitored carefully in individual patients.[69–72] Ideally the transducer of the arterial pressure monitor should be zeroed at the level of the external acoustic meatus, which approximates the zero point for ICP, and not the right atrium, to measure true cerebral perfusion pressure.

Maintaining adequate perfusion pressure is critical. Low cerebral perfusion pressure will lead to ischaemia and consequently increase cytotoxic oedema. However, moderately low cerebral perfusion pressure can also increase intracranial pressure due to autoregulation: in patients with intact autoregulation, decreases in cerebral perfusion pressure will lead to vasodilatation which, especially in patients with low intracranial compliance, leads to an increase in ICP. In patients with lost autoregulation, increases in cerebral perfusion pressure will be mirrored by increases in ICP. Excessively high cerebral perfusion pressure will increase vasogenic oedema. There is no consensus as to the level of cerebral perfusion pressure which is appropriate in an individual patient. For head-injured adults values ranging from 50 to ≥ 90 mmHg are found in the literature.[73-76] The guidelines of the Brain Trauma Foundation list a cerebral perfusion pressure target of 70 mmHg as an option, other authors suggest 60 mmHg as a target. In this context the "Lund concept" needs to be mentioned. This concept is based on the assumption that vasogenic oedema is the major cause of post-traumatic brain oedema and focuses on prevention and reduction of oedema. Therefore cerebral perfusion pressure is not augmented but arterial blood pressure is normalised with metoprolol and clonidine. A cerebral perfusion pressure as low as 50 mmHg is tolerated. Plasma oncotic pressure is corrected through administration of albumin. Dihydroergotamine is used to further reduce the intracerebral blood volume.[73] Good results have been reported with this approach.[77] However, there has never been a controlled trial in which this concept was directly compared to a more traditional approach, and possibly the fact that contusions are removed surgically whenever possible may confound the issue. Irrespective of the targeted cerebral perfusion pressure, hypovolaemia must be corrected. The evidence for this is most clear cut in patients after head injury and subarachnoid haemorrhage: a negative fluid balance exceeding –594 ml during the first 96 hours after head injury was associated with an adverse effect on outcome.[78] Patients with CT evidence of raised ICP are at greater risk of hypovolaemia after subarachnoid haemorrhage,[79] and hypovolaemic patients after subarachnoid haemorrhage, particularly when coupled with hyponatraemia, have an increased risk of cerebral infarction.[80] Hypovolaemia may be revealed only when the patient is given a sedative agent such as propofol. A stable circulation must be maintained, with normal saline, colloids, and if necessary vasoactive drugs. In this context it is useful to briefly comment on hyponatraemia, which is a frequent finding in patients with brain injury and is associated with extracellular volume depletion and cerebral ischaemia. Most neurosurgical patients with hyponatraemia do *not* have inappropriate secretion of antidiuretic hormone (SIADH), which is characterised by a hypervolaemic or euvolaemic state. Cerebral salt wasting, defined as the loss of sodium during intracranial disease leading to hyponatraemia and volume depletion, is the alternative cause of hyponatraemia. Possible mechanisms leading to this syndrome are secretion of atrial and brain natriuretic peptides as well as ouabain-like compounds. The two syndromes are differentiated by the volume status of the patient. Cerebral salt wasting is treated with fluid and sodium substitution (for a detailed review see Harrigan[81]). Overenthusiastic hypertensive-hypervolaemic therapy remains very controversial, especially in the context of head injury with its multiple pathology and uncertainty over the integrity of the blood–brain barrier.[82–84] It carries the risk of development of vasogenic oedema but also of adult respiratory distress syndrome[85] and cardiac dysfunction.[86] The question whether systemic hypertension should be treated in the context of appropriate cerebral perfusion pressure remains controversial and there are no recommendations. In stroke patients it has been suggested that arterial hypertension should be treated if mean arterial pressure exceeds 130 mmHg or systolic pressure exceeds 220 mmHg.[87] If arterial blood pressure is to be lowered vasodilators such as sodium nitroprusside or nitroglycerine are to be avoided. All cerebral vasodilators will increase ICP and some such as sodium nitroprusside impair autoregulation, and this drug has also been shown to increase the risk of boundary zone infarction.[88] If easily corrected causes for hypertension such as pain or urinary retention are excluded and the decision to treat hypertension is made, labetalol, esmolol, or other short acting beta-blockers or clonidine are potentially useful drugs.

Adequate ventilation is critical. Hypoxia must be avoided, as it is one of the most important secondary insults to the injured brain.[89] There is no role for *prophylactic* hyperventilation and $Pa\text{CO}_2$ should be kept in the normal range. Chest infections are a common complication in patients on a neurointensive care unit. Typically they are either a consequence of aspiration or are associated with mechanical ventilation (ventilator associated pneumonia), especially if neuromuscular blockers are used.

Pyrexia not only increases cerebral metabolism and hence cerebral blood volume but also cerebral oedema. Patients should be kept normothermic either by the administration of paracetamol, non-steroidal anti-inflammatory drugs, or surface cooling. It is important to note that brain temperature is approximately 0·5°C higher than core temperature.

Hyperglycaemia should be treated aggressively. There is considerable evidence that cerebral ischaemia and infarction are made worse by hyperglycaemia and the use of high concentration glucose solutions is contraindicated unless there is significant evidence of benefit in a particular metabolic encephalopathy.[90,91] Glucose containing solutions should also be avoided because they are hypo-osmotic once the glucose has been metabolised. Because of concerns about increasing brain oedema by infusing fluids with low osmolarity most units also avoid Ringer's lactate in brain-injured patients and use normal saline as a maintenance fluid.

Adequate sedation and analgesia are essential to control ICP. Coughing, straining, and "fighting the ventilator" all lead to considerable increases in ICP. Sedation not only alleviates stress but also suppresses cerebral metabolism, therefore improving the supply–demand balance. Propofol is widely used because of its cerebral vasoconstrictor effect and its relatively short duration of action. Care has to be taken to avoid hypotension which is likely to occur in hypovolaemic patients due to the propofol induced reduction in preload. An interesting and potentially beneficial side effect of propofol is its free radical scavenging effect.[92] There is some concern about the long term use of propofol for sedation, and it should not be used for this purpose in children as deaths have been linked to long term infusions of this drug ("propofol infusion syndrome").[93] This syndrome has recently also been reported in adults.[94] Furthermore, a substantial amount of long chain fatty acids is infused with propofol and, especially in hypothermic patients, lipid levels need to be checked at regular intervals. Alternatively, midazolam or lorazepam can be used for sedation.

Epilepsy has long been known to raise ICP and increase the risk of cerebral ischaemia as a result of a massive increase in cerebral electrical activity and oxidative metabolism, resulting in an increase in oxygen demand and at the same time a cerebral perfusion pressure decrease. Seizures must be treated aggressively but may be difficult to recognise when the patient is paralysed and ventilated. Episodes of pupillary dilatation with increases in arterial blood pressure and intracranial pressure are suggestive. Some units use continuous EEG monitoring to detect occult seizures. Prophylactic administration of anticonvulsants has been advocated for patients with large haemorrhagic strokes involving the cortex, cortical tumours, and head-injured patients with acute subdural haematomas (evacuated and non-evacuated), depressed skull fractures, and penetrating missile injuries.[95] In this context it should be noted that many antibiotics including carbapenems, fluoroquinolones, and metronidazole have proconvulsant properties through GABA antagonism.

If despite these measures ICP exceeds 20–25 mmHg active treatment should be instigated. If no CT scan has been performed recently, a repeat scan is advisable to exclude conditions that are amenable to surgical interventions.

Continuous CSF drainage and surgical decompression

External ventricular drainage via a catheter or reservoir is a rapid procedure to reduce raised ICP not only in patients with hydrocephalus but also in head-injured patients. In all cases of external drainage, CSF should be drained gradually against a positive pressure of 15–25 cmH$_2$O to avoid unrestrained drainage. In patients with diffuse brain swelling, the ventricles are small and not always easy to cannulate. Even when cannulation is successful, catheters in very tight ventricles readily become blocked. Lumbar CSF drainage may be used after head injuries, provided the basal cisterns remain patient on CT scanning.[96] However, this is not without risk and coning is a potential complication. CSF drainage alone is the optimal method of controlling intracranial hypertension in patients with subarachnoid haemorrhage where the cause is often disturbance of the CSF circulation, but there is probably an increased risk of rebleeding. CSF drainage is also used as a diagnostic technique to assess patients with poor grade subarachnoid haemorrhage. If they improve, early surgery should be considered. Biventricular drainage is required for third ventricular lesions, which occlude both foramina of Munro. Patients with communicating hydrocephalus or benign intracranial hypertension may be temporarily controlled by lumbar drainage through an indwelling catheter. It is unkind and less effective to use repeated lumbar punctures. It is becoming recognised that permanent CSF drainage via lumbar peritoneal shunts may be complicated by secondary descent of the cerebellar tonsils in patients with no previous evidence of a Chiari malformation.[97] In the case of a posterior fossa tumour, upward coning may be precipitated if the supratentorial ventricles are drained too precipitately. In patients with a hemispherical mass causing midline shift and contralateral hydrocephalus, drainage of that ventricle may make the shift worse. Colloid cysts are best treated surgically as the primary procedure unless the patient is *in extremis*.

Removal of bone flaps or subtemporal decompressions is becoming more popular.[98,99] There is a place for decompressive craniotomy following head injury but there is the potential to do considerable harm,[98–100] and it has not been shown that craniectomies improve outcome.[101] A multicentre trial to evaluate the role of craniectomy in head injury is planned. With a very tight brain, opening the dura induces herniation through the defect. Cerebral venous drainage from the herniated brain obstructs and further brain swelling ensues with infarction. Craniectomy may be considered in young patients without evidence of diffuse axonal injury (high Glasgow Coma Scale score on admission) and evidence of diffuse swelling.[102] In large ischaemic strokes of the middle cerebral artery territory, mortality is reduced by extensive craniectomy.[103] Benign intracranial hypertension can be treated by lumbar peritoneal or cisternoperitoneal shunting: subtemporal decompressions are sometimes indicated. Optic nerve fenestration has lost its former popularity. The new procedure of cerebral venous sinus stenting for patients with transverse sinus stenosis has recently been introduced.[104] Patients with large meningiomas may have a smoother postoperative course if a flap is removed electively at the end of the operation rather than as an emergency a few hours later. Babies with complex forms of craniosynostosis may require craniofacial surgery to expand the volume of the skull. For paediatric encephalopathies it was recommended to perform decompression earlier rather than later and certainly before the EEG disappears.[105]

Mannitol and hypertonic saline

Intravenous mannitol is invaluable as a first aid measure in a patient with brain herniation as a result of raised ICP. In practice, mannitol tends to be given as an intermittent bolus (2 ml/kg of a 20% solution over 15–20 minutes) whenever the individual patient's ICP rises significantly above the threshold of 20–25 mmHg. Effects last for up to four hours. As osmotic diuresis may lead to hypovolaemia it is crucial to avoid dehydration and latent hypotension with careful attention to fluid balance. Another dose of mannitol should not be given if osmolarity exceeds 320 mosm/L for fear of tubular damage and renal failure. Repeated doses of mannitol should not be given unless an ICP monitor is in place. Overenthusiastic bolus administration of an osmotic diuretic may cause abrupt systemic hypertension, an increase in cerebral blood volume if autoregulation is defective or its upper limit is exceeded, and promote herniation rather than the reverse.[106]

Much uncertainty remains concerning the mechanisms of action of mannitol and its prolonged use. Many attempts have been made to rationalise how much mannitol may be given, and when, for more prolonged effects.[107,108] Studies indicate that mannitol, given time, removes water from both normal and oedematous brain, be it intracellular (cytotoxic) or interstitial (vasogenic) oedema.[109–111] The oedematous area around many mass lesions may still have an intact blood–brain barrier, at least to the conventional high molecular weight tracers. The time course of this effect is slow and does not account for the immediate effect of mannitol on ICP. In patients with peritumoral oedema, mannitol causes withdrawal of water mainly from brain areas where the barrier is impaired as judged by T1 weighted MRI and *in vitro* measurements of brain water content.[112] Mannitol, however, may accumulate in oedematous white matter with repeated doses.[113]

The more immediate effects of intravenous mannitol include a fall in whole blood viscosity with reduced red cell rigidity and corpuscular volume, an increase in brain compliance, and possibly cerebral vasoconstriction.[114–116] The cerebral vasoconstriction with intravascular bolus administration is short lived: in the cat, both pial arteriolar diameter and ICP returned to normal within 30 minutes and, thereafter, both increased at the same rate as changes in blood viscosity.[116] Administration over 15 minutes produced no change in pial arteriolar or venular diameter in another study.[117] Why should a sudden change in blood viscosity evoke acute transient vasoconstriction? Chronic changes in blood viscosity, without alterations in haemoglobin or arterial oxygen content, do not change steady state cerebral blood flow in humans.[118] Patients with high plasma viscosity or with high viscosity due to large numbers of white cells do not have low cerebral blood flow values. In a series of patients with haematological diseases but no evidence of cerebrovascular disease, arterial oxygen content was the major determinant of cerebral blood flow; blood viscosity per se had no significant effect on cerebral blood flow.[119] If a single blood vessel is considered, the apparent viscosity of blood diminishes in proportion to its radius as a result of the marginal sheath of low viscosity and axial flow of red cells.[120] The width of this sheath is relatively greatest in small vessels. Furthermore, apparent viscosity increases with falling velocity. Hence with pial arterial dilatation, local blood viscosity will rise both because of the increased proportion of red cells and as a result of the reduction in flow velocity if tissue perfusion remains constant. Simplistically, according to Poiseuille, as viscosity is reduced the pressure gradient along the pial arteriole falls. Hence, the distal intravascular pressure increases if the proximal pressure remains constant. The distal end of the arteriole therefore constricts if autoregulatory mechanisms are intact. "Viscosity" autoregulation should depend on pressure autoregulation unless there is a separate endothelial mechanism that is flow or viscosity sensitive. Alternatively, mannitol may transiently increase cerebral blood flow, increase oxygen delivery, or wash out local vasodilators such as adenosine.[116] All these mechanisms would lead to vasoconstriction. Therefore, if the viscosity mechanism is relevant, it will depend upon the distribution gradient of intravascular pressures along the cerebrovascular tree, which may not be easy to predict with different pathologies and cerebral perfusion pressures. *Extracellular* hyperosmolarity is a potent cerebral vasodilator and it is remarkable that the intravenous vasoconstrictor effect of mannitol so completely dominates the acute cerebrovascular effect. Certainly the reported clinical effects of mannitol on cerebral blood flow are not easy to rationalise.[121–125] In patients with severe head injuries, in whom autoregulation was absent, intravenous mannitol caused an increase in cerebral blood flow and no reduction in ICP.[125] In those patients where autoregulation was intact ICP was reduced. In patients with unruptured aneurysms, however, in most of whom autoregulation was presumably intact, mannitol (bolus or infusion) increased cerebral blood flow for many hours.[124] More regional assessments of cerebral blood flow suggest that mannitol may stabilise pH and cerebral blood flow in regions of moderate but not severe ischaemia.[126] Other suggested mechanisms for the effect of mannitol include movement of water from CSF into capillaries and scavenging of free radicals.[127]

Hypertonic saline has recently received much interest for the treatment of cerebral oedema and intracranial hypertension. Hypertonic saline solutions ranging from 1·6% to 29·2% have been used. In humans, so far only case series and results from small controlled groups of patients have been published. Despite a low frequency of side effects and reproducible reduction of intracranial pressure, more data are needed. Dose–response curves are lacking and future studies should not only compare hypertonic saline to mannitol but also address the question whether bolus injections or continuous infusions are more beneficial. Administrations of 250 ml of NaCl 7·5% as a bolus or 30–60 ml of NaCl 23·4% have been recommended. The action of hypertonic saline is augmented if colloids are administrered at the same time. Durations of action of approximately two hours have been reported.[128] The mechanism of action is due to the osmotic action of hypertonic saline that leads to a removal of water from the interstitial and intracellular compartment in areas with intact blood–brain barrier and an increase in regional cerebral blood flow most likely caused by a reduction in size of swollen endothelial cells. However, this effect has not been observed by all investigators.

Hypothermia

Moderate hypothermia (33–36°C) has been shown to be neuroprotective, that is, to reduce secondary brain injury and infarction size and to improve neurological outcome in animal models with both focal and global ischaemia. In humans hypothermia has been shown to reduce cerebral blood flow, arteriojugular venous oxygen difference, and cerebral metabolic rate of oxygen.[129] Much excitement has followed early reports of ICP reduction[130] and improvement of outcome in head-injured patients.[130,131] However, a large randomised multicentre trial has failed to demonstrate an improvement in outcome,[132] but there have been many criticisms of this study and the effects of hypothermia on the outcome of head-injured patients will be re-examined in a further large trial. For subarachnoid haemorrhage a trial to prove the efficacy of intraoperative hypothermia (IHAST) is currently under way. Cooling can be achieved by surface cooling or with various exchanger devices that are inserted into a large vein. It is to be remembered that brain temperature will be ~0·5°C higher than core temperature. Rewarming is a very important issue and no recommendations on how rapidly patients should be rewarmed are available. However, in animals it has been shown that rapid rewarming can reverse the beneficial effects of hypothermia.[133] Hypothermia has relevant side effects: ventricular ectopy and fibrillation limit the extent of hypothermia, but this is known to occur only at temperatures below 30°C. A recent study found a significantly higher rate of pneumonia, electrolyte abnormalities, thrombocytopenia, and increased amylase serum in hypothermic patients when compared to normothermic patients.[134] Other side effects of hypothermia (which have been shown in animal studies) are clotting abnormalities and coagulopathy. In the human, the enzymatic reactions of the coagulation cascade were shown to be strongly inhibited by hypothermia. Although an elevation of serum amylase and lipase levels is frequently observed, the association between hypothermia and pancreatitis is still poorly understood.

Hyperventilation and THAM (tris-hydroxy-methyl-amino-methane)

Neurosurgical patients with healthy lungs and systemic circulation often hyperventilate spontaneously down to a Pa_{CO_2} of 30 mmHg.[8,65] Hyperventilation reduces ICP via a reduction of cerebral blood volume. Unfortunately this reduction in cerebral blood volume also causes a reduction in cerebral blood flow, and therefore the main concern when patients are hyperventilated is whether there is a risk of inducing cerebral ischaemia or not. *Prophylactic hyperventilation* of head-injured patients to a Pa_{CO_2} of 3·4 kPa has been shown to be detrimental to outcome[135] and aggressive hyperventilation to below a Pa_{CO_2} of ~3·5 kPa is not recommended. There is an ongoing controversy about the risk of moderate hyperventilation (Pa_{CO_2} 4·5–3·5 kPa) causing ischaemia.[136,137] Our means to monitor critical reductions of cerebral blood flow during hyperventilation are very limited. Jugular bulb venous oxygen saturation or arteriojugular oxygen content differences are generally used to avoid overaggressive hyperventilation. Despite a single study showing good results with such an "optimised hyperventilation" approach[138] there is evidence that the sensitivity of these methods to detect ischaemia is very limited as approximately 15% of brain tissue need to be ischaemic to reduce jugular bulb oxygen saturation below the generally used critical threshold of 50%. The duration of the cerebral vasoconstrictor effect of hypocapnia is uncertain. While in healthy volunteers cerebral blood flow returns rapidly to baseline despite continued hyperventilation, in head-injured patients the variability of recovery is large, with some patients recovering within a few hours whereas others still have reduced cerebral blood flow after more than a day of hyperventilation.[139] Recovery of cerebral blood flow is brought about because the bicarbonate buffering mechanisms within the brain and cerebrovascular smooth muscle readjust to return extracellular and intracellular pH nearer to the original values.[140] This mechanism is also responsible for the "rebound" intracranial hypertension when the arterial partial pressure of CO_2 increases after a phase of hyperventilation as the brain's buffering mechanisms have to readjust back again. Finally, cerebrovascular reactivity to carbon dioxide is a prognostic factor after head injury and is completely lost in very severe injuries.[139,141,142] There is growing awareness that hyperventilation should be used sparingly, for example, to treat intracranial pressure plateau waves. For head-injured patients the Brain Trauma Foundation guidelines recommend moderate hyperventilation as a short term measure only, except when other forms of medical intracranial pressure treatment have failed.[68]

CSF lactate accumulation and CSF acidosis occur after head injury.[143,144] Both severity of injury and the proportion of patients with a poor outcome are related to high and increasing CSF lactate levels. Cerebral tissue lactic acidosis is related to secondary brain damage following a primary insult such as cerebral ischaemia even if moderate acidosis per se has no persisting effect on normal neurons. Akiota et al.[145] found that the intravenous buffer THAM ameliorated both the CSF acidosis and brain swelling following epidural balloon compression of the brain in dogs. THAM, after intravenous administration, equilibrates with the intracellular and extracellular spaces in the body as well as with CSF. Evidence is accumulating both experimentally and in humans that THAM is at least as effective as mannitol in reducing experimental oedema in the brain and lowering ICP after head injury.[146-148] THAM reduces the demand for mannitol and CSF drainage. In the most recently published randomised prospective clinical trial,[148] a total of 149 patients with severe head injury (Glasgow Coma Scale ≤ 8) were randomly assigned to either a control or a THAM group. THAM was administered as a 0·3 mol/L solution in an initial loading dose (body weight × blood acidity deficit) given over two hours, followed by constant infusion of 1 ml/kg hourly for five days. Both groups of patients were matched in terms of clinical parameters. All patients were treated by standard management protocols and Pa_{CO_2} was maintained in the range 4·3–4·7 kPa for five days. Although analysis indicated no significant difference in outcome between the two groups at three months, six months, or one year, there was a difference regarding ICP. The time that ICP was above 20 mmHg in the first 48 hours after injury was less in patients treated with THAM. Also, the number of patients requiring barbiturate coma was significantly less in the THAM group (5·5% versus 18·4%). The authors concluded that THAM ameliorated the deleterious effects of prolonged hyperventilation, was beneficial in ICP control, and further study of dose and timing of administration was warranted.

Cerebral metabolic suppression

Hypnotic agents, such as propofol, barbiturates, or etomidate, depress cerebral oxidative metabolism and hence lower cerebral blood flow and volume, and ICP. The brain depends on ATP to uphold its structural integrity (~40% of O_2 consumption) and to produce electrical activity (60% of O_2 consumption). Only electrical activity can be suppressed with these drugs. Barbiturates are commonly used for this purpose. Cerebral electrical activity and normal coupling mechanisms between metabolism and flow must be present if barbiturates are to lower ICP.[21,22,65] Flow–metabolism coupling mechanisms may be assessed by the cerebrovascular response to carbon dioxide and barbiturates are only effective if some carbon dioxide reactivity is retained.[22] For thiopentone repeated boluses of 250 mg (up to 3–5 g) are recommended followed by an infusion of 4–8 mg/kg/h. Barbiturate therapy should be targeted to a predefined EEG burst suppression ratio. Unfortunately all agents that depress cerebral metabolism have side effects. For propofol and barbiturates the most relevant is systemic hypotension, which is often exacerbated by hypovolaemia. Etomidate has very little effect on haemodynamics but interferes with endogenous steroid synthesis and its prolonged use in intensive care has been abandoned. Synergy with even moderate hypothermia may be helpful provided mean arterial pressure is maintained.[65] After initial reports of the effectiveness of short acting barbiturates in lowering ICP after head injury, three controlled trials have failed to show any overall significant improvement of outcome or reduction in a number of patients dying with intracranial hypertension.[149-151] Such trials involved heterogeneous groups of patients, however, and a treatment benefit in a subgroup may have been missed. The ideal hypnotic agent awaits development. Elimination of thiopentone takes several days and interferes with establishing brain death.

Other therapies

The mechanism of the remarkable effect of glucocorticoids such as dexamethasone on focal, relatively chronic, cerebral lesions remains incompletely understood. Patients deteriorating with a cerebral tumour or an abscess rapidly improve within 24 hours of administration of dexamethasone. Much controversy has surrounded the use of very high dose steroids in head injury, but carefully controlled trials have shown no benefit and in one study the outcome of the treatment group was worse.[152-156] Currently the use of steroids in head-injured patients is not recommended.[68] A megatrial (CRASH) of methylprednisolone in head injury has recently started in the UK.[157] One purported mechanism of action for steroids involves inhibition of lipid peroxidation and generation of free radicals.[157,158] Up to 2% of oxygen consumed by the brain is used to form semireduced oxygen intermediates: superoxide, hydrogen peroxide, and hydroxyl free radicals. These may be used as part of normal biochemistry or if the safety mechanisms fail then such reactive oxygen species may attack nucleic acids, proteins, carbohydrates, and particularly lipids in the brain. Ferrous iron from blood clots is also active along with such reactive oxygen species. Cerebrovascular effects of acute hypertension and subarachnoid haemorrhage may involve free radical mechanisms damaging the endothelium. Non-glucocorticoid steroid analogues of methylprednisolone as well as methylprednisolone itself weakly inhibit lipid peroxidation. Tirilazad, a 21-amino-steroid, is a potent inhibitor of lipid peroxidation and has a vitamin E sparing effect.[159] Various experimental models of head and spinal injury and focal or global ischaemia have shown a variable degree of protection after treatment with Tirilazad or related compounds.[160] However, large scale clinical trials in head injury,[161] stroke,[162] and subarachnoid haemorrhage have failed to show efficacy.[163,164]

Indometacin is a potent cerebral vasoconstrictor and reduces ICP effectively. In five patients with injury with cerebral contusion and oedema, in whom it was not possible to control ICP by hyperventilation and barbiturate sedation, indometacin (bolus injection of 30 mg, followed by 30 mg/h for seven hours) reduced ICP below 20 mmHg for several hours.[165] Cerebral blood flow was reduced at two hours without any changes in cerebral arteriovenous oxygen or lactate differences. Rectal temperature also fell from 38·6 to 37·3°C. However, because of the intense vasoconstriction, and evidence from primates, there is serious concern about the possibility that indometacin will cause ischaemia. Certainly, cerebral oxygen delivery is seriously impaired when indometacin is given to very early preterm infants undergoing treatment for patent ductus arteriosus.[166] At present indometacin can only be considered an experimental treatment in head-injured patients.

It is interesting that the iron chelator desferrioxamine may be helpful in treating the coma of cerebral malaria and experimental vasogenic oedema. Results in severe head injuries with the oxygen radical scavenger polyethylene glycol conjugated superoxide dismutase have recently been reported, but a much larger trial is required to establish efficacy.[167] Impressive experimental data have led to phase III trials of glutamate receptor antagonists in patients after severe head injury, but the results have been negative.[168,169] Finally, intravenous lidocaine (lignocaine) (1·5 mg/kg) may have a place in lowering ICP.[170] This dose is as effective as 3 mg/kg of intravenous thiopentone.

Children

The management of raised ICP in childhood must take account of a number of factors.[4,171] The critical values for ICP, arterial pressure, and cerebral perfusion pressure are lower the younger the child. The normal intracranial pressure in the newborn is probably of the order of 2–4 mmHg. Arterial pressure at birth is approximately 55/40 mmHg, 80/55 mmHg by one year, and 90/60 mmHg during the early school years. Cerebral perfusion pressure rises from 28 mmHg at 28–32 weeks of gestational age to 38 mmHg at normal full term. In the neonate, much lower cerebral blood flow values may be tolerated for longer. Many of the pathologies differ from the adult, including birth asphyxia, posthaemorrhagic ventricular dilatation, craniocerebral disproportion, and the many metabolic and infective encephalopathies. The skull may expand due to high ICP in children where fusion of the sutures has not occurred. Hyperaemia plays a greater role as a cause of raised ICP in children after head injury than in adults.[172,173] The NIH Traumatic Data Bank of severe head injuries revealed that diffuse brain swelling occurs twice as often in children (aged 16 years or younger) as in adults. A total of 53% of children with diffuse swelling died compared with a mortality rate of 16% in those without. It has recently been suggested that ICP should be treated above a threshold of 15 mmHg in infants, 18 mmHg in children younger than eight years, and 20 mmHg in older children and teenagers.[174] In a retrospective study it has been shown that overall outcome is better when cerebral perfusion pressure is kept above 40 mmHg.[175] In another study analysing data from 24 children with a mean age of 6·3 years, all survivors had had a cerebral perfusion pressure of 50 mmHg or higher.[176] Based on these studies a recent review has suggested that cerebral perfusion pressure should be maintained above 40–45 mmHg in infants and young children and above 50–55 mmHg in older children and adolescents.[174] Seizures are more frequent in head-injured children than in adults.[177] Early seizures may occur in up to a third of the patients.[178] Children with non-accidental injury ("shaken baby syndrome") suffer from very severe injury with poor prognosis and a high morbidity in survivors.[178] Controlled trials of therapy in the various conditions are made difficult by the very small numbers of patients seen in each centre. As with adults, there is a wide diversity of opinion on the use of barbiturate coma, steroids, and mannitol. Mannitol induced hyperosmolarity greater than 320 mosm/L seems to be well tolerated in children.[174]

Management of raised intracranial pressure – conclusions

Conscious patient

- Diagnosis based on suspicious history (novel headaches, nausea, vomiting, visual blurring/obscurations, diplopia) with or without papilloedema on examination

Any patient with drowsiness or fluctuation in level of consciousness or visual obscurations merits emergency referral to neurosurgery

- Definitive investigation by CT scan combined with general medical assessment including chest radiograph

Never perform a lumbar puncture in a patient with suspected raised ICP, even if papilloedema is absent, until a CT scan has shown no evidence of either a mass lesion or diffuse brain swelling

- Management depends on the presumptive diagnosis after CT and proceeds in consultation with neurosurgery; for example, space occupying lesion:

  - tumours: dexamethasone, tissue diagnosis and excision, radiotherapy, chemotherapy as appropriate
  - abscess: aspiration/excision

- Hydrocephalus: CSF shunt with or without prior ICP monitoring/ CSF infusion studies
- Benign intracranial hypertension: referral to combined neurosurgery/neuro-ophthalmology service for CSF monitoring, diuretics/steroids/diet for mild cases. CSF shunt/optic nerve sheath fenestration for severe/refractory cases

Unconscious patient where intracranial catastrophe suspected (for causes see Box 7.1)
Emergency resuscitation for patients no longer obeying commands

- Intubation and ventilation
- Intravenous mannitol (0·2 ml/kg) when patient deteriorating
- Definitive investigation:

  - CT scan in combination with general medical assessment and consideration of any available history
  - intracranial pressure monitoring

Management of raised intracranial pressure

- Institute specific treatment for aetiology (Box 7.1)
- Mass lesions:

- — "lumpectomy"
- — aspiration of cysts/abscesses

- Hydrocephalus: external ventricular drainage:

  - — establish CSF drainage if possible even where no hydrocephalus despite technical difficulties

- Cerebral oedema and brain swelling:

  - — dexamethasone for tumours only, not for trauma
  - — occasionally abscesses

- Maintain cerebral perfusion pressure ≥70 mmHg
- Maintain intracranial pressure ≤25 mmHg:

  - — avoid problems exacerbating raised intracranial pressure (Box 7.4)
  - — nurse at 30 degrees head up
  - — sedation, analgesic, neuromuscular blockade
  - — optimal ventilation ($Pa\text{CO}_2$ 4·5–4·0 kPa)
  - — check for positive end expiratory pressure/venous obstruction
  - — treat seizure activity vigorously
  - — mild hypothermia
  - — boluses of 20% mannitol 2 ml/kg (to plasma osmolality of 310 mmol/L)
  - — consider intravenous anaesthetic to reduce cerebral metabolic rate of oxygen, such as propofol 2–5 mg/kg per hour
  - — consider surgical decompression (remove bone flap/contused temporal or frontal lobe)

- Ensure adequate mean arterial pressure:

  - — adequate hydration
  - — avoid excessive sedation
  - — optimal volume status (right arterial pressure/pulmonary capillary wedge pressure monitoring)
  - — consider vasoactive agents (norepinephrine, dopamine, or phenylephrine)

- Does the patient need rescanning? Reaccumulation of clot/hydrocephalus

Acknowledgement

We are indebted to Dr JM Turner, Mr E Guazzo, and Mr P Kirkpatrick for their comments on the manuscript.

References

1 Jennett B, Teasdale G. *Management of head injuries*. Philadelphia: FA Davies, 1981.
2 Miller JD, Jones PA, Dearden NM, Tocher JL. Progress in the management of head injury. *Br J Surg* 1992;**79**:60–4.
3 Pickard JD, Bailey S, Sanderson H, Rees M, Garfield JS. Steps towards cost–benefit analysis of regional neurosurgical care. *Br Med J* 1990;**301**: 629–35.
4 Minns RA. Problems of intracranial pressure in childhood. *Clinics in developmental medicine*, 113/114. London: MacKeith Press, 1991.
5 Marmarou A, Maset AL, Ward JD, *et al*. Contribution of CSF and vascular factors to elevation of intracranial pressure in severely head-injured patients. *J Neurosurg* 1987;**66**:883–90.
6 Saul TG, Ducker TB. Effect of intracranial pressure monitoring and aggressive treatment on mortality in severe head injury. *J Neurosurg* 1982;**56**:498–503.
7 Langfitt TW. Increased intracranial pressure. *Clin Neurosurg* 1969;**16**: 436–71.
8 Miller JD, ed. Normal and increased intracranial pressure. In: *Northfield's surgery of the central nervous system*, 2nd edn. London: Blackwell, 1987;7–57.
9 Miller JD, Dearden NM. Measurement, analysis and the management of raised intracranial pressure. In: Teasdale GM, Miller JD, eds. *Current neurosurgery*. Edinburgh: Churchill Livingstone, 1992;119–56.
10 Czosnyka M, Richards HK, Czosnyka Z, Piechnik S, Pickard JD. Vascular components of cerebrospinal fluid compensation. *J Neurosurg* 1999;**90**: 752–9.
11 Welch K. The intracranial pressure in infants. *J Neurosurg* 1980;**52**:693–9.
12 Lundberg N. Continuous recording and control of ventricular fluid pressure in neurosurgical practice. *Acta Psych Neurol Scand* 1960;**36**(suppl 149):1–193.
13 Avezaat CJJ, von Eijndhoven JHM, Wyper DJ. Cerebrospinal fluid pulse pressure and intracranial volume–pressure relationships. *J Neurol Neurosurg Psychiatry* 1979;**42**:687–700.
14 Lofgren J, von Essen C, Zwetnow NN. The pressure–volume curve of the cerebrospinal fluid space in dogs. *Acta Neurol Scand* 1973;**49**:557–74.
15 Rosner MJ, Becker DP. Origins and evolution of plateau waves. Experimental observations and theoretical model. *J Neurosurg* 1984;**60**: 312–24.
16 Czosnyka M, Smielewski P, Piechnik S, *et al*. Hemodynamic characterisation of intracranial pressure plateau waves in head injured patients. *J Neurosurg* 1999;**91**:11–19.
17 Newell DW, Aaslid R, Stooss R, Reulen HJ. The relationship of blood flow velocity fluctuations to intracranial pressure B waves. *J Neurosurg* 1992;**76**:415–21.
18 Kirkham FJ, Levin SD, Padaychee TS, *et al*. Transcranial pulsed Doppler ultrasound findings in brainstem death. *J Neurol Neurosurg Psychiatry* 1987;**50**:1504–13.
19 Hassler W, Steinmetz H, Pirschel J. Transcranial Doppler study of intracranial circulatory arrest. *J Neurosurg* 1989;**71**:195–201.
20 Obrist WD, Langfitt TW, Jaggi JL, *et al*. Cerebral blood flow and metabolism in comatose patients with acute head injury. Relationship to intracranial hypertension. *J Neurosurg* 1984;**61**:241–55.
21 Bingham RM, Procaccio F, Prior PF, Hinds CJ. Cerebral electrical activity influences the effects of etomidate on cerebral perfusion pressure in traumatic coma. *Br J Anaesth* 1985;**57**:843–8.

22   Nordstrom CH, Messeter K, Sundbarg G, et al. Cerebral blood flow, vasoreactivity and oxygen consumption during barbiturate therapy in severe traumatic brain lesions. *J Neurosurg* 1988;**68**:424–31.

23   Czosnyka M, Piechnik S, Richards HK, Kirkpatrick P, Smielewski P, Pickard JD. Contribution of mathematical modelling to the bedside tests of cerebrovascular autoregulation. *J Neurol Neurosurg Psychiatry* 1997;**63**:721–31.

24   Piechnik SK, Czosnyka M, Harris NG, Minhas PS, Pickard JD. A model of the cerebral and cerebrospinal fluid circulations to examine asymmetry in cerebrovascular reactivity. *J Cereb Blood Flow Metab* 2001; **21**:182–92.

25   Ursino M. A mathematical study of human intracranial hydrodynamics. Part 1: The cerebrospinal fluid pulse pressure. *Ann Biomed Eng* 1988;**16**:379–401.

26   Czosnyka M, Harris NG, Pickard JD. Carbon dioxide cerebrovascular reactivity as a function of perfusion pressure – a modelling study. *Acta Neurochir (Wien)* 1993;**121**:159–65.

27   Guillaume J, Janny P. Manometrie intracranienne continué interest de la methode et premiers resultants. *Revue Neurol* 1951;**84**:131–42.

28   Katzman R, Hussey F. A simple constant-infusion manometric test for measurement of CSF absorption. I Rationale and method. *Neurology* 1970;**20**:534–44.

29   Borgesen SE, Gjerris F. The predictive value of conductance to outflow of CSF in normal pressure hydrocephalus. *Brain* 1982;**105**:65–86.

30   Avezaat CJJ, Eijndhoven JHM. Cerebrospinal fluid pulse pressure and craniospinal dynamics. A theoretical, clinical and experimental study (thesis). The Hague: Jongbloed A, 1984.

31   Ekstedt J. CSF hydrodynamic studies in man. Method of constant pressure CSF infusion. *J Neurol Neurosurg Psychiatry* 1977;**40**:105–19.

32   Marmarou A, Shulman K, Rosende RM. A non-linear analysis of CSF system and intracranial pressure dynamics. *J Neurosurg* 1978;**48**:332–44.

33   Czosnyka M, Whitehouse H, Smielewski P, Simac S, Pickard JD. Testing of cerebrospinal compensatory reserve in shunted and non-shunted patients: a guide to interpretation based on observational study. *J Neurol Neurosurg Psychiatry* 1996;**60**:549–58.

34   Boon AJ, Tans JT, Delwel EJ, et al. Dutch normal-pressure hydrocephalus study: prediction of outcome after shunting by resistance to outflow of cerebrospinal fluid. *J Neurosurg* 1997;**87**:687–93.

35   Frieden H, Ekstedt J. Instrumentation for cerebrospinal fluid hydrodynamic studies in man. *Med Biol Eng Comput* 1982;**20**:167–80.

36   Raabe A, Czosnyka M, Piper I, Seifert V. Monitoring of intracranial compliance: correction for a change in body position. *Acta Neurochir (Wien)* 1999;**141**:31–6.

37   Pickard JD, Teasdale G, Matheson M, et al. Intraventricular pressure waves – the best predictive test for shunting in normal pressure hydrocephalus. In: Shulman K, Marmarou A, Miller JD, et al. eds. *Intracranial pressure*, IV. Berlin: Springer-Verlag, 1980;498–500.

38   Symon L, Dorsch NWC, Stephens RJ. Pressure waves in so-called low-pressure hydrocephalus. *Lancet* 1972;**ii**:1291–2.

39   Robertson C, Narayan R, Contant C, et al. Clinical experience with continuous monitoring of intracranial compliance. *J Neurosurg* 1989;**71**:673–80.

40   Piper I, Miller JD, Dearden M, et al. System analysis of cerebrovascular pressure transmission: an observational study in head injured patients. *J Neurosurg* 1990;**73**:871–80.

41   Miller JD, Garibi J, Pickard JD. Induced changes in cerebrospinal fluid volume. Effects during continuous monitoring of ventricular fluid pressure. *Arch Neurol* 1973;**28**:265–9.

42　Smielewski P, Czosnyka M, Kirkpatrick P, Pickard JD. Evaluation of transient hyperaemic response test in head injured patients. *J Neurosurg* 1997;**86**:773–8.

43　Czosnyka M, Smielewski P, Kirkpatrick P, Menon DK, Pickard JD. Monitoring of cerebral autoregulation in head-injured patients. *Stroke* 1996;**27**:829–34.

44　Czosnyka M, Smielewski P, Kirkpatrick P, Laing RJ, Menon D, Pickard JD. Continuous assessment of the cerebral vasomotor reactivity in head injury. *Neurosurgery* 1997;**41**:11–19.

45　Czosnyka M, Guazzo E, Whitehouse H, *et al*. Significance of intracranial pressure waveform analysis after head injury. *Acta Neurochir (Wien)* 1996;**138**:531–42.

46　Aaslid R, Markwalder T-M, Nornes H. Non-invasive transcranial Doppler ultrasound recording of flow velocity in basal cerebral arteries. *J Neurosurg* 1982;**57**:769–74.

47　Newell DW, Aaslid R. *Transcranial Doppler*. New York: Raven Press, 1992.

48　Martin JL, Perry S, Pickard JD. Cerebral blood flow and Doppler flow velocity: different responses to three vasodilators. *J Cereb Blood Flow Metab* 1991;**11**(suppl 2):S455.

49　Chan KH, Miller JD, Dearden NM, Andrews PJD, Midgley S. The effect of cerebral perfusion pressure upon changes in middle cerebral artery flow velocity and jugular venous bulb oxygen saturation after severe head injury. *J Neurosurg* 1992;**77**:55–61.

50　Dewey RC, Pieper HP, Hunt WE. Experimental cerebral hemodynamics. Vasomotor tone, critical closing pressure, and vascular bed resistance. *Neurosurgery* 1974;**41**:597–606.

51　Czosnyka M, Smielewski P, Piechnik S, *et al*. Critical closing pressure in cerebrovascular circulation. *J Neurol Neurosurg Psychiatry* 1999;**66**:606–11.

52　Aaslid R, Lundar T, Lindegaard K-F, *et al*. Estimation of cerebral perfusion pressure from arterial blood pressure and transcranial Doppler recordings. In: Miller JD, Teasdale GM, Rowan JO, Galbraith SL, Mendelow AD, eds. *Intracranial pressure*, VI. Berlin: Springer Verlag, 1986;229–31.

53　Czosnyka M, Matta BF, Smielewski P, Kirkpatrick P, Pickard JD. Cerebral perfusion pressure in head-injured patients: a non-invasive assessment using transcranial Doppler ultrasonography. *J Neurosurg* 1998;**88**:802–8.

54　Schmidt EA, Czosnyka M, Gooskens I, *et al*. Preliminary experience of the estimation of cerebral perfusion pressure using trascranial Doppler ultrasonography. *J Neurol Neurosurg Psychiatry* 2001;**70**:198–204.

55　Schmidt B, Czosnyka M, Schwarze JJ, *et al*. Cerebral vasodilatation causing acute intracranial hypertension: a method for non-invasive assessment. *J Cereb Blood Flow Metab* 1999;**19**:990–6.

56　Schoser BG, Riemenschneider N, Hansen HC. The impact of raised intracranial pressure on cerebral venous hemodynamics: a prospective venous transcranial Doppler ultrasonography study. *J Neurosurg* 1999;**91**: 744–9.

57　Petkus V, Ragauskas A, Jurkonis R. Investigation of intracranial media ultrasonic monitoring model. *Ultrasonics* 2002;**40**:829–33.

58　Torikoshi S, Wilson MH, Ballard RE, *et al*. Ultrasound measurement of transcranial distance during head-down tilt. *J Gravit Physiol* 1995;**2**:145–6.

59　Reid A, Marchbanks RJ, Martin R, Pickard JD, Bateman N, Brightwell R. Mean intracranial pressure monitoring by an audiological technique – a pilot study. *J Neurol Neurosurg Psychiatry* 1989;**52**:610–12.

60　Wyatt JS, Cope M, Delpy DT, Wray S, Reynolds EOR. Quantification of cerebral oxygenation and haemodynamics in sick newborn infants by near infrared spectroscopy. *Lancet* 1986;**ii**:1063–6.

61 Filippi R, Reisch R, Mauer D, Perneczky A. Brain tissue po_2 related to $Sjvo_2$, ICP, and CPP in severe brain injury. *Neurosurg Rev* 2000;**23**:94–7.

62 Goodman JC, Valadka AB, Gopinath SP, Uzura M, Grossman RG, Robertson CS. Simultaneous measurement of cortical potassium, calcium, and magnesium levels measured in head injured patients using microdialysis with ion chromatography. *Acta Neurochir Suppl (Wien)* 1999;**75**:35–7.

63 Reinert M, Khaldi A, Zauner A, Doppenberg E, Choi S, Bullock R. High level of extracellular potassium and its correlates after severe head injury: relationship to high intracranial pressure. *J Neurosurg* 2000;**93**:800–7.

64 Guidelines of the Brain Trauma Foundation. Part 1: Guidelines for the management of penetrating brain injury. Introduction and methodology. *J Trauma* 2001;**51**:S3–6.

65 Campkin TV, Turner JM. *Neurosurgical anaesthesia and intensive care*, 2nd edn. London: Butterworth, 1986.

66 Eisenberg HM, Frankowski RF, Contant CF, Marshall LF, Walker MD. High-dose barbiturate control of elevated intracranial pressure in patients with severe head injury. *J Neurosurg* 1988;**69**:15–23.

67 Marmarou A, Anderson R, Ward J, *et al*. Impact of ICP instability and hypotension on outcome in patients with severe head trauma. *J Neurosurg* 1991;**75**:S159–66.

68 Bullock RM, Chesnut RM, Clifton GL, Ghajar J, Marion DW. Guidelines for the management of severe traumatic brain injury. *J Neurotrauma* 2000; **17**:451–554.

69 Ropper AH, O'Rourke D, Kennedy SK. Head position, intracranial pressure and compliance. *Neurology* 1982;**32**:1288–91.

70 Rosner MJ, Coley IB. Cerebral perfusion pressure, intracranial pressure and head elevation. *J Neurosurg* 1986;**65**:636–41.

71 Feldman Z, Kanter MJ, Robertson CS, *et al*. Effect of head elevation on intracranial pressure, cerebral perfusion pressure and cerebral blood flow in head injured patients. *J Neurosurg* 1992;**76**:207–11.

72 Kanter MJ, Robertson CS, Sheinberg MA, *et al*. Changes in cerebral hemodynamics with head elevated vs head flat. In: Avezaat C, ed. *Intracranial pressure*, VIII. Berlin: Springer-Verlag, 1993;429–32.

73 Asgeirsson B, Grande PO, Nordstrom CH. A new therapy of post-trauma brain oedema based on haemodynamic principles for brain volume regulation. *Intensive Care Med* 1994;**20**:260–7.

74 Juul N, Morris GF, Marshall SB, Marshall LF. Intracranial hypertension and cerebral perfusion pressure: influence on neurological deterioration and outcome in severe head injury. The Executive Committee of the International Selfotel Trial. *J Neurosurg* 2000;**92**:1–6.

75 Robertson CS. Management of cerebral perfusion pressure after traumatic brain injury. *Anesthesiology* 2001;**95**:1513–17.

76 Rosner MJ, Rosner SD, Johnson AH. Cerebral perfusion pressure: management protocol and clinical results. *J Neurosurg* 1995;**83**:949–62.

77 Eker C, Asgeirsson B, Grande PO, Schalen W, Nordstrom CH. Improved outcome after severe head injury with a new therapy based on principles for brain volume regulation and preserved microcirculation. *Crit Care Med* 1998;**26**:1881–6.

78 Clifton GL, Miller ER, Choi SC, Levin HS. Fluid thresholds and outcome from severe brain injury. *Crit Care Med* 2002;**30**:739–45.

79 Nelson RJ, Roberts J, Rubin C, Walker V, Ackery DM, Pickard JD. Association of hypovolaemia after subarachnoid haemorrhage with computer tomographic scan evidence of raised intracranial pressure. *Neurosurgery* 1991;**29**:178–82.

80 Hasan D, Vermeulen M, Wijdicks EFM, *et al*. Effect of fluid intake and hypertensive treatment on cerebral ischaemia after subarachnoid haemorrhage. *Stroke* 1989;**20**:1511–15.

81 Harrigan MR. Cerebral salt wasting syndrome: a review. *Neurosurgery* 1996;**38**:152–60.

82 Muizelaar JP. Induced arterial hypertension in the treatment of high intracranial pressure. In: Hoff JT, Betz AL, eds. *Intracranial pressure* VII. Berlin: Springer Verlag, 1989;508–10.

83 Rosner MJ, Rosner SD. Cerebral perfusion pressure management of head injury. In: Avezaat C, ed. *Intracranial pressure*, VIII. Berlin: Springer Verlag, 1993;540–3.

84 Shimoda M, Oda S, Tsugane R, Sato O. Intracranial complications of hypervolemic therapy in patients with delayed ischemic deficit attributed to vasospasm. *J Neurosurg* 1993;**78**:423–9.

85 Contant CF, Valadka AB, Gopinath SP, Hannay HJ, Robertson CS. Adult respiratory distress syndrome: a complication of induced hypertension after severe head injury. *J Neurosurg* 2001;**95**:560–8.

86 Kassell NF, Peerless SJ, Durward QJ, Beck DW, Drake CG, Adams HP. Treatment of ischemic deficits from vasospasm with intravascular volume expansion and induced arterial hypertension. *Neurosurgery* 1982;**11**:337–43.

87 Adams HP Jr, Brott TG, Crowell RM, *et al*. Guidelines for the management of patients with acute ischemic stroke. A statement for healthcare professionals from a special writing group of the Stroke Council, American Heart Association. *Circulation* 1994;**90**:1588–601.

88 Fitch W, Pickard JD, Tamura A, Graham DI. Effects of hypotension induced with sodium nitroprusside on the cerebral circulation before, and one week after, the subarachnoid injection of blood. *J Neurol Neurosurg Psychiatry* 1988;**51**:88–93.

89 Chesnut RM, Marshall LF, Klauber MR, *et al*. The role of secondary brain injury in determining outcome from severe head injury. *J Trauma* 1993; **34**:216–22.

90 Myers RE. Anoxic brain pathology and blood glucose. *Neurology* 1976; **34**:345.

91 Marie C, Bralet J. Blood glucose level and morphological brain damage following cerebral ischaemia. *Cerebrovasc Brain Metab Rev* 1991;**3**:29–38.

92 Murphy PG, Myers DS, Davies MJ, *et al*. The antioxidant potential of propofol (2,6-diisopropylphenol). *Br J Anaesth* 1992;**68**:613–18.

93 Wolf A, Weir P, Segar P, Stone J, Shield J. Impaired fatty acid oxidation in propofol infusion syndrome. *Lancet* 2001;**357**:606–7.

94 Cremer OL, Moons KG, Bouman EA, Kruijswijk JE, de Smet AM, Kalkman CJ. Long-term propofol infusion and cardiac failure in adult head-injured patients. *Lancet* 2001;**357**:117–18.

95 Varelas PN, Mirski MA. Seizures in the adult intensive care unit. *J Neurosurg Anesthesiol* 2001;**13**:163–75.

96 Munch EC, Bauhuf C, Horn P, Roth HR, Schmiedek P, Vajkoczy P. Therapy of malignant intracranial hypertension by controlled lumbar cerebrospinal fluid drainage. *Crit Care Med* 2001;**29**:976–81.

97 Sullivan LP, Stears JC, Ringer SP. Resolution of syringomyelia and chiari malformation by ventriculo-atrial shunting in a patient with pseudotumour cerebri and a lumbo-peritoneal shunt. *Neurosurgery* 1988;**22**:744–7.

98 Editorial. Cranial decompression. *Lancet* 1988;**i**:1204.

99 Guerra WK, Gaab MR, Dietz H, *et al*. Surgical decompression for traumatic brain swelling: indications and results. *J Neurosurg* 1999;**90**:187–96.

100 Gower DJ, Lee KS, McWhorter JM. Role of subtemporal decompression in severe closed head injury. *Neurosurgery* 1988;**23**:417–22.

101 Munch E, Horn P, Schurer L, Piepgras A, Paul T, Schmiedek P. Management of severe traumatic brain injury by decompressive craniectomy. *Neurosurgery* 2000;**47**:315–22; discussion 322–13.

102 Rittierodt M, Gaab MR. Traumatic brain swelling and operative decompression: a prospective investigation. In: Avezaat C, ed. *Intracranial pressure,* VIII. Berlin: Springer Verlag, 1993.

103 Schwab S, Steiner T, Aschoff A, *et al.* Early hemicraniectomy in patients with complete middle cerebral artery infarction. *Stroke* 1998;**29**: 1888–93.

104 Higgins JN, Owler BK, Cousins C, Pickard JD. Venous sinus stenting for refractory benign intracranial hypertension. *Lancet* 2002;**359**:228–30.

105 Kirkham FJ, Neville BGR. Successful management of severe intracranial hypertension by surgical decompression. *Dev Med Child Neurol* 1986;**28**:506–9.

106 Ravassin P, Abou-Madi M, Archer D, *et al.*Changes in CSF pressure after mannitol in patients with and without elevated CSF pressure. *J Neurosurg* 1988;**69**:869–76.

107 Smith HP, Kelly DL, McWhorter JM, *et al.* Comparison of mannitol regimes in patients with severe head injury undergoing intracranial pressure monitoring. *J Neurosurg* 1986;**65**:820–4.

108 Roberts PA, Pollay M, Engles C, Pendleton B, Reynolds E, Stevens FA. Effect on intracranial pressure of furosemide combined with varying doses and administration rates of mannitol. *J Neurosurg* 1987;**66**: 440–6.

109 James HE, Harbaugh RD, Marshall LF, Shapiro HM. The response to multiple therapeutics in experimental vasogenic edema. In: Shulman K, Marmarou A, Miller JD, *et al.*, eds. *Intracranial pressure,* IV. Berlin: Springer Verlag, 1980;272–6.

110 Rosenberg GA. *Brain fluids and metabolism.* Oxford: Oxford University Press, 1990.

111 Inao S, Kuchiwaki H, Wachi A, *et al.* Effect of mannitol on intracranial pressure – volume status and cerebral haemodynamics in brain oedema. *Acta Neurochir (Wien)* 1990;**51**(suppl):401–3.

112 Bell BA, Smith MA, Kean DM, *et al.* Brain water measured by magnetic resonance imaging: correlation with direct estimation and change following mannitol and dexamethasone. *Lancet* 1987;**i**:66–9.

113 Kaufmann AM, Cardoso ER. Delayed cerebral accumulation of mannitol in vasogenic edema. In: Avezaat C, ed. *Intracranial pressure,* VIII. Berlin: Springer Verlag, 1993;592–5.

114 Burke AM, Quest DO, Chien S, *et al.* The effects of mannitol on blood viscosity. *J Neurosurg* 1981;**55**:550–3.

115 Miller JD, Leech P. Effects of mannitol and steroid therapy in intracranial volume pressure relationships. *J Neurosurg* 1975;**42**:274–81.

116 Muizelaar JP, Wei EP, Kontos HA, Becker DP. Mannitol causes compensatory cerebral vasoconstriction and vasodilatation in response to blood viscosity changes. *J Neurosurg* 1983;**59**:822–8.

117 Auer LM, Haselsberger K. Effect of intravenous mannitol on cat pial arteries and veins during normal and elevated intracranial pressure. *Neurosurgery* 1987;**21**:142–6.

118 Harrison MJG. Influence of haemocrit in the cerebral circulation. *Cerebrovasc Brain Metab Rev* 1989;**1**:55–67.

119 Brown MM, Wade JPH, Marshall J. Fundamental importance of arterial oxygen content in the regulation of cerebral blood flow in man. *Brain* 1985;**108**:81–93.

120 Purves MJ. *The physiology of the cerebral circulation.* Cambridge: Cambridge University Press, 1972.

121 Bruce DA, Langfitt TW, Miller JD, *et al*. Regional cerebral blood flow, intracranial pressure, and brain metabolism in comatose patients. *J Neurosurg* 1973;**38**:131–44.

122 Johnston IH, Harper AM. The effect of mannitol on cerebral blood flow. An experimental study. *J Neurosurg* 1973;**38**:461–71.

123 Mendelow AD, Teasdale GM, Russell T, *et al*. Effect of mannitol on cerebral blood flow and cerebral perfusion pressure in human head injury. *J Neurosurg* 1985;**63**:43–8.

124 Jafar JJ, Johns LM, Mullan SF. The effect of mannitol on cerebral blood flow. *J Neurosurg* 1986;**64**:754–9.

125 Muizelaar JP, Lutz HA, Becker DP. Effect of mannitol on intracranial pressure and cerebral blood flow and correlation with pressure autoregulation in severely head-injured patients. *J Neurosurg* 1984;**61**:700–6.

126 Meyer FB, Anderson RE, Sundt TM, Yaksh TL. Treatment of experimental focal cerebral ischaemia with mannitol. Assessment by intracellular pH, cortical blood flow and EEG. *J Neurosurg* 1987;**66**:109–15.

127 Takagi H, Saito T, Kitahara T, Morii SM, Ohwada J, Yada K. The mechanism of the intracranial pressure reducing effect of mannitol. In: Ishii S, Nagai H, Brock M, eds. *Intracranial pressure, V.* Berlin: Springer Verlag, 1983;729–33.

128 Qureshi AI, Suarez JI. Use of hypertonic saline solutions in treatment of cerebral edema and intracranial hypertension. *Crit Care Med* 2000;**28**: 3301–13.

129 Shiozaki T, Sugimoto H, Taneda M, *et al*. Effect of mild hypothermia on uncontrollable intracranial hypertension after severe head injury. *J Neurosurg* 1993;**79**:363–8.

130 Marion DW, Penrod LE, Kelsey SF, *et al*. Treatment of traumatic brain injury with moderate hypothermia. *N Engl J Med* 1997;**336**:540–6.

131 Jiang J, Yu M, Zhu C. Effect of long-term mild hypothermia therapy in patients with severe traumatic brain injury: 1-year follow-up review of 87 cases. *J Neurosurg* 2000;**93**:546–9.

132 Clifton GL, Miller ER, Choi SC, *et al*. Lack of effect of induction of hypothermia after acute brain injury. *N Engl J Med* 2001;**344**:556–63.

133 Matsushita Y, Bramlett HM, Alonso O, Dietrich WD. Posttraumatic hypothermia is neuroprotective in a model of traumatic brain injury complicated by a secondary hypoxic insult. *Crit Care Med* 2001;**29**: 2060–6.

134 Shiozaki T, Hayakata T, Taneda M, *et al*. A multicenter prospective randomized controlled trial of the efficacy of mild hypothermia for severely head injured patients with low intracranial pressure. Mild Hypothermia Study Group in Japan. *J Neurosurg* 2001;**94**:50–4.

135 Muizelaar JP, Marmarou A, Ward JD, *et al*. Adverse effects of prolonged hyperventilation in patients with severe head injury: a randomized clinical trial. *J Neurosurg* 1991;**75**:731–9.

136 Diringer MN, Videen TO, Yundt K, *et al*. Regional cerebrovascular and metabolic effects of hyperventilation after severe traumatic brain injury. *J Neurosurg* 2002;**96**:103–8.

137 Coles JP, Minhas PS, Fryer TD, *et al*. Effect of hyperventilation on cerebral blood flow in traumatic head injury: clinical relevance and monitoring correlates. *Crit Care Med* 2002;**30**:1950–9.

138 Cruz J. The first decade of continuous monitoring of jugular bulb oxyhemoglobinsaturation: management strategies and clinical outcome. *Crit Care Med* 1998;**26**:344–51.

139 Obrist WD, Langfitt TW, Jaggi JL, Cruz J, Gennarelli TA. Cerebral blood flow and metabolism in comatose patients with acute head injury. Relationship to intracranial hypertension. *J Neurosurg* 1984:**61**:241–53.

140   Muizelaar JP, van der Poel HG, Li Z, Kontos HA, Levasseur JE. Pial arteriolar vessel diameter and CO_2 reactivity during prolonged hyperventilation in the rabbit. *J Neurosurg* 1988;**69**:923-7.

141   Enevoldsen EM, Jensen FT. Autoregulation and CO_2 responses of cerebral blood flow in patients with acute severe head injury. *J Neurosurg* 1978;**48**:689-703.

142   Paolin A, Rodriguez G, Betetto M, Simini G. Cerebral hemodynamic response to CO_2 after severe head injury: clinical and prognostic implications. *J Trauma* 1998;**44**:495-500.

143   Enevoldsen EM, Cold G, Jensen FT, *et al.* Dynamic changes in regional cerebral blood flow, intraventricular pressure, CSF pH and lactate levels during the acute phase of head injury. *J Neurosurg* 1976;**44**:191-214.

144   De Salles AAF, Kontos HA, Becker DP, *et al.* Prognostic significance of ventricular CSF lactic acidosis in severe head injury. *J Neurosurg* 1986;**65**:615-24.

145   Akiota T, Ota K, Matsumato A, *et al.* The effect of THAM on acute intracranial hypertension. An experimental and clinical study. In: Beks JWF, Bosch DA, Brock M, eds. *Intracranial pressure, III.* Berlin: Springer Verlag, 1976;219-33.

146   Gordan E, Rossanda M. Further studies in cerebrospinal fluid acid-base status in patients with brain lesions. *Acta Anaesth Scand* 1970;**14**:97-109.

147   Gaab MR, Seegers K, Goetz C. THAM (tromethamine, "tris-buffer"): effective therapy of traumatic brain swelling. In: Hoff JT, Betz AL, eds. *Intracranial pressure, VII.* Berlin: Springer Verlag, 1989;616-19.

148   Wolf AL, Levi L, Marmarou A, *et al.* Effect of THAM upon outcome in severe head injury: a randomized prospective clinical trial. *J Neurosurg* 1993;**78**:54-9.

149   Schwartz M, Tator CH, Rowed DW, *et al.* The University of Toronto Head Injury Treatment Study: a prospective randomized comparison of pento-barbitat and mannitol. *Can J Neurol Sci* 1984;**11**:434-40.

150   Ward JD, Becker DP, Miller JD, *et al.* Failure of prophylactic barbiturate coma in the treatment of severe head injury. *J Neurosurg* 1985;**62**:383-8.

151   Eisenberg HM, Frankowski RF, Condant CG, *et al.* High dose barbiturate control of elevated intracranial pressure in patients with severe head injury. *J Neurosurg* 1988;**69**:15-23.

152   Cooper PR, Moody S, Clark WK, *et al.* Dexamethasone and severe head injury: a prospective double blind trial. *J Neurosurg* 1979;**51**:307-16.

153   Saul TF, Ducker TB, Salomon M, *et al.* Steroids in severe head injury. A prospective randomized clinical trial. *J Neurosurg* 1981;**54**:596-600.

154   Braakman R, Schouten HJD, Dishoeck BMV, Minderhoud JM. Megadose steroids in severe head injury: results of a prospective double blind clinical trial. *J Neurosurg* 1983;**58**:326-30.

155   Giannotta SL, Weiss MH, Apuzzo MLJ, Martin E. High dose glucocorticoids in the management of severe head injury. *Neurosurgery* 1984;**15**:497-501.

156   Dearden NM, Gibson JB, McDowall DG, *et al.* Effect of high dose dexamethasone on outcome from severe head injury. *J Neurosurg* 1986;**64**:81-8.

157   Alderson P, Roberts I. Corticosteroids in acute traumatic brain injury: systematic review of randomised controlled trials. *Br Med J* 1997;**314**:1855-9.

158   Floyd RA, Carney JM. Protection against oxidative damage to CNS by α-phenyl-tert-butyl nitrone and other spin-trapping agents: a novel series of non-lipid free radical scavengers. In: Marangos PJ, Lal H, eds. *Emerging strategies in neuroprotection.* Boston: Birkauser, 1992;252-72.

159   Halliwell B, Gutteridge JMC. *Free radicals in biology and medicine.* Oxford: Clarendon Press, 1985.

160 Hall ED. Lazaroids: novel cerebroprotective antioxidants. In: Marangos PJ, Lal H, eds. *Emerging strategies in neuroprotection*. Boston: Birkauser, 1992;224–37.

161 Roberts I. Aminosteroids for acute traumatic brain injury. *Cochrane Database Syst Rev* 2000;CD001527.

162 Bath PM, Iddenden R, Bath FJ, Orgogozo JM. Tirilazad for acute ischaemic stroke. *Cochrane Database Syst Rev* 2001;CD002087.

163 Marshall LF, Maas AIR, Marshall SB, *et al*. A multicentre trial on the efficacy of using tirilazad mesylate in cases of head injury. *J Neurosurg* 1998;**89**:519–25.

164 Kassell NF, Haley EC Jr, Apperson-Hansen C, Alves WM. A randomised double-blind, vehicle controlled trial of tirilazad mesylate in patients with aneurysmal subarachnoid haemorrhage: a comparative study in Europe/Australia/New Zealand. *J Neurosurg* 1996;**84**:221–8.

165 Jensen K, Öhrstrom J, Cold GE, Astrup J. The effects of indomethacin on intracranial pressure, cerebral blood flow and cerebral metabolism in patients with severe head injury and intracranial hypertension. *Acta Neurochir (Wien)* 1991;**108**:116–21.

166 Edwards AD, Wyatt JS, Richardson C, *et al*. Effects of indomethacin on cerebral haemodynamics in very preterm infants. *Lancet* 1990;**335**:1491–5.

167 Muizelaar JP, Marmarou A, Young HA, *et al*. Improving the outcome of severe head injury with the oxygen radical scavenger polyethylene glycol-conjugated superoxide dismutase: a Phase II trial. *J Neurosurg* 1993;**78**:375–82.

168 MRC. *Neuroprotection in acute brain injury after trauma and stroke*. London: MRC 1998;1–61.

169 Teasdale GM, Graham DI. Craniocerebral trauma: protection and retrieval of the neuronal population after injury. *Neurosurgery* 1998;**43**:723–38.

170 Bedford RF, Persing JA, Pobereskin L, Butler A. Lidocaine or thiopental for rapid control of intracranial hypertension? *Anaesth Analg* 1980;**59**:435–7.

171 Levene M. *Neonatal neurology*. Edinburgh: Churchill Livingstone, 1987.

172 Brace DA, Alavi A, Bilaniuk L, *et al*. Diffuse cerebral swelling following head injuries in children: the syndrome of "malignant brain edema". *J Neurosurg* 1981;**54**:170–8.

173 Aldrich EF, Eisenberg HM, Saydjari C, *et al*. Diffuse brain swelling in severely head-injured children. *J Neurosurg* 1992;**76**:450–4.

174 Mazzola CA, Adelson PD. Critical care management of head trauma in children. *Crit Care Med* 2002;**30**:S393–401.

175 Downard C, Hulka F, Mullins RJ, *et al*. Relationship of cerebral perfusion pressure and survival in pediatric brain-injured patients. *J Trauma* 2000;**49**:654–8; discussion 658–9.

176 Kaiser G, Pfenninger J. Effect of neurointensive care upon outcome following severe head injuries in childhood – a preliminary report. *Neuropediatrics* 1984;**15**:68–75.

177 Ong LC, Dhillon MK, Selladurai BM, Maimunah A, Lye MS. Early post-traumatic seizures in children: clinical and radiological aspects of injury. *J Paediatr Child Health* 1996;**32**:173–6.

178 Duhaime AC, Christian C, Moss E, Seidl T. Long-term outcome in infants with the shaking-impact syndrome. *Pediatr Neurosurg* 1996;**24**:292–8.

8: Management of subarachnoid haemorrhage

THOMAS A KOPITNIK, CAROL CROFT,
SHAWN MOORE, JONATHAN A WHITE

Introduction

The brain is unique in its structure and development. Unlike other organ systems in which the vascular tree arborises within the organs they perfuse, the cerebral blood vessels form a collateral network along the base of the brain with only the smaller vessels penetrating the brain substance. The larger vessels are contained within the subarachnoid space, a well formed compartment which contains circulating cerebrospinal fluid (CSF).[1-3] Sheets of arachnoid partition the subarachnoid space into distinct chambers called cisterns. It is within this fragile network of arachnoidal reflections that a subarachnoid haemorrhage may occur.

Aetiologies

Subarachnoid haemorrhage (SAH) is a multiaetiological condition. The 1966 Cooperative Study recorded 6368 patients with spontaneous SAH over an eight year period. Of these, 51% had cerebral aneurysms.[4] Stehbens reviewed 11 series from 1950 to 1969 and found cerebral aneurysms to be the cause of SAH in 18–76% of cases.[5] Other aetiologies included trauma, cerebral and spinal vascular malformations, intrinsic and extrinsic cranial and spinal neoplasms, pathological and iatrogenic coagulopathy, vasculitis, collagen vascular disease, sickle cell anaemia, cerebral infarction, and drug abuse.

Incidence

The reported incidence of SAH varies considerably on a geographic basis. In the United States SAH is the cause of death in 16 per 100 000 population,[6] while Japan reports rates of 25 deaths per 100 000 people.[7] Zimbabwe (formerly Rhodesia) reported only 3·5 deaths from SAH per 100 000 people per year.[8]

Demographics

The 1966 Cooperative Study of intracranial aneurysms and SAH found that 50% of subjects with aneurysmal SAH were female. Subarachnoid haemorrhage occurs more commonly in males under 40 and females over 50.[9] Regardless of aetiology, SAH most frequently occurs between ages 40 and 60, with the peak between 55 and 60 years of age. The peak incidence of SAH secondary to aneurysms occurred at slightly older ages than SAH from arteriovenous malformations (AVM), with 63% of first haemorrhagic episodes from AVMs occurring between 30 and 40.[10]

Timing

While SAH does not appear to have a consistent seasonal prevalence,[11] some authors have reported an increased incidence in spring and autumn.[12,13] Ohno reported a peak seasonal incidence in Japan in the winter months.[14-17] One third of patients develop SAH while asleep, one third during routine daily activities, and one third during strenuous activity. The International Cooperative Study on Intracranial Aneurysms found that from a statistical standpoint, bending and lifting activities have the highest association with SAH among those activities considered strenuous.[10]

Mortality

Ruptured cerebral aneurysm is the most common cause of non-traumatic SAH, although hypertensive SAH was the most common cause of early death in the Cooperative Study. Death rates from the initial aneurysmal haemorrhage range from 40% to 60%.[18-20] Freytag reported 250 consecutive deaths from

SAH and found that 60% were immediate while 20% were within 24 hours of the ictus. Only 11% of patients lived beyond 24 hours.[19]

Diagnosis

For the purposes of discussion we will divide SAH into two distinct categories of aneurysmal and non-aneurysmal SAH. Although some overlap exists in the medical management of SAH in both categories, aneurysmal SAH presents unique surgical management circumstances that will be discussed separately.

Signs and symptoms

Headaches occur in 85–95% of patients with SAH.[21–23] At least one third of patients have a minor leak, referred to as a sentinel haemorrhage, which may occur hours or days prior to a major aneurysmal haemorrhage.[24] Many authors have emphasised that a sudden and unusual headache may herald a haemorrhage in the near future.[21–27] In 2621 cases reviewed by the 1966 Cooperative Study, the following signs and symptoms were present immediately prior to a major SAH: headache (48%), orbital pain (7%), diplopia (4%), ptosis (3%), visual loss (4%), seizures (4%), motor or sensory deficit (6%), dysphasia (2%), bruit (3%), dizziness (10%), and other (13%).[10,20]

A significant SAH usually presents with the sudden onset of intense headache followed by pain radiating into the occipital or cervical region. As blood enters the spinal canal, cervical pain or nuchal rigidity develops. The duration and intensity of nuchal rigidity varies between patients, but usually relates to the magnitude of the SAH. Signs and symptoms similar to infectious meningitis are typically seen with SAH, due to an inflammatory reaction of the leptomeninges to extravasated blood. Kernig's or Laségue's sign may be present if substantial meningeal irritation exists.

Other symptoms of SAH include photophobia, nausea, vomiting, lethargy, and altered mental status. Brief or permanent loss of consciousness occurs in the majority of patients suffering SAH. After the haemorrhage the patient may either regain normal mentation or remain lethargic, confused, or obtunded. Altered consciousness can be related to haematoma formation, hydrocephalus, increased intracranial pressure (ICP), post-haemorrhagic vasospasm, or electrolyte imbalances.[28] Other signs of neurological involvement include motor or sensory deficits, upper motor neuron reflex changes, visual field deficits, abnormal brain stem reflexes, and abnormal motor posturing. Less common causes of motor deficits include emboli from the aneurysm sac, brain compression by a large or giant aneurysm, or seizures. Seizures occur at the time of SAH in approximately 10% of patients,[29-32] but may be confused with tonic motor posturing during a severe SAH. Additional clinical signs of SAH that often accompany the presenting symptoms include mild hyperpyrexia, hypertension, and ophthalmological findings. Intraocular haemorrhages may occur in the vitreous or retina, but subhyaloid or preretinal haemorrhages are more indicative of SAH.[33,34] Subhyaloid haemorrhages appear as bright red, sharply demarcated regions adjacent to the optic disc.

Cranial nerve palsies can accompany SAH, especially in cases of posterior communicating and superior cerebellar artery aneurysms and less frequently with aneurysms of the carotid and basilar bifurcation, and the posterior cerebral and anterior choroidal arteries. Third cranial nerve palsy associated with aneurysmal SAH and aneurysm induced compression typically results in a dilated pupil, ptosis, and/or deficits in ocular motility. Compression of the third nerve within the cavernous sinus may present with a midpoint pupil secondary to compression of sympathetic fibres en route to the iris. Pain in the trigeminal distribution can result from SAH or aneurysmal nerve compression, but is rare and more commonly seen in association with cavernous carotid aneurysms. Abducens nerve palsy is frequently seen following SAH and is thought to be related to increased intracranial pressure and subsequent nerve traction from downward brain stem herniation.

A high level of suspicion is important when considering SAH. Shields noted that minor bleeds were often misdiagnosed as influenza, migraine, sinusitis, headache, stiff neck, and malingering.[35] Nearly 50% of patients with SAH enrolled in a recent international cooperative study had delays in excess of three days from onset of SAH to transfer to a

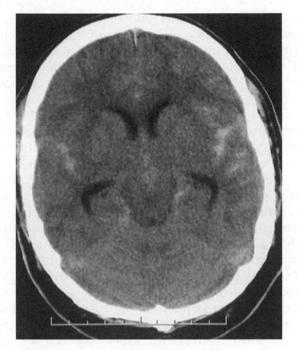

Figure 8.1   CT scan demonstrating diffuse SAH from ruptured basilar apex aneurysm

neurosurgical centre.[36] Kassell studied 150 consecutive patients with proven aneurysm rupture and found that only 38% were referred to neurosurgeons within 48 hours of the first symptoms of SAH. The most common cause for delay was physician misdiagnosis (37%), followed by administrative referral delays (23%).[37] Because delayed referral to a neurosurgical centre seriously affects patient outcome, education of primary care physicians towards rapid diagnosis and triage seems warranted.

Diagnostic tests

CT scanning of the brain is the procedure of choice for the diagnosis of SAH. The CT scan can demonstrate the magnitude and location of the SAH, give clues to probable aneurysm location, and assess ventricular size (Figure 8.1).

CT's success in detecting SAH is dependent upon the length of time between SAH and scan acquisition. Eighty-five per cent of patients scanned within 48 hours of SAH and 75% of patients scanned within five days will have detectable subarachnoid blood.[38-41] The distribution of blood on the CT scan may suggest the probable aneurysm location. Acute blood within the interhemispheric and supratentorial ventricular system is often the consequence of a ruptured anterior communicating artery aneurysm. Focal blood within the fourth ventricle suggests a vertebral or posterior inferior cerebellar artery (PICA) aneurysm. Intracerebral haematomas are most frequently seen with ruptured middle cerebral, internal carotid bifurcation, or distal anterior cerebral artery aneurysms. Inferior frontal lobe and interhemispheric flame shaped haematomas commonly occur with ruptured anterior communicating artery aneurysms and are a highly accurate CT scan finding for localising the source of the SAH.[42,43]

In 1980, Fisher developed a grading scale for the CT scan appearance of SAH dependent upon the severity and location of subarachnoid blood.[44] Grade I had no blood detectable, whereas grade II patients had a layer of blood less than 1 mm thick diffusely spread throughout the subarachnoid cisterns. Grade III patients had CT appearance of SAH greater than 1 mm thick and grade IV patients had intraventricular or intracerebral blood without significant subarachnoid blood. The Fisher grading system is used to relate the amount of subarachnoid blood on a CT scan to the probability of developing delayed ischaemia secondary to vasospasm. Grade I, II, and IV patients had no or minimal incidence of clinically significant vasospasm while grade III patients had a 95·8% incidence. These findings implicate blood breakdown products in the genesis of cerebral vasospasm. The greater the magnitude of subarachnoid clot, the higher the likelihood that delayed cerebral ischaemia from vasospasm will occur.

Visual examination of CSF obtained by lumbar puncture can confirm the diagnosis of SAH when the CT scan is negative. In 1901, Sicard found that yellow discoloration of CSF after centrifugation was a reliable diagnostic sign of previous SAH.[45] The term xanthochromia (xanthochromie) was first used in 1902 to describe the yellow colour of CSF in a case of pneumococcal meningitis and was later used in the 1920s to refer to the colour of CSF several hours after SAH.[46-50] The CSF supernatant does not demonstrate discoloration immediately following SAH, but only after red blood cells haemolyse and release oxyhaemoglobin. Xanthochromia can usually be detected four hours after SAH, becomes maximal one week after haemorrhage, and is usually undetected at three weeks.[51] If xanthochromia is present in the CSF, SAH has probably occurred. If a traumatic lumbar puncture is suspected, partial or total clearing of the CSF may occur during collection. In addition, bloody CSF allowed to stand undisturbed in a test tube will form a clot while blood from SAH will generally not. Repeat lumbar puncture hours following a traumatic tap will be of little diagnostic value, since blood contaminating the CSF will produce xanthochromia.

Lumbar puncture after SAH is not without risk. Duffy found that 13% of patients undergoing post-SAH lumbar puncture had significant neurological deterioration.[52] Whether or not these changes were directly related to the lumbar puncture is unknown, but because lumbar puncture carries the risk of brain herniation or aneurysm rebleeding, the procedure should only be performed if the diagnosis remains in question following the CT scan or when CT scanning is unavailable. Lumbar puncture is also useful in ruling out infectious meningitis, which may mimic SAH.

After making a diagnosis of SAH, four-vessel cerebral angiography should be performed as soon as possible. The angiographic investigation must visualise the full course of all intracranial vessels in at least two planes, including both posterior inferior cerebellar arteries. The angiographer's goal is to demonstrate the cause of the SAH, define the aneurysm's neck and projection, delineate the vessels arising adjacent to the aneurysm, determine whether multiple aneurysms are present (20% incidence), and assess the degree of any concomitant vasospasm. If no aneurysmal bleeding source is detected, common carotid injections must be performed to rule out the possibility of a dural arteriovenous fistula with retrograde cortical venous drainage as the aeteology of the haemorrhage. In 1977, Nibbelink reported a significant complication rate for cerebral angiography in acute SAH.[53] Complications and their frequencies were: transient hemiparesis 2%; permanent neurological deficits 2·5%; death 2·6%; worsening of ischaemic deficit 3%; and aneurysmal rebleeding 1·5%. The present day complication rate for cerebral angiography should be less than 1%, with an experienced neuroradiologist,[54-56] and is approximately 0·4% in our institution. Aneurysm rupture during angiography has been reported, but is fortunately an infrequent occurrence.[57-61]

With the advent of rapid scanning helical CT technology, three-dimensional CT angiography has become more widely used in the detection and investigation of cerebral aneurysms.[62,63] We currently use CT angiography to augment the information provided by arterial angiography in the analysis of complicated aneurysms. The CT images help detect the position of afferent and efferent vessels and the relationship of the lesion to surrounding structures. CT angiography is also useful to investigate the possibility of arterial dissection when a patient presents with SAH and a negative or equivocal cerebral arteriogram.

MRI is not useful in the acute diagnosis of SAH because of the difficulty in imaging blood products immediately following SAH. MRI has proven valuable in the localisation of subarachnoid clot beyond the time the blood is detectable with CT scanning.[64] We have found MRI invaluable in the evaluation of giant intracranial aneurysms. Because giant aneurysms are often partially thrombosed, they often opacify incompletely during angiography, and MRI can demonstrate the magnitude and location of these lesions. We have used MR angiography, and occasionally CT angiography, to follow the size of untreated giant aneurysms in which no treatment was performed due to medical issues.[65-70]

Serial CT scans are performed periodically for the first several days following SAH to detect hydrocephalus or rebleeding. Hydrocephalus may present with headache, drowsiness, confusion, or agitation. The incidence of acute hydrocephalus following SAH varies extensively among reported series. Bohn and Hugosson found that 1% of their patients operated on for ruptured cerebral aneurysms ultimately required shunting for hydrocephalus.[71] Modesti and Binet found a 63% incidence of abnormal ventricular enlargement on CT scanning within 24 hours of SAH.[72] In 1985, van Gijn reported a series of 174 patients who suffered SAH. Thirty-four (20%) developed acute hydrocephalus within 72 hours of the haemorrhage. Although intraventricular blood was closely associated with the development of hydrocephalus, the extent of cisternal haemorrhage was not. The mortality rate among those patients with acute hydrocephalus was significantly higher than in those without this complication.[73] If hydrocephalus develops following SAH, clinical judgement should be used to assess its severity and the need for CSF diversion. We have found that some patients will exhibit transient, asymptomatic ventricular enlargement following SAH. If hydrocephalus causes clinical manifestations, continuous external ventricular or lumbar drainage is instituted until the ventricular size and intracranial pressure normalise. One exception to this strategy is the existence of an unsecured ruptured aneurysm. In these cases CSF drainage, if required, is carefully controlled so as not to reduce ventricular size or intracranial pressure to a point that the tamponade effect on the aneurysm is lost and re-rupture is promoted.[74] Continuous external ventricular drainage can usually be performed with little additional morbidity or mortality.[75] If the external ventriculostomy cannot be weaned without the recurrence of hydrocephalus, a permanent ventriculo-peritoneal shunt is placed.

Clinical classification

After the diagnosis of SAH has been established, patients are assigned a clinical grade based on one of the accepted grading systems. Grading systems for SAH have been reported since the 1930s, when Bramwell labelled patients either apoplectic or paralytic.[76] Botterell and coworkers introduced a useful scale in 1956 which has undergone several modifications, including one in 1973 by Lougheed and Marshall.[77,78] One of the more universally accepted grading systems is that of Hunt and Hess (1968),[79] which was later modified by Hunt in 1974 (Box 8.1).[80] Both Botterell and Hunt grading scales drop the patient into the next worse grade if serious systemic disease or vasospasm is present. Neither system is felt to be relevant in the face of a moribund patient with a significant intracranial haematoma.

While the Hunt and Hess grading remains the most widely used system for patient assessment, others have considered using new systems to improve predictive value. Oshiro *et al.* developed a grading system based on the Glasgow Coma Scale (GCS) with GCS scores of 15, 12–14, 9–11, 6–8, and 3–5 replacing the Hunt and Hess scores of 1–5, respectively.[81]

> **Box 8.1 Hunt and Hess grading system**
>
> Grade 0   Unruptured aneurysm without symptoms
>
> Grade 1   Asymptomatic or minimal headache and slight nuchal rigidity
>
> Grade 1a No acute meningeal or brain reaction, but with fixed neurological deficit
>
> Grade 2   Moderate to severe headache, nuchal rigidity, no neurological deficit
>
> Grade 3   Drowsy, confused, or mild focal deficit
>
> Grade 4   Stupor, moderate to severe hemiparesis, possible early decerebrate rigidity and vegetative disturbances
>
> Grade 5   Deep coma, decerebrate rigidity, moribund appearance

These authors felt their system was at least equal to, if not better than, the Hunt and Hess system at predicting patient outcome while at the same time being more reproducible across observers.

No matter what system of grading is used, it is important to pay close attention to the name and date of the classification system used to ensure comparability of various patients or patient series reported.[82]

Non-aneurysmal subarachnoid haemorrhage

Approximately 75% of patients who suffer a non-traumatic, spontaneous SAH will be found to have a cerebral aneurysm.[83] An AVM will be discovered in another 5%. Twenty per cent of SAH patients will have various other causes to which the haemorrhage is attributed. When the initial angiogram does not demonstrate an aetiology, further investigation with MRI and CT angiography is warranted. While past studies have found that a significant number of patients with initially negative arteriograms had an aneurysm ultimately demonstrated on a second angiogram or at autopsy, the use of repeat angiography is controversial.[84–86] As angiographic techniques have improved, the yield of repeat angiography has decreased. Forster reported only one patient in whom a second angiogram diagnosed a previously occult cerebral aneurysm out of 56 SAH patients with initially negative studies.[87] Others have reported higher diagnostic yields of 3–22%.[88–93] It has been our policy to tailor each diagnostic evaluation to the patient's specific findings. If the initial angiogram fails to demonstrate a cause of the SAH but shows focal vasospasm, the angiogram is repeated five to seven days later. We also advocate repeat angiography if a portion of the cerebral vasculature is not adequately visualised on the initial study or in patients who have a large amount of subarachnoid blood visualised on CT scanning.

The differential diagnoses that must be considered in cases of non-aneurysmal SAH are extensive. Trauma is the most frequent cause of non-aneurysmal SAH and at times it can be difficult to determine if the SAH was the result or the cause of the patient's injuries. Other aetiologies include angiographically demonstrable and angiographically occult vascular malformations and arteriovenous fistulas, coagulopathies, granulomatous angiitis, venous thrombosis, small arterial and venous tears, central nervous system infection, intra- and extra-axial tumours, hypertension, drug abuse, and various aetiologies within the spinal canal.[94–96] SAH of spinal origin occurs most commonly from spinal AVMs.

The management goals in spontaneous SAH are similar to those in patients with head trauma, namely diagnose the condition and minimise the potential for further injury. The treatment of SAH of unknown aetiology is aimed at preventing secondary injury and providing relief of symptoms. Patients are initially placed on bedrest under close observation. Blood pressure is controlled with antihypertensives and the patients are well hydrated. Headache and cervical pain are treated with analgesics as needed and prophylactic anticonvulsants are administered. Corticosteroids, in the form of dexamethasone 4 mg every six hours, are used to alleviate symptomatically signs of blood induced meningitis. While symptomatic vasospasm occurs in a small percentage of patients who present with SAH of undetermined aetiology, we administer an oral calcium channel blocking agent, nimodipine, 60 mg every four hours, to reduce the effects of cerebral vasospasm, should it occur. The incidence of vasospasm is less than in those patients found to have aneurysmal SAH and may be related to the magnitude of the haemorrhage seen on the presenting CT scan.[89] We have observed angiographic vasospasm in non-aneurysmal SAH, although clinically symptomatic vasospasm in this specific group of patients is rare in our experience. The treatment of symptomatic vasospasm will be discussed further in the following section on aneurysmal SAH.

Patients who present with non-aneurysmal SAH are typically in better neurological condition than those patients with SAH from ruptured aneurysms.[97-100] Although the source of SAH remains undiscovered in 20% of patients, the mortality rate for this group of patients is less than 3%. The incidence of rebleeding is 4% in the first six months and ranges from 0·2% to 0·86% per year after six months.[101] The outcomes of a number of reported series concerning SAH with negative angiography have found that 80% of patients with SAH of undetermined aetiology will have a good outcome and return to gainful employment, as opposed to less than 50% of patients who survive aneurysmal SAH.[83,100] The patient's clinical status usually corresponds to the amount of subarachnoid blood present on the CT scan.[90] The magnitude of the haemorrhage seen on CT scan relates to the development of complications secondary to the haemorrhage. These complications include cerebral vasospasm, hydrocephalus, seizures, memory disturbances, headache, and psychological disturbances. Stober has reviewed the blood distribution on CT scans following both aneurysmal and non-aneurysmal SAH and determined that SAH of unknown aetiology is unlikely to result in blood in the Sylvian or interhemispheric fissures.[102] The interpeduncular or perimesencephalic cisterns often demonstrate focal blood collections when SAH of unknown aetiology occurs.[43,103,104]

Aneurysmal subarachnoid haemorrhage

General considerations

Ruptured cerebral aneurysms account for 77% of SAH cases.[105] Chason and Hindman demonstrated 137 cerebral aneurysms, a 5% incidence, in an autopsy study of 2786 patients who died of causes unrelated to SAH. Forty-two per cent of these aneurysms had evidence of prior rupture. This would be consistent with other reports that have demonstrated a history of prior haemorrhage in 60% of aneurysms discovered in people under 60 years of age.[106,107]

Autopsy studies demonstrate a higher incidence of ruptured aneurysms than clinical or radiological studies because aneurysm rupture is a frequent cause of sudden death. Although many series reflect widely variable epidemiological statistics, an approximate occurrence rate for aneurysm rupture is 10 per 100 000 population per year. There is an average prevalence rate of unruptured aneurysms of 5% in the adult population.

Three basic theories attempt to explain the pathogenesis of cerebral aneurysms. One theory proposes that a congenital weakness in the muscular layer of cerebral arteries allows the intimal layer to herniate and eventually distend and destroy the elastic membrane, leading to outpouching of an aneurysmal sac. Other theories have attributed aneurysm formation to postnatal degeneration within the vessel wall that leads to deterioration of the internal elastic lamina and resultant aneurysm formation. Others have postulated that it is a combination of congenital and degenerative effects that lead to aneurysm formation.[108] The law of LaPlace relates wall stress to radius and transmural pressure and can be used to show that as the radius of the aneurysm enlarges, significantly less force is required to cause further enlargement or rupture of the sac.[109]

Aneurysms tend to occur at vascular bifurcations, although they may occur unassociated with vessel branches.[110] Forbus used a rigid glass model to demonstrate that the point of greatest stress on the artery wall occurs at the apex of a vascular bifurcation in line with the direction of flow.[111]

The average size of ruptured aneurysms is 7·5 mm. Two per cent of aneurysms under 5 mm rupture, in contrast to 40% of those between 6 mm and 10 mm in external diameter.[112–114] Unruptured but symptomatic giant aneurysms (2·5 cm) carry a grave prognosis related to both mass effect and future rupture. The commonly held perception that giant aneurysms do not bleed and can be managed conservatively is dangerously misleading. Between 30% and 70% of giant aneurysms that become symptomatic are associated with SAH.[115,116]

Approximately 20% of SAH patients demonstrate multiple aneurysms.[6] This makes it imperative to visualise all cerebral vessels on diagnostic angiography when SAH is investigated. The presence of multiple aneurysms will significantly affect surgical planning. When multiple aneurysms are present, the most proximal, irregularly shaped, and largest will be the most likely source of SAH.[117] Aneurysms with small secondary outpouchings are thought to be particularly prone to rupture and these outpouchings may actually be false sacs from previous haemorrhages.[118] DuBoulay has hypothesised that secondary aneurysm bulges are regions where the aneurysm wall is most unstable. Asymptomatic aneurysms rarely had secondary protuberances. He also found the mortality rate of such aneurysms to be twice that of smooth walled lesions.[119]

To help determine which of multiple aneurysms is the most likely source of SAH, one must correlate the history of the ictal event, clinical examination, CT scan, angiogram, and MRI study. The patient may lateralise the initial headache when bilateral aneurysms are present and the clinical exam may demonstrate unilateral weakness or cranial nerve palsy. When multiple aneurysms are diagnosed, CT localisation of subarachnoid blood, ventricular shift, and the site of an intraparenchymal haematoma are helpful findings. Local vasospasm may be present near the ruptured lesion on angiography. The aneurysm most likely to have bled will often be the largest, have the most irregular contour, or have a nipple-like secondary bulge. Nehls found statistical evidence that aneurysms associated with the anterior communicating complex, the basilar apex, and the posterior inferior cerebellar artery–vertebral junction were the most likely aneurysms to bleed when multiple aneurysms were diagnosed.[120] MRI can be valuable in detecting subarachnoid clot beyond the time clot is visible on the CT scan and in localising the causative source of haemorrhage in cases with multiple aneurysms. Focal increased signal intensity is often found around a ruptured aneurysm on T2 weighted MR scans.[64]

After the diagnosis of ruptured cerebral aneurysm has been confirmed as the cause of SAH, treatment plans need to be considered. The treatment for SAH secondary to a ruptured aneurysm is a complex decision depending upon multiple factors. Treatment in the past has been primarily surgical, however, the development of Guglielmi Detachable Coils (GDC) (Target Therapeutics, Fremont, CA) has made interventional neuroradiologic management a viable option in selected cases.[121-131] In general, aneurysms with a small neck to fundus ratio are more favourable for endovascular therapy than wide-necked lesions.[132,133] Endovascular technology continues to improve, however, and techniques are evolving that further the spectrum of endovascular therapy options.[132,134-137] The long-term durability of GDC embolisation of aneurysms is still largely unknown.[138,139] The decision between surgical or endovascular therapy for any given aneurysm must be tailored to the specific patient, and this is best performed by a cerebrovascular team composed of cerebrovascular neurosurgeons, endovascular neurosurgeons, and interventional neuroradiologists.[140,141]

Surgical clipping versus endovascular coiling

The International Subarachnoid Aneurysm Trial (ISAT) was a prospective, randomised trial comparing surgical clipping of ruptured cerebral aneurysms to endovascular coiling and was published in *The Lancet*.[141] This study demonstrated that for a *carefully pre-selected subgroup of patients*, cared for in designated study centres, patients with ruptured aneurysms treated with coiling fared better at one year follow up than patients treated with surgical clipping at those designated centres. Unfortunately, we believe that the ISAT study results have been misrepresented in the international media and that very specific data have been inappropriately generalised to all patients with intracranial aneurysms. The reported ISAT data relate that patients with aneurysmal SAH treated with craniotomy and aneurysm clipping at the study centres had a 30·6% incidence of poor outcome at one year follow up. Patients with ruptured aneurysms treated by endovascular coiling at these centres had 23·7% chance of poor outcome at one year follow up. The absolute risk reduction at one year follow up when comparing coiling versus clipping at the study centres was 6·9%. The majority of the centres involved in the study were located in Europe (particularly England), Australia, and Canada. Only two patients were entered into the study from a single centre within the United States, where practice patterns and neurovascular subspecialisation, particularly in major academic centres, is very different. The number of procedures performed per neurosurgeon/endovascular specialist participating in the ISAT trial heretofore has not been published and is critical in determining the relative expertise between the different treatment modalities.

More importantly, of 9278 patients with ruptured intracranial aneurysms considered for the ISAT study, only 2143 patients were randomised, with the majority of the remaining 7135 patients undergoing craniotomy for aneurysm clipping. As well, during the short follow-up period of the report, 2·6% of the patients who underwent coiling suffered a haemorrhage after treatment, compared to 0·9% of the surgical group. In addition, more than four times more patients treated with aneurysm coiling in the ISAT study required additional treatment for their ruptured aneurysms than did patients treated by microsurgical clipping. The 2143 patients randomised in the ISAT study will need to be closely followed for many years before legitimate conclusions regarding the durability of endovascular coiling and the comparative outcomes of coiling versus clipping can be deduced.

Surgical treatment

When surgical treatment is pursued, the primary surgical approach is aimed at repairing the ruptured lesion and treating any asymptomatic aneurysms that are accessible through the same surgical exposure. There appears to be a poorly understood phenomenon of enlargement and rupture of previously asymptomatic aneurysms in patients who undergo surgery to clip the ruptured lesion.[142,143] A possible explanation may relate to increased haemodynamic stress in the perioperative period producing an increase in the transmural pressure gradient within asymptomatic aneurysms. Despite these statements, haemorrhage from a previously asymptomatic aneurysm following surgery to treat the ruptured aneurysm is an extremely rare occurrence. Others have reported that postoperative volume expansion and induced hypertension following surgery for a ruptured aneurysm are both safe and efficacious and do not appear to promote rupture of asymptomatic lesions.[144,145]

While some authors have reported good results in moribund individuals, in our practice we reserve non-operative/ non-interventional treatment for those patients in the poorest grades who are not expected to survive.[146] Yasargil retrospectively compared surgical and non-surgical management in patients with ruptured aneurysms in one specific region of Switzerland. Of 624 proven ruptured aneurysms, 349 (55·9%) underwent operation with five (1·4%)

deaths. Two hundred and seventy-five (44·1%) patients did not undergo surgery and only four (0·6%) patients survived, resulting in a mortality rate of 98·5% in the non-operated patients.[147] SAH from a ruptured cerebral aneurysm clearly has a high mortality. In our opinion, therefore, expectant management should only be confined to poor grade patients who are not expected to survive.

Patient selection and timing of treatment are important factors determining outcome. The dilemma of which patient should undergo surgery and when surgery should be performed in relation to the onset of SAH or vasospasm remains an unresolved issue. Current trends in neurosurgery and our own results support early intervention in patients with good clinical grades. The goal of early surgery is to secure the ruptured aneurysm, prevent rebleeding, and remove as much subarachnoid clot as possible in order to potentially reduce the risk of vasospasm. We generally offer surgery or embolisation in Hunt and Hess grades 1–3 patients as soon as they are fully radiologically and medically evaluated.[82] Grade 4 and 5 patients are treated interventionally or, if not good interventional candidates, non-operatively until their clinical condition improves.[82] Hunt and Hess grades 0–3 patients are selected for coiling on a case by case basis depending upon their medical history and aneurysm geometry and location.

Diagnosis and treatment of acute posthaemorrhagic hydrocephalus by external ventricular drainage will often result in patient improvement by one grade. In a similar fashion, patients who are in a poor grade but who harbour a significant intraparenchymal haematoma may demonstrate significant improvement with surgery that obliterates the aneurysm and reduces the haematoma induced mass effect.

The rationale for conservative management of poor grade patients stems from previous studies evaluating surgical results related to the patient's preoperative status. Hunt and Hess categorised patients into grades to investigate prognosis of the preoperative neurological status, and found that operative mortality approached 75% in poor grade (grades 4 and 5) patients.[79] The explanation for dismal surgical results in poor grade patients is probably multifactorial. Elevated intracranial pressure, reduced cerebral blood flow, poor tissue tolerance to manipulation, and poor tolerance to temporary occlusion all contribute to poor surgical results. Some have seen encouraging results with aggressive surgical treatment of poor grade patients,[146–148] although our experience and that of others has reaffirmed that, in general, these patients have poor surgical outcomes.[112,149–152]

Once a patient with aneurysmal SAH is deemed a surgical candidate, timing becomes an important issue. The overall management morbidity and mortality must be a consideration in the surgical planning. Major factors include:

- rate of aneurysm rebleeding
- risk of vasospasm induced delayed ischaemia
- the procedure's technical considerations.

The predominant historical opinion has been that if surgery was intentionally delayed for one to two weeks following SAH, the surgical outcomes were much more favourable compared with those of early surgery. Norlen and Olivecrona published the results of 100 consecutive anterior communicating artery aneurysms managed in this fashion and reported a remarkable 3% mortality rate.[153] It was presumed that technical difficulties associated with early surgery would negate any potential benefit early surgery afforded in preventing rebleeding and facilitating the management of vasospasm. There was also concern that early surgery could worsen the effects of vasospasm in the face of disturbed autoregulation.[154,155] Because of improvements in neuroanaesthesia and neurosurgical instrumentation and the advent of the operative microscope, investigators have readdressed the optimal timing of aneurysm surgery.

Recent studies investigating the timing of surgery for ruptured intracranial aneurysms have shown that early surgery was not significantly more difficult than delayed surgery from a technical standpoint, as perceived by the operating surgeons. Although the results of surgery delayed until after postbleed day 10 were superior to results of early surgery, the morbidity and mortality of rebleeding and other complications associated with delayed surgery negated any benefit of delaying the procedure. Early surgery did result in a decreased incidence of aneurysm rebleeding but did not significantly affect the incidence of subsequent vasospasm.[36,156]

The overall results of these contemporary studies show that overall management morbidity and mortality of early versus delayed surgical therapy are not significantly different.

Nevertheless, one must keep in mind that such studies included patients treated prior to the advent of triple-H therapy (Hypertension, Hypervolaemia, Haemodilution), calcium channel blockers, and non-steroidal medications which may improve patients' outcome. The possible exception to the above statement may be patients who are alert and in excellent grade upon admission, for this group has had the most favourable results with early surgery. The surgeon must weigh all factors, including his/her technical capabilities, the risk of rebleeding, and potential management difficulties, including vasospasm, when deciding on the best time to perform the surgical procedure. Timing may be less of an issue for aneurysm coiling as this procedure may be performed along with the diagnostic arteriogram, thus theoretically securing the aneurysm immediately upon presentation.

SAH from aneurysms is further complicated by a concurrent pregnancy. Because surgical management reduces both maternal and fetal death, it is generally recommended. In cases of unruptured aneurysms, caesarean section has not been shown to reduce the risk of SAH.[157]

Preoperative management of aneurysmal subarachnoid haemorrhage

Evaluation

We believe in early surgical repair of ruptured aneurysms followed by aggressive medical therapy, if necessary, for vasospasm. It is preferable that patients be transferred to a neurosurgical centre as soon as possible following their haemorrhage. The thought that patients need to be observed for a period prior to transfer is an erroneous concept and only serves to delay treatment unnecessarily and place patients at risk of rebleeding. We have found that immediate transfer once the diagnosis of SAH is suspected provides the best chance for optimal patient outcome. It is imperative that pertinent radiographic studies, including arteriograms, be sent along with the patient. Sending poor quality copies of radiographs or not sending the complete angiogram because of individual hospital administrative policy results in needless and dangerous repetition of vital diagnostic examinations.

We admit patients with SAH directly to the surgical intensive care unit, where further assessment is performed. Patients are graded according to the Hunt–Hess grading scale and accompanying radiographic studies are evaluated.[79,80] If not previously obtained, angiography is performed as soon as possible after admission, with each case individualised for the patient. Early angiography is beneficial for early diagnosis, even if patients are not offered immediate surgery. An angiogram obtained early after SAH will confirm the diagnosis and allow for preoperative planning or immediate surgery or coil embolisation. Preoperative preparation usually includes routine blood tests, type and crossmatch of packed red blood cells, placement of central venous access and radial arterial monitoring catheters, and premedication. All patients are assessed for peri-SAH cardiac ischaemia. In our experience of using preoperative serum cardiac troponin levels (cTnl), 17% of patients with SAH had evidence of cardiac ischaemia. The presence of ischaemia leads to echocardiographic evaluation, the result of which may affect the type of treatment and anaesthetic utilised.[158]

Medical management

Preoperative medication and fluid management is an important aspect of SAH care. We initially attempt to normalise the patient's intravascular volume status and do not prophylactically induce hypervolaemia since its institution has been shown to be potentially hazardous and offers no clear benefit.[159] Administered medications include anticonvulsants, corticosteroids, calcium channel blockers, antihypertensives, and analgesics. Strict attention to blood pressure control prior to aneurysm surgery has been shown to reduce the rate of aneurysm rebleeding.[160] For patients who are hypertensive and have risk factors for coronary artery disease, the addition of a beta-blocker perioperatively will significantly reduce the risk of perioperative cardiac complications. The effect of calcium channel blockers on outcome is less clear. Reports show that prophylactic use of these agents does not prevent angiographic vasospasm but may decrease the overall management morbidity following SAH.[161–163] In light of the referenced reports on calcium channel blocking agents, we place all patients on this drug immediately upon admission to the hospital. Further studies need to be performed on this important issue.

The administration of antifibrinolytics designed to minimise clot lysis is controversial.[164-167] Epsilon-aminocaproic acid (AMICAR) is one of the more widely used medications which primarily inhibits the conversion of plasminogen into plasmin, the main function of which is to digest fibrin and aid in clot lysis. Intravenous injection of AMICAR provides a peak plasma level within 20 minutes. The drug crosses the blood–brain barrier and achieves maximal antifibrinolytic activity within the CSF 48 hours after therapy is initiated.[167] Patients are given 2 g per hour intravenously for 48 hours, then 1·5 g per hour for the duration of therapy or until surgery is performed. Review of the 1966 Cooperative Study found a reduction in rehaemorrhage and death at 14 days from 21% to 10% with the use of antifibrinolytics.[168] Although antifibrinolytic therapy decreases rebleeding by 50% during the first two weeks following SAH, there is an increase in associated medical complications, the most frequent of which is diarrhoea, occurring in 24% of patients. Communicating hydrocephalus is 25% more frequent with antifibrinolytic therapy.[169] The greatest concern over use of antifibrinolytic agents is the associated increase in ischaemic neurological deficits that has negated its benefits in some studies.[164] Our feeling is that antifibrinolytics have little role in acute aneurysmal SAH if surgery is anticipated within two days of admission. These agents may be of value if an operative procedure is delayed longer than 48 hours. Their efficacy when used in conjunction with calcium channel blockers has yet to be studied.

Surgical planning

Aneurysm rebleeding is a catastrophic event that may occur relatively soon after the initial SAH.[144] The frequency of rebleeding is 4% within the first 48 hours following the initial SAH and 1·5% each day for the next 12 days. The mortality rate from aneurysm rebleeding is at least 70%. Surgical or interventional treatments offer the best protection against rebleeding and its attendant complications.

Some neurosurgeons are concerned that surgery soon after acute SAH is technically more difficult due to brain swelling and obscuration of vital structures by acute blood within the subarachnoid space. Despite the above considerations, the majority of our grade 1–3 patients undergo surgery early after SAH to minimise the incidence of rebleeding. Although this surgery can be technically more demanding, we have not found patient morbidity and mortality to be adversely affected. We have found intraoperative ventricular puncture and aggressive gravity drainage of CSF to be an extremely useful adjunct in overcoming an initially swollen brain soon after SAH.[170] The results of the most recent Cooperative Study confirm that although most surgeons report the brain to be significantly more swollen during early surgery, the majority feel early surgery is not significantly more difficult.[156] In this Cooperative Study, early surgery reduced the incidence of rebleeding but had no effect in decreasing the incidence of vasospasm.[171–174] Nevertheless, most patients were treated prior to the widespread use of triple H therapy and calcium channel blockers.

Surgical considerations and complications

The goals of aneurysm surgery following SAH are: (1) aneurysm obliteration with preservation of normal vasculature; and (2) minimisation of brain tissue disruption (Figures 8.2, 8.3). Our patients undergoing uncomplicated aneurysm repair following SAH had morbidity and mortality rates of approximately 10%. When intraoperative rupture occurred, the morbidity and mortality rates increased to approximately 20%. Factors such as the phase of the dissection, the use of blunt versus sharp dissection techniques, and complete aneurysm neck dissection play key roles in minimising intraoperative rupture. Adequate depth of anaesthesia, strict blood pressure control, ventricular drainage at the time of surgery, aggressive sphenoid wing removal, and appropriately situated craniotomies which permit minimal brain retraction will aid in reducing the incidence of aneurysm rupture prior to subarachnoid dissection.

The most frequent time for intraoperative aneurysm rupture is during subarachnoid dissection prior to clip application.[175–177] In our experience, ill advised blunt dissection techniques are the most frequent cause of intraoperative rupture. Aneurysm rupture produced by blunt

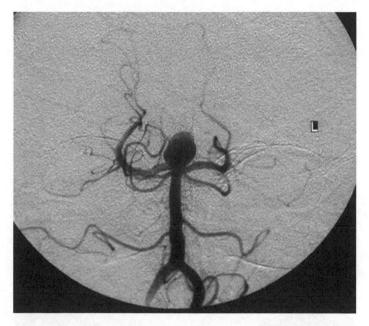

Figure 8.2 AP vertebral arteriogram demonstrating basilar apex aneurysm

dissection typically produces a large tear at the aneurysm sac–neck junction and the amount of bleeding is usually torrential. Bleeding from sharp dissection is usually from punctate holes and, therefore, more controllable. To reduce the risk of rupture, dense clot surrounding the vessels and the aneurysm should be sharply divided with microscissors or microarachnoid knives. Dissection should also hug the normal vasculature when working in the aneurysm's vicinity. Early proximal and distal vascular control prior to aneurysm dissection is mandatory in all cases. Definitive neck dissection prior to clip application will also reduce the likelihood of clip induced aneurysm rupture which is similar to aneurysm rupture from blunt dissection.

Intraoperative aneurysm rupture is an inevitable complication of aneurysm surgery. Close blood pressure control, basal craniotomy flaps, minimal brain retraction, strict use of sharp dissection techniques, dissection along normal vascular anatomy, temporary occlusion of parent

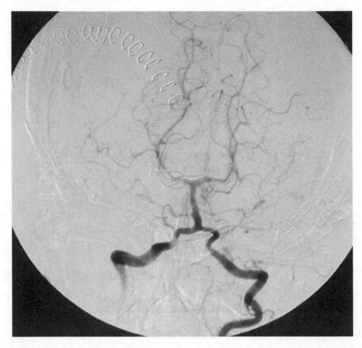

Figure 8.3 AP vertebral arteriogram of basilar apex aneurysm which has been successfully clipped with sparing of both posterior cerebral arteries

vessels, and appropriate use of available clips can minimise the incidence of intraoperative rupture and provide the optimal chance for a good surgical outcome.

In the event of intraoperative aneurysm rupture, temporary occlusion of afferent and efferent vessels is one of the most useful measures. We utilise pentothal induced electroencephalographic burst suppression during temporary occlusion to theoretically optimise cerebral protection.[178] We do not use induced hypotension to control intraoperative aneurysm rupture because of the theoretically deleterious effects of hypotension on patients specifically susceptible to acute ischaemia. Giannotta found that induced hypotension negatively influenced outcomes when used to control intraoperative aneurysm rupture.[177]

During surgery, we attempt to remove as much subarachnoid clot as is deemed safe. The variable consistency of acute and subacute subarachnoid blood at various stages of fibrinolysis renders success of clot removal unpredictable. Previous reports have found some potential benefit in preventing vasospasm or lessening its severity by aggressive subarachnoid clot removal.[172,173] Recent reports have focused on the use of topical thrombolytic agents such as tissue-type plasminogen activator (tPA) instilled into the subarachnoid space during surgery. Use of tPA has been reported to show some effect on chemical thrombolysis of subarachnoid clot in the postoperative period.[166,169,179-184] In our limited experience, tPA does appear to aid in the clearance of subarachnoid blood seen on CT scan. Whether this chemically induced thrombolysis will be beneficial in decreasing the morbidity and mortality of vasospasm remains to be demonstrated. The addition of tPA at surgery carries some risk of increased bleeding in the operative site postoperatively.

Management of aneurysms using Guglielmi Detachable Coils (GDC)

Background

The GDC coil system was developed by Italian neurosurgeon Guido Guglielmi and Target Therapeutics, Fremont, California. The device gives the surgeon the ability to insert a coil into an aneurysm or blood vessel, assess its position, and withdraw it if the result is less than satisfactory.[121-127] Other coil systems are not detachable but rather pushed or injected into position. Once these coils leave the catheter they are difficult, if not impossible, to retrieve.

In order to treat an aneurysm with GDC coils, the surgeon must first place a microcatheter into the aneurysm fundus. Once properly positioned, a coil is inserted through the catheter and into the aneurysm. If the operator does not like the coil's configuration he or she can remove it and reposition it or choose another size coil. The GDC system consists of a soft platinum coil soldered to a stainless steel delivery wire. When the coil is properly positioned within the fundus a 1 mA current is applied to the delivery wire. The current dissolves the stainless steel delivery wire proximal to the platinum coil by means of electrolysis. At the same time, the positively

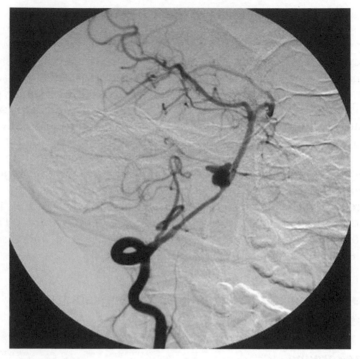

Figure 8.4 Oblique vertebral arteriogram demonstrating vertebrobasilar junction aneurysm

charged platinum theoretically attracts the negatively charged blood elements such as white and red blood cells, platelets, and fibrinogen, thus inducing intraaneurysmal thrombosis. Once electrolysis occurs the delivery wire can be removed, leaving the coil in place. Another coil can now be introduced into the fundus. The process is continued until the aneurysm is densely packed with platinum and no longer opacifies during diagnostic contrast injections (Figures 8.4, 8.5).

The mechanism by which GDC coils occlude aneurysms is still debated. We have made observations at surgery on recently coiled aneurysms that lead us to question the theory that the positive charge within the aneurysm during electrolysis induces significant thrombus formation. Coils probably provide immediate protection against rehaemorrhage by reducing blood flow within the aneurysm sac, buffering arterial pulsations within the fundus, and sealing the weak

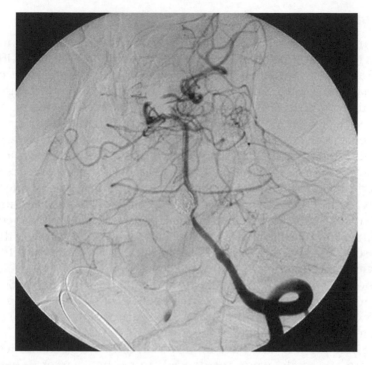

Figure 8.5 AP vertebral arteriogram of vertebrobasilar junction aneurysm which has been successfully treated with endovascular coiling

portion of the wall or hole. Eventually organised thrombus does form within the aneurysm and the aneurysm is excluded from the parent vessel by the formation of an endothelialised layer of connective tissue that covers the neck's ostium. This has been demonstrated by Mawad in experimental dog models and in our own human autopsy studies.[124,185]

While the indications for GDC coils are continually expanding as surgeons become more skilful in their placement and new products are developed, they tend to be most successful in cases of aneurysms with small necks or necks that are smaller in diameter than the maximal aneurysm diameter and aneurysms without significant intrafundal thrombus. Nevertheless, decisions concerning their applications are made on a case by case basis and few dogmatic rules exist.

Outcomes

In 1995 Fernando Vinuela (personal communication) reviewed the USA Multicenter GDC Study Group's results with 753 aneurysms treated in 715 patients. Complete occlusion of small aneurysms with small necks occurred in 62% of cases while complete occlusion in small aneurysms with wide necks was 33%. Large aneurysms with small necks and giant aneurysms with thrombus each had a 37% occlusion rate and giant aneurysms alone had 35% occlusion rates. Technical complications occurred in 11% of cases and included aneurysm perforation (1·5%), parent artery narrowing (0·5%), parent artery occlusion (3·8%), embolisation (3·7%), and coil migration (1·1%) (Figures 8.6, 8.7). Complications that had permanent clinical implications, however, occurred in only 4·4% of the cases. The procedure related mortality rate was 1·12% and the overall mortality rate for the entire study population was 5·2%. The postembolisation aneurysm haemorrhage rate was 1·26%. Aneurysm recanalisation occurred in 7·7% of small aneurysms, 15% of large aneurysms, 29% of giant aneurysms, and 31% of giant/partially thrombosed lesions.

Since 1994, results have improved as different sized and less traumatic coils were introduced into the market. These advances allow for denser fundus packing and improved obliteration rates with reduction in delayed recanalisation. More recent publications have provided some follow-up data relating to GDC results in the intermediate follow-up period.[186–188] Debrun recently reported his group's results in 144 patients treated between 1994 and 1997. When aneurysms with fundus to neck ratios of 2 were specifically analysed the mortality and permanent morbidity rate was 1·0%. Complete occlusion rates in this group for acutely ruptured aneurysms and non-acute aneurysms were 72% and 80%, respectively.[128] Keuther et al. reported a series of 74 aneurysms managed with GDC embolisation over a 4·5 year period with average angiographic follow up of 1·4 years.[129] Complete aneurysm obliteration was demonstrated in 40% of cases with an additional 52% of lesions showing 90–99% occlusion. Procedure related morbidity was 9·1%. No completely occluded lesions rehaemorrhaged in the follow-up period and 2·6% of partially occluded aneurysms rebled. Vinuela et al. published results for 403 coiled patients with

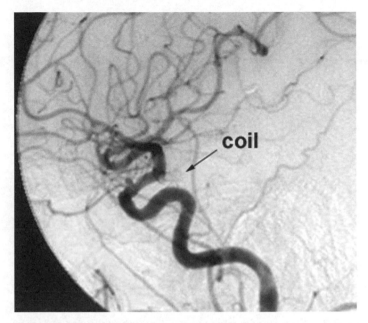

Figure 8.6 Lateral carotid arteriogram of posterior communicating aneurysm which was appreciated to be completely obliterated by endovascular coiling

SAH in the Multicenter Study.[130] Complete occlusion was demonstrated in 71% of small aneurysms with a small neck, 35% of large aneurysms, and 50% of giant aneurysms. Procedure related morbidity was 8·9% and procedure related mortality was 1·7%.

Aneurysm embolisation using the GDC system offers an alternative to traditional surgical clipping in selected cases. The results of such treatment are not yet as effective as those of open surgery and delayed aneurysm recurrence may be a significant problem (Figures 8.6, 8.7). Nevertheless, in certain instances coiling is a viable option. Decisions must be made on a case by case basis. At our institution considerations include patient preference, age, medical condition, aneurysm geometry, and location. While the particular surgeon's and interventionalist's skills are not as relevant at institutions where both disciplines are practised at the highest level, such considerations are relevant where discrepancies exist.

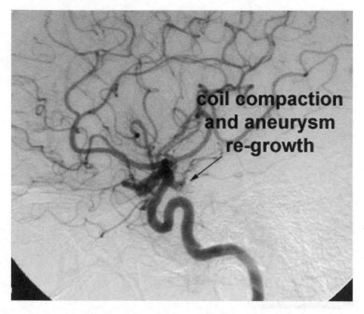

Figure 8.7 Lateral carotid arteriogram six months following successful endovascular aneurysm coiling demonstrating coil compaction and re-growth of aneurysm neck

Postoperative management

Patient care following surgery to obliterate a ruptured cerebral aneurysm is complex and must be based on many considerations. Major immediate postoperative problems include brain swelling, bleeding into the operative site, fluid and electrolyte disturbances, hydrocephalus, and the onset of cerebral vasospasm. Complicating the picture is the fact that many postoperative complications present with similar symptoms but require entirely different treatments. Along with the neurological examination, frequent CT scanning, evaluation of vital signs, blood electrolyte determination, transcranial Doppler (TCD) evaluations, and cerebral blood flow determinations are particularly helpful in differentiating these various processes.

Patients who have undergone surgery to repair a ruptured aneurysm are predisposed to develop brain swelling and oedema. Irritation of the brain surface and vessels by subarachnoid clot, disturbance of cerebral vascular autoregulation, elevation of intracranial pressure, and infarction related to iatrogenic vessel occlusion or vasospasm all contribute to postoperative brain swelling. Patients are typically maintained on 16 mg/day of dexamethasone during the first postoperative week. While no studies prove any benefit from corticosteroid therapy with SAH, we believe their inhibitory effects on phospholipase A2, inhibition of complement activation, depression of leucocyte migration, and inhibition of lymphocyte function may be beneficial in the prevention of vasospasm.[189] For diabetics, glucose control with sliding scale or continuous infusion insulin may be necessary in the setting of SAH and corticosteroid use. Intravascular volume status is closely assessed with either central venous access monitors or pulmonary artery catheters, depending on the patient's condition. Judicious euvolaemic to very slight hypervolaemic fluid management can minimise cerebral swelling by avoiding systemic overload. Repletion of potassium and magnesium will decrease the incidence of arrhythmias, particularly in those patients being treated with induced hypertension for vasospasm. Monitoring of chest radiographs for signs of volume overload and nosocomial pneumonia is prudent during induced hypertensive therapy or for those patients who require prolonged mechanical ventilation. At the time of surgery the degree of brain swelling and the necessity for frontal or temporal lobectomy are assessed. In a similar fashion, lobectomy is considered postoperatively if clinical deterioration occurs concomitant with CT evidence of brain swelling.

Fluid and electrolyte disturbances are relatively common following SAH and surgery to repair a ruptured aneurysm. Takaku found an 8·8% incidence of electrolyte disturbances following aneurysm surgery.[190] Hyponatraemia is the most common abnormality, occurring in 53%, whereas hypernatraemia had the highest mortality rate (42%). Hyponatraemia can be due to either inappropriate secretion of antidiuretic hormone or true natriuresis as a result of cerebral salt wasting.[191,192] Both syndromes are characterised by a decrease in plasma sodium levels and osmolality, associated with increased urine sodium concentration greater than 25 mmol/L. Clinical differentiation of these syndromes is important because patients with primary salt wasting syndrome are hypovolaemic and require sodium and fluid replacement. Conversely, true inappropriate antidiuretic hormone secretion is treated with "free water" restriction.

As previously discussed, communicating hydrocephalus both before and after surgery can be seen in SAH patients. There have been some reports that early operation and subarachnoid clot removal may decrease the incidence of postoperative hydrocephalus.[193] Others have proposed that preoperative antifibrinolytics contribute to the development of hydrocephalus.[194] Regardless of the cause, hydrocephalus should be ruled out in any patient with a decline in mental status prior to and following aneurysm surgery.

Delayed ischaemic deficit secondary to cerebral vasospasm is the greatest cause of morbidity in patients surviving the initial SAH. Angiographic vasospasm occurs in 70% of patients, with 20% having clinically significant narrowing. Cerebral vasospasm has a peak incidence around the sixth to eighth day following SAH, although it can occur at any time up to about 14 days postbleed, beyond which it is extremely rare.[195,196] When vasospasm develops, it may last several days to several weeks.[195,197] The most reliable predictor of those patients predisposed to develop vasospasm is the amount and distribution of subarachnoid blood on the CT scan. Thick blood in the basal cisterns carries a higher risk of vasospasm than diffuse or focal loculations. Lobar haematomas and interhemispheric blood are associated with a low risk of vasospasm. Subarachnoid blood in the sylvian fissure appears to carry an intermediate vasospasm risk.[198,199] Clinical vasospasm develops gradually over hours or days and is typically associated with gradual, progressive decline in neurological status. Headache, fever, and leucocytosis are often present and may herald the onset of vasospasm prior to neurological deterioration. Permanent neurological deficit or death occurs in approximately 12% of patients who develop severe clinical vasospasm.[195,200]

At present, the mainstay of treatment for clinically significant cerebral vasospasm is the induction of hypervolaemia and systemic hypertension, often referred to as hyperdynamic therapy. The neurological deficits seen with vasospasm are the result of arterial narrowing and increased cerebrovascular resistance. Because autoregulation is usually impaired after SAH, manoeuvres that increase cerebral perfusion pressure can increase cerebral blood flow in the ischaemic regions.[201,202] Patients undergoing induced hypertension and intravascular volume expansion are best treated in an intensive care unit with arterial and central venous pressure monitoring. An indwelling arterial catheter assesses blood pressure, a Swan–Ganz catheter monitors pulmonary capillary wedge pressure, and transcutaneous pulse oximeters monitor oxygen saturation. Desaturations may indicate early pulmonary decompensation from hypervolaemic therapy. Fluid balance is assessed hourly.

As mentioned above, the initial therapy for symptomatic vasospasm consists of volume expansion with plasma protein fractionate to create a positive fluid balance. Pulmonary artery wedge pressure is usually maintained between 14 and 18 mmHg and central venous pressure is kept at approximately 10 mmHg. If clinical improvement is not seen soon after volume expansion, arterial blood pressure is elevated with dopamine, dobutamine, and/or noradrenaline (norepinephrine), and typically maintained with systolic pressures between 180 and 220 mmHg. Kassell has reported 58 patients treated for cerebral vasospasm with volume expansion and induced arterial hypertension in which he demonstrated reversal of neurological symptoms in 75%. He found neurological improvement to be permanent in 74%.[144] As intravascular volume is expanded, patients may undergo a secondary diuresis which can make artificial elevation of the pulmonary capillary wedge pressure difficult. Use of low dose vasopressin can help minimise the diuresis and maintain an elevated intravascular fluid volume. Hypervolaemic and hypertensive therapy is continued until the neurological symptoms resolve, vasospasm clears as demonstrated by arteriography, or Doppler monitoring or complications from therapy require re-evaluation of the risk/benefit ratio of continuing this type of treatment. Complications include pulmonary oedema, congestive heart failure, brain oedema, hypertensive cerebral haemorrhage, systemic complications of prolonged vasopressor use, and myocardial infarction. Relative contraindications to hyperdynamic therapy include cerebral oedema, cerebral infarction, myocardial dysfunction, pulmonary oedema, adult respiratory distress syndrome, and increased intracranial pressure.[203]

When hyperdynamic therapy has proven unsuccessful or is contraindicated, we have found other manoeuvres helpful.

Selective intra-arterial infusion of papaverine hydrochloride (300 mg/100 ml normal saline over one hour) into the symptomatic vascular territory may reverse angiographic vasospasm in some patients. The results of this therapy can be clinically dramatic, but, in a similar fashion, may be extremely fleeting or completely unsuccessful.[204–206] Further investigation needs to be performed in order to clarify both the role of intra-arterial infusions of vasodilator substances for treatment of cerebral vasospasm and the necessity for superselective infusion.[207,208]

Another potentially useful adjunct in the treatment of posthaemorrhagic cerebral vasospasm is transluminal balloon angioplasty of the large intracranial vessels (intracranial carotid artery, M1 segment of middle cerebral artery, vertebral and basilar arteries). A number of investigators have reported encouraging results with the use of this technique.[209–214] We have witnessed marked improvement in cerebral perfusion following transluminal angioplasty but have also seen fatal complications due to vessel dissection or rupture. Linskey reported a fatal SAH that was produced by rupture of residual aneurysm neck by the angioplasty catheter.[215] Despite the risks, however, we now routinely rely on angioplasty for those patients with vasospastic neurological deficit who do not respond quickly to medical therapy. Our own complication rate for this procedure over a four year period was 2·9% permanent neurological deficit and 6% death.

New pharmaceutical products may improve SAH patient outcome. Calcium channel blockers have been discussed earlier (nimodipine, 60 mg orally every four hours for 10–21 days). Their efficacy in reducing the detrimental effects of vasospasm has been shown in controlled studies,[159–163] although the true mechanism of action remains elusive. A second drug currently under intense investigation is the free radical scavenger 21-aminosteroid U74006F (tirilazad, Upjohn Co., Kalamazoo, MI, USA). Four controlled studies have demonstrated a reduction in post-SAH morbidity in men administered this medication.[216–219] Tirilazad has been shown to decrease the incidence of symptomatic vasospasm in patients with aneurysmal SAH, although the impact on overall patient mortality has been less impressive.[220,221] The use of intraventricular sodium nitroprusside in patients with symptomatic vasospasm improved cerebral oxygenation and blood flow in preliminary studies, although further investigation into the efficacy of this therapy is needed.[222]

A frequently overlooked complication of SAH is Terson's haemorrhage (vitreous haemorrhage) and retinal haemorrhage, which are reported to occur in up to 40% of patients with ruptured cerebral aneurysms.[223] Careful screening will permit detection and treatment with vitrectomy when necessary so that visual acuity is maximised in all patients in the long run.

A final consideration in the postoperative management of SAH patients is nutrition. SAH increases resting energy expenditures significantly, especially in patients with Hunt and Hess grades 3–5. Understanding of these metabolic derangements makes attention to nutritional supplementation of major importance.[224]

Management following hospital discharge

Patients who have survived SAH and are ultimately discharged from the hospital require close follow up to detect and treat latent complications. Communicating hydrocephalus, manifested by increasing headache, lethargy, confusion, or regression of a previously improving neurological status, may develop following discharge. Fluid and electrolyte disturbances may not become evident until after discharge and may only be suspected with a patient history of abnormal fluid intake coupled with mental status changes. Seizures following SAH occur in 10–30% of patients, with the highest incidence associated with middle cerebral artery aneurysms. Most occur within 18 months of the haemorrhage and 83% of patients have fewer than three events. The most important risk factors determining the development of a seizure disorder are poor neurological grade and focal neurological deficits. There is no evidence that seizures during the initial haemorrhage are likely to persist or recur. Hart was unable to demonstrate the benefit of prophylactic anticonvulsant therapy after acute SAH.[31] Patients in our practice suffering SAH are usually placed on prophylactic anticonvulsants when they present to the hospital and are postoperatively maintained on medications for 7–10 days following surgery. Patients who undergo significant brain resection or had large intracerebral haematomas are maintained on anticonvulsants for three to six months.

An important consideration in SAH survivors is the disease's neuropsychiatric sequelae.[225,226] Even patients with good Glasgow Outcome Scores will have deficits 12 months posthaemorrhage. Short term memory is reduced in 53% and long term memory is reduced in 21%. Visuospatial construction and memory, mental flexibility, and psychomotor speed remain abnormal in 28–62%. Ten per cent have dysphasic language performance and up to 50% remain unemployed.

Because latent complications may develop, our protocol is to follow patients on a monthly basis following discharge with CT scans and laboratory testing as necessary. Patients who have remained on anticonvulsants are weaned approximately three to six months postoperatively and are followed with clinic visits until they are neurologically stable for one year.

Management of subarachnoid haemorrhage

Subarachnoid haemorrhage is a complex medical event. Among the multiple aetiologies, one of the most common relates to bleeding from a cerebral aneurysm. The optimal management of this life threatening condition relies on a systematic and organised approach leading to the correct diagnosis and timely referral to a neurosurgeon capable of treating this condition. The following is a brief summary of the steps that should be initiated when SAH is suspected.

- The clinician should have a high index of suspicion that a sudden, severe, unexplained headache in any patient could represent an acute subarachnoid haemorrhage.
- A CT scan should be obtained immediately after the diagnosis is suspected.
- If the CT scan is positive, lumbar puncture is unnecessary and dangerous due to the risks of aneurysm rebleeding or transtentorial brain herniation. If the CT scan is negative, lumbar puncture may be helpful if the history of the ictal headache is not typical of subarachnoid haemorrhage, insidious in onset, or of migrainous character. If the patient relates a history typical of SAH, a cerebral arteriogram should be performed despite a negative CT scan. Up to 15% of CT scans obtained within 48 hours of SAH will be negative.
- Once the diagnosis is confirmed with a CT scan, a neurosurgeon who can ultimately treat the patient should be contacted immediately. Delays in transfer may prove fatal because of the potential for aneurysm rebleeding prior to intervention. It is often

best to allow the surgeon who will be caring for the patient to arrange for the diagnostic arteriogram to be performed at the institution where the patient will undergo surgery to repair the aneurysm. Arteriography performed by institutions infrequently treating SAH may be technically inadequate and require repetition upon transfer to the neurosurgeon.

- Blood pressure must be closely monitored and controlled following SAH. Hypertension will increase the chance of catastrophic rebleeding. Blood pressure control should be initiated immediately upon diagnosis of SAH.
- Preoperative medications include prophylactic anticonvulsants, calcium channel blockade, corticosteroids, and antihypertensives as needed. We do not initiate antifibrinolytic therapy unless surgery is not considered within 48 hours of the initial SAH. Medications that can be initiated prior to transfer to a neurosurgeon include:

  - dexamethasone, 4 mg IV six hourly
  - nimodipine, 60 mg orally four hourly
  - phenytoin, 10 mg/kg IV load, then 100 mg orally/IV three times daily.

A frequent source of diagnostic difficulty for the neurosurgeon lies in the use of excessive amounts of narcotic analgesics prior to transfer to the neurosurgical service. Although pain control facilitates blood pressure control, the ability to grade accurately the patient's level of consciousness has significant impact on the timing of surgery. Clinical grading obscured by large doses of narcotic analgesics makes surgical planning more difficult.

- Send all x ray films, MRI scans, and lab work with the patient to avoid needless repetition.
- We perform surgery or endovascular coiling to obliterate the ruptured aneurysm as soon as possible after the onset of SAH. Poor grade patients, grades 4 and 5, are treated non-operatively or neurointerventionally until their clinical condition improves.
- Postoperative care is directed towards supportive care and complication recognition and treatment. Frequent postoperative complications include brain oedema, bleeding into the operative site, fluid and electrolyte disturbances, hydrocephalus, and cerebral vasospasm.
- Cerebral vasospasm may occur at any time, with a peak incidence around the sixth to eighth day following SAH, and should be suspected for any unexplained decline in neurological status.
- CT scans are useful to detect haematomas, acute hydrocephalus, or the development of subclinical ischaemic infarcts.
- Current treatments for cerebral vasospasm include calcium channel blockers, induced hypervolaemia and systemic hypertension, transluminal angioplasty, intra-arterial vasodilator infusion, and investigational systemic medications such as tirilizad.

References

1 Clemente CD. *Anatomy, a regional atlas of the human body*, 3rd edn. Baltimore: Urban and Schwarzenberg, 1987;572–3.
2 Liliequist B. The subarachnoid cisterns. An anatomic and roentgenologic study. *Acta Radiol (Stockh)* 1959;(suppl):185.
3 Haines DE, Harkey HL, Al-Mefty O. The "subdural" space: a new look at an outdated concept. *Neurosurgery* 1993;**32**:111–20.
4 Sahs AL. Randomized treatment study. Introduction. In: Sahs AL, Nibbelink DW, Turner JC, eds. *Aneurysmal subarachnoid hemorrhage. Report of the Cooperative Study*. Baltimore: Urban and Schwarzenberg, 1981;19–20.
5 Stehbens WE. Subarachnoid hemorrhage. In: *Pathology of the cerebral blood vessels*. St Louis: CV Mosby, 1972;252–83.
6 Sahs A, Perret GE, Locksley HB, Nishioka H. *Intracranial aneurysms and sub-arachnoid hemorrhage*. Philadelphia: JB Lippincott, 1969.
7 Shokichi U, Masumichi I, Munesuke S, Masayoshi S. Subarachnoid hemorrhage as a cause of death in Japan. *Z Rechtsmed* 1973;**72**:151–60.
8 Levy LE, Rachman L, Castle WM. Spontaneous primary subarachnoid hemorrhage in Rhodesian Africans. *J Afr Med Sci* 1973;**4**:77–86.
9 Locksley HB. Report on the cooperative study of intracranial aneurysms and subarachnoid hemorrhage, Sect 5, Pl. Natural history of subarachnoid hemorrhage, intracranial aneurysms, and arteriovenous malformations. *J Neurosurg* 1966;**25**:219–39.
10 Locksley HB. Natural history of subarachnoid hemorrhage, intracranial aneurysms and arteriovenous malformations. Part 1. In: Sahs AL, Perret GE, Locksley HB, Nishioka H, eds. *Intracranial aneurysms and subarachnoid hemorrhage. A cooperative study*. Philadelphia: JB Lippincott, 1969;37–57.
11 Talbot S. Epidemiological features of subarachnoid and cerebral haemorrhages. *Postgrad Med J* 1973;**49**:300–4.
12 Crompton MR. The coroner's cerebral aneurysm: a changing animal. *J Forensic Sci Soc* 1975;**15**:57–65.
13 Murphy JP. Subarachnoid hemorrhage; intracranial aneurysm. In: *Cerebrovascular disease*. Chicago: Year Book, 1954;199–241.
14 Ohno Y. Biometeorologic studies on cerebrovascular diseases. I. Effects of meteorologic factors on the death from cerebrovascular accident. *Jpn Circ J* 1969;**33**:1285–98.
15 Ohno Y. Biometeorologic studies on cerebrovascular diseases. II. Seasonal observation on effects of meteorologic factors on the death from cerebrovascular accident. *Jpn Circ J* 1969;**33**:1299–308.
16 Ohno Y. Biometeorologic studies on cerebrovascular diseases. III. Effects by the combination of meteorologic changes on the death from cerebrovascular accident. *Jpn Circ J* 1969;**33**:1309–14.
17 Chyahe D, Chen T, Bronstein K, Brass LM. Seasonal fluctuation in the incidence of intracranial aneurysm rupture and its relationship to changing climate conditions. *J Neurosurg* 1994;**81**:525–30.
18 Pakarinen S. Incidence, aetiology, and prognosis of primary subarachnoid hemorrhage. *Acta Neurol Scand* 1967;**29**(suppl):1–128.
19 Freytag E. Fatal rupture of intracranial aneurysms. Survey of 250 medicolegal cases. *Arch Pathol* 1966;**81**:418–24.
20 Locksley HB. Natural history of subarachnoid hemorrhage, intracranial aneurysms and arteriovenous malformations. Part II. In: Sahs AL, Perret GE, Locksley HB, Nishioka H, eds. *Intracranial aneurysms and subarachnoid hemorrhage. A cooperative study*. Philadelphia: Lippincott, 1969;58–108.

21 Adams HP, Jergenson DD, Sahs AL. Pitfalls in the recognition of subarachnoid hemorrhage. *JAMA* 1980;**244**:794–6.
22 Leblanc R. The minor leak preceding subarachnoid hemorrhage. *J Neurosurg* 1987;**66**:35–9.
23 Leblanc R, Winfield JA. The warning leak in subarachnoid hemorrhage and the importance of its early diagnosis. *Can Med Assoc J* 1984;**131**:1235–6.
24 Calvert JM. Premonitory symptoms and signs of subarachnoid hemorrhage. *Med J Aust* 1966;**53**:651–7.
25 Richardson JC, Hyland HH. Intracranial aneurysm. A clinical and pathological study of subarachnoid and intracerebral hemorrhage caused by berry aneurysms. *Medicine* 1984;**20**:1–83.
26 Berman AJ. The problem of the intracranial aneurysm. *Angiology* 1958;**9**:136–53.
27 Gillingham FJ. The management of ruptured intracranial aneurysm. *Ann R Coll Surg* 1958;**23**:89–117.
28 Ito Z, Matsuoka S, Moriyama T, *et al.* Factors related to level of consciousness in the acute stage of ruptured intracranial aneurysms. *Brain Nerve (Tokyo)* 1975;**27**:895–901.
29 Austin DC. A review of intracranial aneurysms. *Henry Ford Hosp Med Bull* 1964;**12**:251–71.
30 Fisher CM. Clinical syndromes in cerebral thrombosis, hypertensive hemorrhage, and ruptured saccular aneurysm. *Clin Neurosurg* 1975;**22**:117–47.
31 Hart RG, Byer JA, Slaughter JR, *et al.* Occurrence and implications of seizures in subarachnoid hemorrhage due to ruptured intracranial aneurysms. *Neurosurgery* 1981;**8**:417–21.
32 Sarner M, Rose FC. Clinical presentation of ruptured intracranial aneurysm. *J Neurol Neurosurg Psychiatry* 1967;**30**:67–70.
33 Tsementzis SA, Williams A. Ophthalmological signs and prognosis in patients with a subarachnoid hemorrhage. *Neurochirurgia* 1984;**27**:133–5.
34 Garfunkle AM, Danys IR, Nicolle DH, Colohan ART, Brem S. Terson's syndrome: a reversible cause of blindness following subarachnoid hemorrhage. *J Neurosurg* 1992;**76**:766–71.
35 Shields CB. Current trends in management of cerebral aneurysms. *J Kentucky Med Assoc* 1977;**75**:529–35.
36 Kassell NF, Torner JC, Haley C, *et al.* The International Cooperative Study on the Timing of Aneurysm Surgery. Part 1: Overall management results. *J Neurosurg* 1990;**73**:18–36.
37 Kassell NF, Kongable GL, Torner JC, Adams HP, Mazuz H. Delay in referral of patients with ruptured aneurysms to neurosurgical attention. *Stroke* 1985;**16**:587–90.
38 Kendall BE, Lee BC, Claveria E. Computerized tomography and angiography in subarachnoid hemorrhage. *Br J Radiol* 1976;**49**:483–501.
39 Liliequist B, Lindquist M, Valdimarsson E. Computed tomography and subarachnoid hemorrhage. *Neuroradiology* 1977;**14**:21–6.
40 Modesti LM, Binet EF. Value of computed tomography in the diagnosis and management of subarachnoid hemorrhage. *Neurosurgery* 1978;**3**:151–6.
41 Scotti G, Ethler R, Melancon D *et al.* Computed tomography in the evaluation of intracranial aneurysms and subarachnoid hemorrhage. *Radiology* 1977;**123**:85–90.
42 Weir B, Miller J, Russell D. Intracranial aneurysms: a clinical, angiographic, and computerized tomographic study. *Can J Neurol Sci* 1977;**4**:99–105.

43 Jafar JJ, Weiner HL. Surgery for angiographically occult cerebral aneurysms. *J Neurosurg* 1993;**79**:674–9.
44 Fisher CM, Kistler JP, Davis JM. Relation of cerebral vasospasm to subarachnoid hemorrhage visualized by computerized tomographic scanning. *Neurosurgery* 1980;**6**:1–9.
45 Sicard J-A. Chromodiagnostic du liquide cephalorachidien dans les hemorragies du nevraxe. Valeur de la teinte jaunatre. *CR Soc Biol* 1901; **3**:1050–3.
46 Milian G, Chiray F. Meningite à pneumocoques. Zanthochromie du liquide cephal-rachidien. *Bull Soc Anat Paris* 1902;**4**:550–2.
47 Froin G. *Les hemorragies sous-arachnoidiennes et le mecanisme de l'hematolyse en general.* Paris: Steinheil, 1904.
48 Collier J, Adie WJ. Cerebral vascular lesions. In: Price FW, ed. *A textbook of the practice of medicine.* London: Henry Frowde and Hodder and Stoughton, 1922;1348–65.
49 Symonds CP. Spontaneous subarachnoid hemorrhage. *Q J Med* 1924–25; **18**:93–122.
50 Greenfield JG, Carmichael EA. *The cerebrospinal fluid in clinical diagnosis.* London, Macmillan, 1925;50–2.
51 Barrows LJ, Hunter FT, Banker BQ. The nature and clinical significance of pigments in the cerebrospinal fluid. *Brain* 1955;**78**:59–80.
52 Duffy GP. Lumbar puncture in spontaneous subarachnoid hemorrhage. *Br Med J* 1982;**285**:1163–4.
53 Nibbelink DW, Torner J, Henderson WG. Intracranial aneurysms and subarachnoid hemorrhage. *Stroke* 1977;**8**:202–18.
54 Hesselink JR. Investigation of intracranial aneurysm. In: Fox JL, ed. *Intracranial aneurysms,* vol 1. New York: Springer Verlag, 1983;497–548.
55 Horowitz MB, Dutton K, Purdy PD. Assessment of complication types and rates related to diagnostic angiography and interventional neuroradiologic procedures. A four year review 1993–1996. *Interventional Neuroradiol* 1998;**4**:27–37.
56 Cloft HJ, Joseph GJ, Dion JE. Risk of cerebral angiography in patients with subarachnoid hemorrhage, cerebral aneurysm, and arteriovenous malformation: a meta-analysis. *Stroke* 1999;**30**:317–20.
57 Teal JS, Wade PJ, Bergeron RT, *et al.* Ventricular opacification during carotid angiography secondary to rupture of intracranial aneurysm. *Radiology* 1973;**106**:581–3.
58 Vines FS, Davis DO. Rupture of intracranial aneurysm at angiography. *Radiology* 1971;**99**:353–4.
59 Goldstein SL. Ventricular opacification secondary to rupture of intracranial aneurysm during angiography. *J Neurosurg* 1967;**27**:265–7.
60 Komiyama M. Aneurysmal rupture during angiography. *Neurosurgery* 1993;**33**:798–803.
61 Saitoh H, Hayakawa K, Nishimura K, *et al.* Rerupture of cerebral aneurysms during angiography. *Am J Neuroradiol* 1995;**16**:539–42.
62 Anderson GB, Findlay JM, Steinke DE, Ashforth R. Experience with computed tomographic angiography for the detection of intracranial aneurysms in the setting of acute subarachnoid hemorrhage. *Neurosurgery* 1997;**41**:522–8.
63 Zouaoui A, Sahel M, Marro B, *et al.* Three-dimensional computed tomographic angiography in detection of cerebral aneurysms in acute subarachnoid hemorrhage. *Neurosurgery* 1997;**41**:125–30.
64 Hackney DB, Lesnick JE, Zimmerman RA, Grossman RI, Goldberg HI, Bilaniuk LT. MR identification of bleeding site in subarachnoid hemorrhage with multiple intracranial aneurysms. *J Comput Assist Tomog* 1986;**10**:878–80.

65 Hope JKA, Wilson JL, Thomson FJ. Three dimensional CT angiography in the detection and characterization of intracranial berry aneurysms. *Am J Neuroradiol.* 1996;**17**:439–45.

66 Ogawa T, Okudera T, Nogushi K, *et al.* Cerebral aneurysms: evaluation with three dimensional CT angiography. *Am J Neuroradiol* 1996;**17**: 447–54.

67 Hsiang JNK, Liang EY, Lam JMK, Zhu XL, Poon WS. The role of computed tomographic angiography in the diagnosis of intracranial aneurysms and emergent aneurysm clipping. *Neurosurgery* 1996;**38**:481–7.

68 Tampier D, Leblanc R, Oleszek J, Pokrupa R, Melancor D. Three dimensional computed tomographic angiography of cerebral aneurysms. *Neurosurgery* 1995;**36**:749–55.

69 Huston J, Nichols DA, Leutmer PH, *et al.* Blinded prospective evaluation of sensitivity of MR angiography to known intracranial aneurysms: importance of aneurysm size. *Am J Neuroradiol* 1994;**15**:1607–14.

70 Masaryk AM, Frayne R, Unal O, *et al.* Utility of CT angiography and MR angiography for the follow-up of experimental aneurysms treated with stents or Guglielmi detachable coils. *Am J Neuroradiol* 2000;**21**: 1523–31.

71 Bohn E, Hugosson R. Experiences of surgical treatment of 400 consecutive ruptured cerebral aneurysms. *Acta Neurochir* 1978;**49**:33–43.

72 Modesti LM, Binet EF. Value of computed tomography in the diagnosis and management of subarachnoid hemorrhage. *Neurosurgery* 1978;**3**: 151–6.

73 van Gijn J, Hijdra A, Wijdicks EF, Vermeulen M, Crevel HV. Acute hydrocephalus after aneurysmal subarachnoid hemorrhage. *J Neurosurg* 1985;**63**:355–62.

74 Pare L, Delfino R, Leblanc R. The relationship of ventricular drainage to aneurysmal rebleeding. *J Neurosurg* 1992;**76**:422–7.

75 Bogdahn U, Lau W, Hassel W, Gunreben G, Mertens HG, Brawanski A. Continuous-pressure controlled, external ventricular drainage for treatment of acute hydrocephalus — evaluation of risk factors. *Neurosurgery* 1992;**31**:898–904.

76 Bramwell E. The etiology of recurrent ocular paralysis (including periodic ocular paralysis and ophthalmoplegic migraine). *Edinburgh Med J* 1933; **40**:209–81.

77 Botterell EH, Lougheed WM, Scott JW, *et al.* Hypothermia, and interruption of carotid, or carotid and vertebral circulation in the surgical management of intracranial aneurysms. *J Neurosurg* 1956;**13**:1–42.

78 Lougheed WM, Marshall BM. Management of aneurysms of the anterior circulation by intracranial procedures. In: Youmans JR, ed. *Neurological surgery,* vol 2. Philadelphia: WB Saunders, 1973;731–67.

79 Hunt WE, Hess RM. Surgical risk as related to time of intervention, in the repair of intracranial aneurysms. *J Neurosurg* 1968;**28**:14–20.

80 Hunt WE, Kosnik EJ. Timing and perioperative care in intracranial aneurysm surgery. *Clinical Neurosurg* 1974;**21**:79–89.

81 Oshiro EM, Walter KA, Piantadosi S, Witham TF, Tamargo RJ. A new subarachnoid hemorrhage grading system based on the Glasgow coma scale: a comparison with the Hunt and Hess and World Federation of Neurological Surgeons' scales in a clinical series. *Neurosurgery* 1997;**41**: 140–8.

82 Hunt WE. Grading of patients with aneurysms. Letter to the Editor. *J Neurosurg* 1977;**47**:13.

83 Friedman AH. Subarachnoid hemorrhage of unknown etiology. In: Wilkins RH, Rengachary SS, eds. *Neurosurgery update II.* New York: McGraw-Hill, 1991;73–7.

84   Nishioka H, Torner JC, Graf CJ, *et al*. Cooperative study of intracranial aneurysms and subarachnoid hemorrhage: a longterm prognostic study. III. Subarachnoid hemorrhage of undetermined etiology. *Arch Neurol* 1984;**41**:1147–51.
85   Perret G, Nichioka H. Cerebral angiography: diagnostic value and complications of carotid and vertebral angiography. In: Sahs AL, ed. *Intracranial aneurysms and subarachnoid hemorrhage: a cooperative study.* Philadelphia: Lippincott, 1969:109–24.
86   Iwanage H, Wakai S, Ochiai C, Narita J, Inoh S, Nagai M. Ruptured cerebral aneurysms missed by initial angiographic study. *Neurosurgery* 1990;**27**:45–51.
87   Forster DMC, Steiner L, Hakanson S. The value of repeat panangiography in cases of unexplained subarachnoid hemorrhage. *J Neurosurg* 1978;**48**:712–16.
88   Biller J, Toffol GJ, Kassell NF, *et al*. Spontaneous subarachnoid hemorrhage in young adults. *Neurosurgery* 1987;**21**:664–7.
89   Juul R, Fredricksen TA, Ringkjob R. Prognosis in subarachnoid hemorrhage of unknown etiology. *J Neurosurg* 1986;**64**:359–62.
90   Giombini S, Burzzone MG, Pluchino F. Subarachnoid hemorrhage of unexplained cause. *Neurosurgery* 1988;**22**:313–16.
91   Suzuki S, Kayama T, Sakurai Y, *et al*. Subarachnoid hemorrhage of unknown cause. *Neurosurgery* 1987;**21**:310–13.
92   Duong H, Melancon D, Tampieri D, *et al*. The negative angiogram in subarachnoid haemorrhage. *Neuroradiology* 1996;**38**:15–19.
93   Urbach H, Zentner J, Solymosi L. The need for repeat angiography in subarachnoid haemorrhage. *Neuroradiology* 1998;**40**:6–10.
94   Smith RP, Miller JD. Pathophysiology and clinical evaluation of subarachnoid hemorrhage. In: Youmans JR, ed. *Neurological surgery.* Philadelphia: WB Saunders, 1990;1644–60.
95   Margolis MT, Newton TH. Methamphetamine ("speed") arteritis. *Neuroradiology* 1971;**2**:179–82.
96   Weir B. Medical, neurologic, and ophthalmologic aspects of aneurysms, Part 2: Neurology of aneurysms and subarachnoid hemorrhage. In: *Aneurysm affecting the nervous system.* Baltimore: Williams and Wilkins, 1987,74–83.
97   Alexander MSM, Dias PS, Uttley D. Spontaneous subarachnoid hemorrhage and negative cerebral panangiography: review of 140 cases. *J Neurosurg* 1986;**64**:537–42.
98   Andrioli GC, Salar G, Rigobello L, *et al*. Subarachnoid hemorrhage of unknown etiology. *Acta Neurochir (Wien)* 1979;**48**:217–21.
99   Beguelin C, Seiler R. Subarachnoid hemorrhage with normal cerebral panangiography. *Neurosurgery* 1983;**13**:409–11.
100   Brismar J, Sundbarg G. Subarachnoid hemorrhage of unknown origin: prognosis and prognostic factors, *J Neurosurg* 1985;**63**:349–54.
101   Nishioka H, Torner JC, Graf CJ, Kassell NF, Sahs AL, Goettler LC. Cooperative study of intracranial aneurysms and subarachnoid hemorrhage: a long-term prognostic study. II. Ruptured intracranial aneurysms managed conservatively. *Arch Neurol* 1984;**41**:1142–6.
102   Stober T, Emde H, Anstatt T, *et al*. Blood distribution in computer cranial tomograms after subarachnoid hemorrhage with and without an aneurysm on angiography. *Eur Neurol* 1985;**24**:319–23.
103   Ildan F, Tuna M, Erman T, *et al*. Prognosis and prognostic factors in nonaneurysmal perimesencephalic hemorrhage: a follow-up study in 29 patients. *Surg Neurol* 2002;**57**:160–5.
104   Schwartz TH, Mayer SA. Quadrigeminal variant of perimesencephalic nonaneurysmal subarachnoid hemorrhage. *Neurosurgery* 2000;**46**:584–8.

105 Pakarinen S. Incidence, aetiology, and prognosis of primary subarachnoid hemorrhage: a study based on 589 cases diagnosed in a defined urban population during a defined period. *Acta Neurol Scand* 1967;**43**(suppl 29):1–128.

106 Drake CG. Giant intracranial aneurysms: experience with surgical treatment in 174 patients. *Clin Neurosurg* 1979;**26**:12–95.

107 Chason JL, Hindman WM. Berry aneurysms of the circle of Willis: results of a planned autopsy study. *Neurology* 1958;**8**:41–4.

108 Sekhar LN, Heros RC. Origin, growth, and rupture of saccular aneurysms: a review. *Neurosurgery* 1981;**8**:248–60.

109 Early CB, Fink LH. Some fundamental applications of the law of LaPlace in neurosurgery. *Surg Neurol* 1976;**6**:185–9.

110 Nakagawa F, Kobayashi S, Takemae T, Sugita K. Aneurysms protruding from the dorsal wall of the internal carotid artery. *J Neurosurg* 1986;**65**: 303–8.

111 Forbus WD. On the origin of the miliary aneurysms of the superficial cerebral arteries. *Bull Johns Hopkins Hosp* 1930;**47**:239–84.

112 McCormick WF, Rosenfield DB. Massive brain hemorrhage. A review of 144 cases and an examination of their causes. *Stroke* 1973;**4**:946–54.

113 Anonymous. Unruptured intracranial aneurysms – risk of rupture and risks of surgical intervention. International Study of Unruptured Intracranial Aneurysms Investigators. *N Engl J Med* 1998;**339**:1725–33.

114 Yasui N, Suzuki A, Nishimura H, *et al.* Long-term follow-up study of unruptured intracranial aneurysms. *Neurosurgery* 1997;**40**:1155–9.

115 Sundt TM, Piepgras DG. Surgical approach to giant intracranial aneurysm. Operative experience with 80 cases. *J Neurosurg* 1979;**51**:731–42.

116 Crompton MR. Mechanism of growth and rupture in cerebral berry aneurysms. *Br Med J* 1966;**1**:138–42.

117 Crompton MR. The natural history of cerebral berry aneurysms. *Am Heart J* 1976;**73**:567–9.

118 Stehbens WE. Aneurysms and anatomical variation of cerebral arteries. *Arch Pathol* 1953;**75**:45–64.

119 DuBoulay GH. The significance of loculation of intracranial aneurysms. *Bull Schweiz Akad Med Wiss* 1969;**24**:480–5.

120 Nehls DG, Flom RA, Carter LP, Spetzler RF. Multiple intracranial aneurysms: determining the site of rupture. *J Neurosurg* 1985;**63**:342–8.

121 Mizoi K, Takahashi A, Yoshimoto T, Fujiwara S, Koshu K. Combined endovascular and neurosurgical approach for paraclinoid internal carotid artery aneurysms. *Neurosurgery* 1993;**33**:986–92.

122 Civit T, Anque J, Marchal JC, Bracard S, Picard L, Hepner H. Aneurysm clipping after endovascular treatment with coils: a report of eight patients. *Neurosurgery* 1996;**38**:948–54.

123 Pierot L, Boulin A, Castaings L, Rey A, Moret J. Selective occlusion of basilar artery aneurysms using controlled detachable coils: report of 35 cases. *Neurosurgery* 1996;**28**:948–54.

124 Mawad M, Mawad J, Cartwright J, Eokaslan Z. Long-term histopathologic changes in canine aneurysms embolized with Guglielmi Detachable Coils. *Am J Neuroradiol* 1995;**16**:7–13.

125 Graves VB, Strother CM, Duff TA, Perl J. Early treatment of ruptured aneurysms with Guglielmi Detachable Coils: effect on subsequent bleeding. *Neurosurgery* 1995;**37**:640–8.

126 Guglielmi E. Electrothrombosis of saccular aneurysms via endovascular approach. *J Neurosurg* 1991;**75**:8–14.

127 Guglielmi E, Vinuela F. Endovascular treatment of posterior circulation aneurysms by electrothrombosis using electrically detachable coils. *J Neurosurg* 1992;**77**:514–24.

128 Debrun GM, Aletich VA, Kehrli P, Mosra M, Ausman JI, Charbel F. Selection of cerebral aneurysms for treatment using Guglielmi detachable coils: the preliminary University of Illinois at Chicago experience. *Neurosurgery* 1998;**43**:1281–97.

129 Keuther TA, Nesbit GM, Barnwell SL. Clinical and angiographic outcomes, with treatment data, for patients with cerebral aneurysms treated with Guglielmi detachable coils: a single center experience. *Neurosurgery* 1998;**43**:1016–25.

130 Vinuela F, Duckwiler G, Mawad M. Guglielmi detachable coil embolization of acute intracranial aneurysm: perioperative anatomical and clinical outcome in 403 patients. *J Neurosurg* 1997;**86**:475–82.

131 Uda K, Murayama Y, Gobin YP, et al. Endovascular treatment of basilar artery trunk aneurysms with Guglielmi detachable coils: clinical experience with 41 aneurysms in 39 patients. *J Neurosurg* 2001;**95**: 624–32.

132 Dovey Z, Misra M, Thornton J, et al. Guglielmi detachable coiling for intracranial aneurysms: the story so far. *Arch Neurol* 2001;**58**:559–64.

133 Shanno GB, Armonda RA, Benitez RP, et al. Assessment of acutely unsuccessful attempts at detachable coiling in intracranial aneurysms. *Neurosurgery* 2001;**48**:1066–72.

134 Kwon OK, Han MH, Lee KJ, et al. A technique of GDC embolization for deeply bilobulated aneurysms. *Am J Neuroradiol* 2002;**23**:693–6.

135 Cottier JP, Pasco A, Gallas S, et al. Utility of balloon-assisted Guglielmi detachable coiling in the treatment of 49 cerebral aneurysms: a retrospective, multicenter study. *Am J Neuroradiol* 2001;**22**:345–51.

136 Nelson PK, Levy DI. Balloon-assisted coil embolization of wide-necked aneurysms of the internal carotid artery: medium-term angiographic and clinical follow-up in 22 patients. *Am J Neuroradiol* 2001;**22**:19–26.

137 Cloft HJ, Joseph GJ, Tong FC, et al. Use of three-dimensional Guglielmi detachable coils in the treatment of wide-necked cerebral aneurysms. *Am J Neuroradiol* 2000;**21**:1312–14.

138 Hayakawa M, Murayama Y, Duckwiler GR, et al. Natural history of the neck remnant of a cerebral aneurysm treated with the Guglielmi detachable coil system. *J Neurosurg* 2000;**93**:561–8.

139 Gruber A, Killer M, Bavinzski G, et al. Clinical and angiographic results of endosaccular coiling treatment of giant and very large intracranial aneurysms: a 7-year, single-center experience. *Neurosurgery* 1999;**45**: 793–803.

140 Sturaitis MK, Rinne J, Chaloupka JC, et al. Impact of Guglielmi detachable coils on outcomes of patients with intracranial aneurysms treated by a multidisciplinary team at a single institution. *J Neurosurg* 2000;**93**:569–80.

141 International Subarachnoid Aneurysm Collaborative Group. International subarachnoid aneurysm trial (ISAT) of neurosurgical clipping versus endovascular coiling in 2143 patients with ruptured intracranial aneurysms: a randomized trial. *Lancet* 2002;**360**:1267–74.

142 Heiskanen O. The identification of ruptured aneurysm in patients with multiple intracranial aneurysms. *Neurochirurgia (Stuttg)* 1965;**8**:102–7.

143 Pool JL, Potts DG. *Aneurysms and arteriovenous anomalies of the brain. Diagnosis and treatment.* New York: Harper and Row, 1965.

144 Kassell NF, Peerless SJ, Durward QJ, et al. Treatment of ischemic deficits from vasospasm with intravascular volume expansion and induced arterial hypertension. *Neurosurgery* 1982;**11**:337–43.

145 Swift DM, Solomon RA. Unruptured aneurysms and postoperative volume expansion. *J Neurosurg* 1992;**77**:908–10.

146 Bailes JE, Speltzer RF, Hadley MN, Baldwin HZ. Management morbidity and mortality of poor-grade aneurysm patients. *J Neurosurg* 1990;72: 559–66.

147 Yasargil MG. Unoperated cases. In: *Microneurosurgery*. Stuttgart: Georg Thieme Verlag, 1984;329–30.

148 Gumprecht H, Winkler R, Gerstner W, *et al*. Therapeutic management of grade IV aneurysm patients. *Surg Neurol* 1997;47:54–8.

149 Chiang VL, Claus EB, Awad IA. Toward more rational prediction of outcome in patients with high-grade subarachnoid hemorrhage. *Neurosurgery* 2000;46:28–35.

150 Duke BJ, Kindt GW, Breeze RE. Outcome after urgent surgery for grade IV subarachnoid hemorrhage. *Surg Neurol* 1998;50:169–72.

151 Le Roux PD, Elliott JP, Newell DW, *et al*. Predicting outcome in poor-grade patients with subarachnoid hemorrhage: a retrospective review of 159 aggressively managed cases. *J Neurosurg* 1996;85: 39–49.

152 Seifert V, Trost HA, Stolke D. Management morbidity and mortality in grade IV and V patients with aneurysmal subarachnoid hemorrhage. *Acta Neurochir* 1990;103:5–10.

153 Norlen G, Olivecrona H. The treatment of aneurysms of the circle of Willis. *J Neurosurg* 1953;10:404–15.

154 Weir B, Aronyk K. Management and postoperative mortality related to time of clipping for supratentorial aneurysms. A personal series. *Acta Neurochir* 1982;63:135–9.

155 Wilkins RH. The role of intracranial arterial spasm in the timing of operations for aneurysm. *Clin Neurosurg* 1977;24:185–207.

156 Kassell NF, Torner JC, Jane JA, *et al*. The International Cooperative Study on the Timing of Aneurysm Surgery. Part 2: Surgical results. *J Neurosurg* 1990;73:37–47.

157 Dias M, Sekhar LN. Intracranial hemorrhage from aneurysms and arteriovenous malformations during pregnancy and puerperium. *Neurosurgery* 1990;72:855–66.

158 Horowitz MB, Willet D, Keffer J. The use of cTnI to determine the incidence of myocardial ischemia and injury in patients with aneurysmal and presumed aneurysmal subarachnoid hemorrhage. *Acta Neurochir (Wien)* 1998;140:87–93.

159 Pickard JD, Murray GD, Illingworth R, *et al*. Effect of oral nimodipine on cerebral infarction and outcome after subarachnoid hemorrhage: British Aneurysm Nimodipine Trial. *Br Med J* 1989;298:636–42.

160 Allen GS, Ahn HS, Preziosi TJ, *et al*. Cerebral arterial spasm: a controlled trial of nimodipine in patients with subarachnoid hemorrhage. *N Engl J Med* 1983;308:619–24.

161 Mee E, Dorrance D, Lowe D, *et al*. Controlled study of nimodipine in aneurysm patients treated early after subarachnoid hemorrhage. *Neurosurgery* 1988;22:484–91.

162 Pretruk KC, West M, Mohr G, *et al*. Nimodipine treatment in poor grade aneurysm patients. Results of a multicenter double-blind placebo-controlled trial. *J Neurosurg* 1988;68:505–17.

163 Barker FG, Ogilvy CS. Efficacy of prophylactic nimodipine for delayed ischemic deficit after subarachnoid hemorrhage: a metaanalysis. *J Neurosurg* 1996;84:405–14.

164 Kassell NF, Torner JC, Adams HP. Antifibrinolytic therapy in the acute period following aneurysmal subarachnoid hemorrhage: preliminary observations from the Cooperative Aneurysm Study. *J Neurosurg* 1984;61:225–30.

165   Adams HP Jr. Current status of antifibrinolytic therapy of patients with subarachnoid hemorrhage. *Stroke* 1982;13:256–9.
166   Mizoi K, Yoshimoto T, Fujiwara S, Sugawara T, Takahashi A, Koshu K. Prevention of vasospasm by clot removal and intrathecal bolus injection of tissue-type plasminogen activator: preliminary report. *Neurosurgery* 1991;28:807–13.
167   Findlay JM, Weir BKA, Steinke D, Tanabe T, Gordon P, Grace M. Effect of intrathecal thrombolytic therapy on subarachnoid clot and chronic vasospasm in a primate model of SAH. *J Neurosurg* 1988;69:723–35.
168   Burchiel JK, Hoffman JN, Bakay FAR. Quantitative determination of plasma fibrinolytic activity in patients with ruptured intracranial aneurysms who are receiving Eaminocaproic acid: relationship of possible complications of therapy to the degree of fibrinolytic inhibition. *Neurosurgery* 1984;14:57–63.
169   Adams HP, Nibbelink DW, Torner JC, Sahs AL. Antifibrinolytic therapy in patients with aneurysmal subarachnoid hemorrhage. In: Sahs AL, Nibbelink DW, Torner JC, eds. *Aneurysmal subarachnoid hemorrhage. Report of the Cooperative Study.* Baltimore: Urban and Schwarzenberg, 1981;331–9.
170   Paine JT, Batjer HH, Samson DS. Intraoperative ventricular puncture – technical note. *Neurosurgery* 1988;22:1107–9.
171   Kassell NF, Torner JC. Aneurysmal rebleeding: a preliminary report from the Cooperative Study. *Neurosurgery* 1983;13:479–81.
172   Mizukami M, Kawase T, Usami T, *et al.* Prevention of vasospasm by early operation with removal of subarachnoid blood. *Neurosurgery* 1982; 10:301–7.
173   Sano K, Saito I. Early operation and washout of blood clots for prevention of cerebral vasospasm. In: Wilkins RH, ed. *Cerebral arterial spasm.* Baltimore: Williams and Wilkins, 1980;510–13.
174   Taneda M. Effect of early operation for ruptured aneurysm on prevention of delayed ischemic symptoms. *J Neurosurg* 1982;57:622–8.
175   Batjer HH, Samson D. Intraoperative aneurysmal rupture: incidence, outcome, and suggestions for surgical management. *Neurosurgery* 1986; 18:701–6.
176   Yasargil MG. *Microsurgery,* vol 2. Stuttgart: Georg Thieme Verlag, 1984;58–9.
177   Giannotta SL, Oppenheimer JH, Levy ML, Zelman V. Management of intraoperative rupture of aneurysm without hypotension. *Neurosurgery* 1991;28:531–6.
178   Batjer HH, Frankfurt AI, Purdy PD, *et al.* Use of etomidate, temporary arterial occlusion, and intraoperative angiography in surgical treatment of large and giant cerebral aneurysms. *J Neurosurg* 1988;68:234–40.
179   Seifert V, Eisert WG, Stolke D, Goetz C. Efficacy of single intracisternal bolus injection of recombinant tissue plasminogen activator to prevent delayed cerebral vasospasm after experimental subarachnoid hemorrhage. *Neurosurgery* 1989;25:590–8.
180   Findlay JM, Weir RILA, Kassell NF, Disney LB, Grace MGA. Intracisternal recombinant tissue plasminogen activator after aneurysmal subarachnoid hemorrhage. *J Neurosurg* 1991;75:181–8.
181   Sasaki T, Ohta T, Kikuchi H, Takakura K, Usui M, Ohnishi H. A phase II clinical trial of recombinant human tissue-type plasminogen activator against vasospasm after aneurysmal hemorrhage. *Neurosurgery* 1994;35: 597–605.
182   Usui M, Saito N, Hoya K, Todo T. Vasospasm prevention with postoperative intrathecal thrombolytic therapy: a retrospective

comparison of uroleinase, tissue plasminogen activator, and cisternal drainage alone. *Neurosurgery* 1994;**34**:235–45.

183 Kawada S, Kinugasa K, Meguro T, *et al.* Experimental study of intracisternal administration of tissue-type plasminogen activator followed by cerebrospinal fluid drainage in the ultra-early stage of subarachnoid haemorrhage. *Acta Neurochir* 1999;**141**:1331–8.

184 Gorski R, Zabek M, Jarmuzek P. Influence of intraoperative using of recombinant tissue plasminogen activator on the development of cerebral angiospasm after subarachnoid haemorrhage in patients with ruptured intracranial aneurysms. *Neurol Neurochir Pol* 2000;**34**:41–7.

185 Stiver SI, Porter PJ, Willinsky RA, *et al.* Acute human histopathology of an intracranial aneurysm treated using Guglielmi detachable coils: case report and review of the literature. *Neurosurgery* 1998;**43**:1203–8.

186 Versari PP, Cenzato M, Tartara F, *et al.* Introduction of GDC embolization in the clinical practice as treatment synergical to surgery: impact on overall outcome of patients with subarachnoid hemorrhage. *Acta Neurochir* 2000;**142**:677–83.

187 Tateshima S, Murayama Y, Gobin YP, *et al.* Endovascular treatment of basilar tip aneurysms using Guglielmi detachable coils: anatomic and clinical outcomes in 73 patients from a single institution. *Neurosurgery* 2000;**47**:1332–9.

188 Uda K, Murayama Y, Gobin YP, *et al.* Endovascular treatment of basilar artery trunk aneurysms with Guglielmi detachable coils: clinical experience with 41 aneurysms in 39 patients. *J Neurosurg* 2001;**95**: 624–32.

189 Lee SH, Heros RC. Principles of management of subarachnoid hemmorhage: steroids. In: Ratctieson RA, Wirth FP, eds. *Concepts in neurosurgery. Ruptured cerebral aneurysms: perioperative management.* Baltimore: Williams and Wilkins, 1994;77–83.

190 Takaku A, Tanaka S, Mori T, Suzuki J. Postoperative complications in 1000 cases of intracranial aneurysms. *Surg Neurol* 1979;**12**:137–44.

191 Nelson PB, Sief SM, Maroon JC, Robinson AE. Hyponatremia in intracranial disease: perhaps not the syndrome of inappropriate secretion of antidiuretic hormone (SIADH). *J Neurosurg* 1981;**55**:938–41.

192 Harrigan MR. Cerebral self wasting syndrome: a review. *Neurosurgery* 1996;**38**:152–60.

193 Yamamoto I. Early operation for ruptured intracranial aneurysms: comparative study with computerized tomography. Presented at the 32nd Annual Meeting, Congress of Neurological Surgeons, Toronto, 1982.

194 Park BE. Spontaneous subarachnoid hemorrhage complicated by communicating hydrocephalus: epsilon amino caproic acid as a possible predisposing factor. *Surg Neurol* 1979;**11**:73–80.

195 Heros R, Zarvas N, Varsos V. Cerebral vasospasm after subarachnoid hemorrhage: an update. *Ann Neurol* 1983;**14**:599–608.

196 Ropper AH, Zervas NT. Outcome 1 year after SAH from cerebral aneurysm. Management, morbidity, mortality, and functional status in 112 consecutive good risk patients. *J Neurosurg* 1984;**60**:909–15.

197 Weir BK. Pathophysiology of vasospasm. *Int Anesthesiol Clin* 1982;**10**: 39–43.

198 Pasqualin A, Rosta L, Da Pian R, Cavazzani P, Scienza R. Role of computed tomography in the management of vasospasm after subarachnoid hemorrhage. *Neurosurgery* 1984;**15**:344–53.

199 Kistler JP, Crowell RM, Davis KR, *et al.* The relation of cerebral vasospasm to the extent and location of subarachnoid blood visualized by CT scan. A prospective study. *Neurology* 1983;**33**:424–36.

200 Fisher CM, Roberson GH, Ojemann RG. Cerebral vasospasm with ruptured saccular aneurysm – the clinical manifestations. *Neurosurgery* 1977;**1**:245–8.

201 Symon L. Disordered cerebro-vascular physiology in aneurysmal subarachnoid hemorrhage. *Acta Neurochir (Wien)* 1979;**41**:7–22.

202 Pritz MB, Giannotta SI, Kindt GW, McGillicuddy JE, Prager RL. Treatment of patients with neurological deficits associated with cerebral vasospasm by intravascular volume expansion. *Neurosurgery* 1978; **3**:364–8.

203 Shimoda M, Oda S, Tsugane R, Sato O. Intracranial complications of hypervolemic therapy in patients with a delayed ischemic deficit attributed to vasospasm. *J Neurosurg* 1993;**78**:423–9.

204 Minami H, Kuwamura K, Tamaki N. Intraarterial infusion of papaverine and change of cerebral hemodynamics in symptomatic cerebral vasospasm. *Kobe J Med Sci* 2001;**47**:169–79.

205 Vajkoczy P, Horn P, Bauhuf C, et al. Effect of intra-arterial papaverine on regional cerebral blood flow in hemodynamically relevant cerebral vasospasm. *Stroke* 2001;**32**:498–505.

206 Wanke I, Dorfler A, Dietrich U, et al. Combined endovascular therapy of ruptured aneurysms and cerebral vasospasm. *Neuroradiology* 2000;**42**: 926–9.

207 Kaku Y, Yonekawa Y, Tsukahara T, Kazekawa K. Superselective intra-arterial infusion of papaverine for the treatment of cerebral vasospasm after subarachnoid hemorrhage. *J Neurosurg* 1992;**77**:842–7.

208 Kassell NF, Helm G, Sommons N, Phillips CD, Cail WS. Treatment of cerebral vasospasm with intra-arterial papaverine. *J Neurosurg* 1992;**77**: 848–52.

209 Higashida RT, Halbach W, Cahan LD, et al. Transluminal angioplasty for treatment of intracranial arterial vasospasm. *J Neurosurg* 1989;**71**: 648–53.

210 Newell DW, Eskridge JM, Maybery MR, et al. Angioplasty for the treatment of symptomatic vasospasm following subarachnoid hemorrhage. *J Neurosurg* 1989;**71**:654–60.

211 Zubkov YN, Nikiforov BM, Shustin VA. Balloon catheter technique for dilatation of constricted cerebral arteries after aneurysmal SAH. *Acta Neurochir* 1984;**70**:65–79.

212 Firlik AD, Kaufmann AM, Jungreis CA, Yonas H. Effect of transluminal angioplasty on cerebral blood flow in the management of symptomatic vasospasm following aneurysmal subarachnoid hemorrhage. *J Neurosurg* 1997;**86**:830–9.

213 Polin RS, Coenen VA, Hansen CA, et al. Efficacy of transluminal angioplasty for the management of symptomatic cerebral vasospasm following aneurysmal subarachnoid hemorrhage. *J Neurosurg* 2000;**92**: 284–90.

214 Morgan MK, Jonker B, Finfer S, et al. Aggressive management of aneurysmal subarachnoid haemorrhage based on a papaverine angioplasty protocol. *J Clin Neurosci* 2000;**7**:305–8.

215 Linskey ME, Horton JA, Rao GF, Yonas H. Fatal rupture of the intracranial carotid artery during transluminal angioplasty for vasospasm induced by subarachnoid hemorrhage. *J Neurosurg* 1991;**74**:985–90.

216 Haley EC, Kassell NF, Alves WM, Weir BKA, Hansen CA. Phase II trial of Tirilizad in aneurysmal subarachnoid hemorrhage. *J Neurosurg* 1995;**82**:786–90.

217 Matsni T, Asano T. Effects of new 21 amino steroid Tirilizad mesylate (U74006F) on chronic cerebral vasospasm in a "two hemorrhage" model of beagle dogs. *Neurosurgery* 1994;**34**:1035–9.

218 Smith S, Scherch HM, Hall ED. Protective effects of Tirilizad mesylate and metabolite U-89678 against blood–brain barrier damage after subarachnoid hemorrhage and lipid peroxidative neuronal injury. *J Neurosurg* 1996;**84**:229–33.

219 Kassell NF, Haley CE, Hansen C, Alves WM. Randomized, double blind, vehicle controlled trial of Tirilizad mesylate in patients with aneurysmal subarachnoid hemorrhage: a cooperative study in Europe, Australia, and New Zealand. *J Neurosurg* 1996;**84**:221–8.

220 Lanzino G, Kassell NF. Double-blind, randomized, vehicle-controlled study of high-dose tirilazad mesylate in women with aneurysmal subarachnoid hemorrhage. Part II. A cooperative study in North America. *J Neurosurg* 1999;**90**:1018–24.

221 Lanzino G, Kassell NF, Dorsch NW, *et al*. Double-blind, randomized, vehicle-controlled study of high-dose tirilazad mesylate in women with aneurysmal subarachnoid hemorrhage. Part I. A cooperative study in Europe, Australia, New Zealand, and South Africa. *J Neurosurg* 1999;**90**: 1011–17.

222 Raabe A, Zimmerman M, Setzer M, *et al*. Effect of intraventricular sodium nitroprusside on cerebral hemodynamics and oxygenation in poor-grade aneurysm patients with severe, medically refractory vasospasm. *Neurosurgery* 2002;**50**:1006–13.

223 Frizzell RT, Kuhn F, Morris R, Quinn C, Fisher WS. Screening for ocular hemorrhages in patients with ruptured cerebral aneurysms; a prospective study of 99 patients. *Neurosurgery* 1997;**41**:529–34.

224 Kasuya H, Kawashima A, Namiki K, Shimizu T, Takakura K. Metabolic profiles of patients with subarachnoid hemorrhage treated by early surgery. *Neurosurgery* 1998;**42**:1268–75.

225 Hutter BO, Eislbach JM. Which neuropsychological deficits are hidden behind a good outcome (Glasgow = 1) after aneurysmal subarachnoid hemorrhage? *Neurosurgery* 1993;**33**:999–1006.

226 Ogden JA, Mee EW, Henning M. A prospective study of impairment of cognition and memory and recovery after subarachnoid hemorrhage. *Neurosurgery* 1993;**33**:572–87.

9: Cerebral infection

J GREIG, MJ WOOD

Broadly, infection within the skull can be categorised clinically under three headings: meningitis, encephalitis, and focal space occupation. These are not mutually exclusive and commonly two – or less commonly all three – clinical syndromes may be found in the same patient. Symptoms and signs common to all three are pyrexia, headache, disturbance of consciousness, and focal neurological signs. With meningitis, photophobia, neck stiffness, vomiting, and a variable degree of altered consciousness are found. Encephalitis implies disease of brain parenchyma and, although there are usually signs of meningitis in addition, the findings are of altered mental state earlier in the evolution of the illness, together with more marked deterioration of conscious level, epileptic seizures, and focal neurology. A focal space-occupying syndrome may occur with local suppuration and abscess or granuloma formation, necrotising encephalitis, or with infarction as a result of arteritis or phlebitis.

With all these syndromes there may or may not be evidence of coexistent systemic or localised infection elsewhere. Raised intracranial pressure (ICP) occurs with all three and is always a significant component of the illness. Failure to recognise this will result in catastrophe. Depression of the conscious level, even just drowsiness, is a common indication that ICP is raised. Neck stiffness may result from cerebellar tonsil impaction at the foramen magnum. Papilloedema, when present, indicates raised ICP but it takes time to develop and its absence does not mean that ICP is normal.

The same clinical syndrome may be caused by different organisms. A meningitic picture may follow infection by viruses, bacteria, fungi, or protozoa. Subarachnoid haemorrhage is an illustration of a non-infectious cause of the same syndrome. Important clues that point to the aetiology are obtained by observation of the speed of onset, progression of the disease, and response to treatment. Knowledge of any pre-existing diseases, current medication, occupation and environment, recent travel and recreational habits, and the state of health of family and colleagues may indicate a potential pathogen.

Acute meningitis is the most common of the brain infectious syndromes. Epidemiology, pathogenesis, and evolution are complex and vary with geography and with age. Presentation occurs within hours or, at most, a few days of the onset of symptoms. These, together with the physical signs, are characteristically headache, fever, photophobia, irritability, neck stiffness, and altered mentation. The causal agent is generally either a virus or a bacterium: fungi and parasites cause acute meningitis only in special circumstances. Viral meningitis is a much more benign illness than the bacterial form.

Viral meningitis

Wallgren coined the term "acute aseptic meningitis" in 1925[1] to describe acute meningeal irritation, benign and self-limiting, with complete recovery and sterile pleocytic cerebrospinal fluid (CSF).

It has become evident that viruses cause at least 70% of such cases. Viral infections of the central nervous system (CNS) are complications of systemic viral infections and the virus gains access to the brain via the bloodstream or, less commonly, by travelling up peripheral nerves.[2] Viral meningitis results from haematogenous infection and, to enter the CNS, the virus must cross the endothelial cell junctions of the blood–brain barrier. The ability to do this is dependent upon surface adhesion molecules on the cells, surface charges and cellular receptors of the virus, and the property of entering infected cells.[3] Certain viruses preferentially infect the meninges, choroid plexus, and ependyma rather than cerebral parenchyma and cause meningitis; others infect neurons and glia to cause encephalitis. There is considerable overlap and some viruses cause meningoencephalitis, incorporating signs of both.

Most cases of viral meningitis occur in children and young adults. Infections occur throughout the year, with a preponderance in summer and autumn in temperate climates. The annual reported incidence varies from 11 to 27 cases per 100 000 and several thousand cases are reported annually in the United States. The actual number of infections is almost

---

Box 9.1 Viral causes of cerebral infection

Meningitis	Encephalitis
Enteroviruses	Herpes simplex
Echo	Varicella zoster virus
Polio	Cytomegalovirus
Coxsackie	Epstein–Barr virus
Herpes simplex 2	HIV
Lymphocytic choriomeningitis virus	Mumps
Varicella zoster virus	Measles
Mumps	Rabies
HIV	Arboviruses

---

certainly several multiples higher because of underreporting. The recent introduction of polymerase chain reaction (PCR) tests for the detection of enteroviral ribonucleic acid (RNA) in CSF has greatly increased the detection of enteroviral CNS infections and it has become apparent that 85–90% of acute viral meningitis is caused by enteroviruses (coxsackie B or echo).[4] Much less commonly meningitis is caused by herpes simplex virus (HSV) type 2, varicella zoster virus (VZV), mumps, lymphocytic choriomeningitis, and HIV (Box 9.1).

The clinical onset is usually rapid over hours, with pyrexia, malaise, headache, neck stiffness, photophobia, myalgia, lethargy, and irritability. Most cases do not progress further and the subject can be roused easily and remains coherent. In approximately 3% of infected people the conscious level falls or focal signs or seizures develop, suggesting encephalitis. Resolution begins within a few days and is complete within two weeks in most. A few will have persistent malaise and myalgia for some weeks. The pathogen can seldom be identified clinically; parotitis and orchitis may point to mumps, arthralgia and lymphadenopathy to HIV, myalgia and myocarditis to coxsackie, and rashes to enterovirus. The illness is not as severe and prolonged as bacterial meningitis and the signs are not so florid.

Differential diagnosis

Conditions from which viral meningitis must be differentiated are: the early stages of (or partially treated) bacterial meningitis; some cases of subarachnoid haemorrhage; other causes of aseptic meningitis caused by fastidious bacteria, fungi, and parasites that do not grow readily in routine culture; parameningeal infection, inflammation, or neoplasia; and collagen/vasculitic disease. To confirm the diagnosis, CSF examination is mandatory. If there are neurological signs suggestive of raised ICP then appropriate imaging (see below) should be undertaken first. CSF pressure is normal or slightly raised and the fluid is clear to the naked eye. White cell counts are in the range of up to 500–1000/mm^3, mainly lymphocytes although, in some, polymorphs may predominate. In such cases it is prudent to re-examine the CSF 12 hours later to identify a developing lymphocytosis and exclude a bacterial cause.[5] CSF protein may be slightly raised, glucose is normal or only slightly reduced. Numerous laboratory tests have been applied to CSF with the claim that they differentiate a bacterial from a viral aetiology, but none has sufficient discrimination to be useful. A similar lack of specificity attaches to the occasional abnormalities, which may be seen in blood counts, blood biochemistry, and the EEG.

In most cases it is not necessary to establish an exact aetiology for treatment purposes, as the disease is benign and self-limiting. To establish the aetiology, the virus may be isolated from CSF or by serological studies of acute and convalescent serum samples, identification of IgM antibody, or viral antigen in CSF. The use of PCR for amplification of viral nucleic acid within CSF has revolutionised the diagnosis of viral infections of the central nervous system.[6,7]

Provided other similar treatable disorders have been excluded, symptomatic treatment with analgesics and antiemetics is all that is required. Antibiotics should not be given. Pleconaril is a novel antiviral agent that integrates into the "pocket" on the surface of the enteroviral capsid into which the cellular receptor normally fits and thus inhibits viral attachment to host cells and uncoating.[8] It has been shown in randomised, placebo controlled trials to be safe and effective in the treatment of enteroviral meningitis in children, adolescents, and adults. It will probably also be useful in the treatment of life threatening and chronic enteroviral meningoencephalitis.[9]

Viral encephalitis

Acute viral encephalitis is due to direct invasion of brain parenchyma and the clinical manifestations are caused by cell dysfunction and associated inflammatory change. At the bedside this may be indistinguishable from postinfectious encephalitis, the pathology of which is perivenous demyelination caused by allergic or immune reactions triggered after a latent period by viral infection.[10,11] Viruses are far and away the most common cause of encephalitis globally, but in certain locations and seasons other organisms such as malaria and other protozoa, rickettsiae, and fungi may induce an encephalitic syndrome. It is therefore of paramount importance to obtain from the patient or a relative a full account of the recent travel history.

As with meningitis, the virus usually reaches the brain by either haematogenous or neuronal routes. The haematogenous route is the most common. Viral entry may be through the skin following an insect bite, as with arbovirus infection, or via the respiratory or gastrointestinal route. Local replication ensues, resulting in transient viraemia and spread to the reticuloendothelial system whence, following further replication, secondary viraemia increases and spread takes place to other sites including the CNS. Here there is inflammation of the capillary and endothelial cortical vessels and, as disease progresses, astrocytosis and gliosis become prominent histopathological findings. Modification of this process by host immune responses may occur and if these are compromised, disease progression may be fulminant. More rarely, virus may ascend neurons centripetally to lodge in brain cells, as with herpes encephalitis and rabies. There is some evidence that the olfactory tract is one route of access of HSV to the brain. Fortunately, encephalitis is a rare complication of common viral infections and most patients with systemic viral infections do not develop neurological signs.

Certain viruses exhibit tropism towards specific cell types – the limbic system in rabies,[12] temporal lobe in herpes simplex encephalitis – and this may produce clinical signs that are diagnostically useful.[11] In most cases of encephalitis, however, signs and symptoms are common to most pathogens and diagnostic clues must be sought elsewhere. Is there evidence of infection elsewhere, such as the characteristic rashes of varicella and measles or the parotitis of mumps? Has there been travel to an area that harbours known insect vectors? Even aircraft stopovers in "at-risk" areas may be important;

cases of "runway" infection have been recorded where the insect vectors have entered the aircraft. Is there evidence of a current or past insect bite? What is the season of the year? Diagnostic tests may help, yet in perhaps as many as a third of all cases no specific aetiology can be established.

Viral encephalitis is not rare and occurs globally.[11] In the United Kingdom and Europe, most cases are sporadic and are caused by herpes simplex and other herpesviruses (Box 9.1). Since the widespread use of childhood measles, mumps, and rubella (MMR) vaccine, encephalitis caused by these viruses is now rare. In the United States, sporadic and epidemic forms are caused by arboviruses (*ar*thropod *bo*rne). Japanese B encephalitis causes most epidemic infections elsewhere. As many as 20 000 cases of encephalitis per annum may occur in the United States.[13]

Patients who develop viral encephalitis often have several days of a prodrome, which includes myalgia, fever, malaise, mild upper respiratory infection, rash, or parotitis. The development of headache, mental change, and drowsiness implies encephalitis, which is usually associated with meningitic features. As the disease progresses, disorientation and disturbance of behaviour and speech worsen and drowsiness merges into coma. Epileptic seizures are common and focal signs may appear appropriate to the area of the brain that suffers the brunt of the infection. For example, hallucinations and memory upset from the temporal lobes, hemiparesis, spasticity, sensory loss and speech upset from the parietal lobes, and coordination problems and dysarthria with cerebellar deficits. There may also be signs of raised intracranial pressure. The very young, the very old, and those with compromised immune systems often have more severe disease. Signs should be sought in other organ systems, which may point to a particular virus. Some forms of encephalitis have specific features that are briefly discussed later.

Differential diagnosis

The list of diseases that may cause a similar clinical picture is large and includes all forms of bacterial meningitis, malaria and other protozoal and fungal infections, intracranial suppuration, septicaemia and endocarditis, metastatic disease, collagen/vascular disease, drug abuse, and metabolic encephalopathies.

Faced with a patient with rapid onset of pyrexia and stupor or coma, the above potentially remediable conditions need to be excluded quickly. Blood counts and biochemical tests are not diagnostic but may be abnormal as a result of inadequate hydration or inappropriate secretion of antidiuretic hormone. If indicated, blood films should be examined for malaria parasites and blood cultures should be set up.

As these results are awaited, the brain should be imaged to determine if there is a space occupying lesion, cerebral oedema, or focal areas of necrosis, such as might occur in the temporal lobes with herpes simplex encephalitis (HSE). Some of the abnormalities are subtle and it is necessary to interpret the scans with close attention to their timing in the evolution of the disease. In the first two or three days there may be no obvious abnormality and repeat scanning may be necessary. MRI scanning is preferable to CT because it may reveal abnormalities missed by CT scanning and cerebral oedema and white matter abnormalities are easier to see.[14] Unfortunately MRI scanning is not always available for emergencies. Furthermore, it is not always appropriate for a seriously ill patient, as the acquisition time for images is quite long, and any movement degrades the images. In patients with encephalitis the EEG is abnormal, most often showing non-specific diffuse slow wave activity, perhaps with seizure activity. Temporal lobe focal abnormality with high voltage spike and slow wave complexes is highly suggestive of HSE.

The CSF should be examined as soon as possible when deemed safe; unfortunately cranial scanning does not convey an accurate picture of intracranial pressure and judgement of the potential safety of lumbar puncture requires experience and not a little luck. The decision to examine CSF in such circumstances should not be taken by a junior doctor. The CSF is often under pressure and there is usually a leucocytosis, with between 10 and several thousand white cells per mm^3. These are principally lymphocytes but polymorphs may predominate in the early stages. Red cells may be found if there is a necrotising component, as in HSE. The glucose content is normal, protein is raised, and organisms are not seen. In 3–5% of patients with severe viral infections of the CNS the CSF may be completely normal.

Treatment

There is no specific therapy for most forms of viral encephalitis in previously healthy individuals. With the success of early therapy with intravenous aciclovir in HSE, it is imperative to identify the organism as quickly as possible. The most sensitive and rapid way of detecting HSV and other viruses is by PCR.[6,7,15] The application of PCR in HSE has a sensitivity of 95% and a specificity of 94%.[16] Brain biopsy no longer has a place in the diagnosis of viral encephalitis, except to determine if a lesion demonstrated by scan is an abscess, granuloma, or tumour. It is safer to begin treatment with aciclovir in essentially all patients with unexplained encephalitis.[17] If another aetiology is subsequently identified, then aciclovir can be stopped. Effective therapy for most other viral encephalitides has not yet been clearly established and generally the treatment of viral encephalitis is symptomatic and requires maintenance of adequate nutrition, hydration, and oxygenation. Some potentially useful treatments are under clinical evaluation, such as pleconaril for enteroviral meningoencephalitis.[9] Seizures are controlled with anticonvulsants and secondary infections are treated as necessary. Intracranial hypertension and cerebral oedema may be a problem but there is no consensus on the correct treatment. Intubation and hyperventilation, glycerol, mannitol, and dexamethasone have all been used, although there are theoretical objections to the last in HSE. The subject has been extensively reviewed.[18]

Specific encephalitides

Herpes simplex virus

Herpes simplex virus (HSV) is the most common cause of non-epidemic acute focal viral encephalitis in Europe and North America, with an incidence of up to 0·5 per 100 000 population per year.[19] This is almost certainly an underestimate as many milder cases pass unrecognised. It occurs throughout the year and except for neonatal infections, almost all cases are caused by HSV type 1. Using serological studies, it is estimated that one-third of these infections occur during primary HSV1 infection and two-thirds result from reactivation of latent virus. It is no more common in those with compromised immune systems and it affects patients of any age. A third are below 20 and half over 50.[20] The clinical presentation is enormously variable. Onset is usually insidious, with a prodrome of 4–10 days with malaise, pyrexia, and irritability, followed by frontal and temporal lobe disturbance manifest by personality change, hallucinations, psychiatric upset, and increasing focal signs, seizures, and deteriorating conscious level. In perhaps as many as 87%, focal signs appear.[20] In a few, the onset is cataclysmic and the evolution is compressed into only a few days. Abscess, tumour, granuloma, vascular disease, and other forms of viral encephalitis are other diagnoses that have been mistaken for HSE.[21] Focal changes on CT, MRI, and EEG are helpful but not pathognomonic. The use of PCR on CSF can provide a rapid, specific, and sensitive diagnosis.

The HSV1 viral load may also provide prognostic information, with high viral loads (greater than 100 HSV copies per microlitre of CSF) correlating with longer illness, greater mortality, and more long term sequelae. Treatment must be given quickly with aciclovir 10 mg/kg eight hourly by intravenous infusion for 14 days. This has been shown to diminish the mortality rate from greater than 70% in untreated patients to below 30%.[22,23] Younger patients and those with a higher Glasgow Coma Score have a better outcome than older patients and those with a markedly disturbed conscious level.

Varicella zoster virus

Encephalitis accounts for 90% of the neurological complications of varicella, which are in themselves rare, affecting only 0·1% of cases.[24,25] In half, the encephalitis is of the cerebellar type with ataxia, dysarthria, headache, and drowsiness coming on about a week after the rash begins, but the neurological onset may precede the rash. Convulsions are common[26] and progression to hemiplegia, cranial nerve palsies, aphasia, and coma may ensue. Patients with the cerebellar form usually recover completely but 10% of those with the general form die. Encephalitis may rarely follow shingles.[27] Management of VZV-associated encephalitis is with aciclovir as described for HSE.

Cytomegalovirus

This is not an important cause of encephalitis except in neonates and immunocompromised patients, recipients of organ transplants, and patients with AIDS.[28] Treatment with ganciclovir or foscarnet has been shown to be helpful in some cases but in neonatal CMV encephalitis, the prognosis is still gloomy.[29]

Epstein–Barr virus

Meningoencephalitis has been described as a rare complication of Epstein–Barr virus (EBV) virus infection.[30,31] There are no specific features and the prognosis is excellent. CSF PCR can be used for diagnosis. Semiquantitative PCR analysis of EBV DNA levels correlates with active infection as compared with latently infected individuals who are seropositive for EBV.

Measles

Acute encephalitis occurring in the course of measles infection is usually caused by a postinfectious, perivenous, demyelination, although in some there may be direct virus induced cellular damage.[32] Clinically the manifestations are the same and occur in up to 1 in 1000 cases of measles in those above the age of two, the frequency increasing with age. With widespread measles vaccination the disease has become extremely rare.

Mumps

Encephalitis is a rare complication of mumps, occurring in less than 1% of cases; it has no specific features. It follows up to two weeks after the development of parotitis, though this may be absent in up to half.[33] Treatment is symptomatic and prognosis is excellent.

Rabies

Rabies is still associated with 100% mortality. It is transmitted by bites or scratches from a variety of mammals, including bats.[12] The incubation period ranges from a few days to several months and then, after a prodromal phase of fever, anxiety, and disturbed sensation at the site of the wound, CNS signs develop. Encephalitic or paralytic signs may predominate but the patient inexorably progresses to coma and cardiorespiratory failure. Other than supportive care, there is no therapy for human rabies.

Epidemic encephalitis

Arboviruses cause epidemic encephalitis in various parts of the world.[11] They are not an important cause of encephalitis in Britain, but with the increasing ease of intercontinental travel, cases are now being recognised here and the frequency is likely to increase. It is imperative therefore that a full travel and recreational history be taken from anyone suspected of neurological infection and arbovirus encephalitis should be suspected if there has been exposure to insect bites in countries known to harbour these viruses.

All these arboviruses are perpetuated by zoonoses of pathologically insignificant infection in birds and smaller vertebrates. Transmission is by an arthropod vector, such as the mosquito or tick. Replication and viraemia develop after a bite. Most people suffer only a mild systemic illness but some go on to develop encephalitis, the severity of which depends upon the strain of the virus. Clinical features are common to all, with some variation in incubation, progression, and severity. They cannot be distinguished on clinical grounds alone. There are no specific features on imaging, EEG, or in the CSF. Diagnosis is by demonstration of antibody titre rise in paired serum samples. Treatment is largely symptomatic.

West Nile Virus

West Nile Virus is a mosquito-borne flavivirus indigenous to Africa, Asia, Europe, and Australia, and has recently been responsible for outbreaks of encephalitis in Romania[34] and the United States.[35] Birds are the natural reservoir of infection. It can cause a distinctive clinical syndrome with flaccid weakness, hyporeflexia, and encephalitis, predominantly of the brain stem. Seroepidemiological studies suggest that up to 200 cases of mild or asymptomatic disease occur for each recognised case of encephalitis. In the Romanian outbreak, mortality was related to age. Although there is no specific therapy, ribavirin has been shown to inhibit West Nile Virus replication in culture. Presently there is no vaccine, so disease prevention depends on vector mosquito control.

Nipah virus

Nipah virus caused an outbreak of severe encephalitis in Singapore and Malaysia in 1998–99.[36] The virus is a previously unrecognised paramyxovirus that chiefly infected pig farmers and those in related industries. Pigs provide a reservoir of infection and the virus is spread to man by the aerosol route. It causes a CNS vasculitis with endothelial cell infection, vascular thrombosis, and tissue infarction. Ribavirin may reduce the mortality. Aggressive culling of pigs has effectively terminated the outbreak.

Eastern equine encephalitis

Birds of the Atlantic and Gulf coasts of America are the reservoir of this rare condition.[11,37] Epidemics may occur in horses. Cases occur at migration time, summer and autumn, and children are most affected. There is acute encephalitis, which may be abrupt and violent and carries a mortality of 70%, with 80% of survivors having neurological sequelae.

Western equine encephalitis

This is less severe and occurs in eastern, central and western United States, Canada, and eastern South America.[37]

St Louis encephalitis

This disease shares the same clinical features as other arboviral encephalitides and is transmitted sporadically in large areas of the United States and in Central America. West of the Mississippi it is endemic and cases occur in epidemics or sporadically from July to October. Most cases are benign and of short duration. The elderly are more likely to get clinical disease after infection.

California and La Crosse viruses

These viruses are similar and cause the same disease in central and midwest United States. The reservoir is small rodents and the vector is the mosquito, *Aedes* sp. Children are affected with a peak in August and September. Clinical onset is sudden and recovery takes place within 10 days.[11,38] Although the mortality is low, 10–15% of survivors have significant neurological defects.

Central European encephalitis

This encephalitis may be contracted from woodlands in Scandinavia through to northern Greece and the former Yugoslavia. Increasing numbers of cases are being reported from Austria. The virus is maintained in small woodland mammals and transmitted to people who enter the forest for recreation or work and are bitten by *Ixodes* ticks. There is a biphasic course with an initial flu-like illness, followed within two weeks by mild meningitis or encephalitis, perhaps with muscle weakness. Management is symptomatic and recovery is usually complete. Diagnosis is serological. Russian spring–summer encephalitis is a similar, more severe condition.

Japanese encephalitis

This is the most common arbovirus encephalitis worldwide and is endemic in Southeast Asia, Japan, China, the Philippines, Borneo, and large areas of the Indian subcontinent.[11,39] Birds and domestic animals are the reservoir, mosquitoes the vector. Encephalitis is seen most commonly in those under 15 years and in the elderly. After an incubation period of one to two weeks there is abrupt onset of encephalitis, often with myalgia. Extrapyramidal features have been noted and a polio-like illness is now recognised. Convalescence may be prolonged and sequelae are common. Although there is no effective antiviral agent for Japanese encephalitis, good supportive management can improve the outcome. Diagnosis is by virus isolation or the demonstration of specific antigen or antibodies in the CSF or blood.[40] Prevention is by vector control and use of effective vaccination.

HIV

Cerebral infection is a frequent accompaniment of HIV infection, with 39–70% of those with AIDS suffering from neurological complications.[41,42] HIV enters the central nervous system soon after primary infection and causes symptoms both as a primary effect of the virus and also secondary to the systemic immune suppression that accompanies AIDS and renders the sufferer liable to opportunistic infections. The manifestations of HIV infection of the brain coexist with opportunistic infection and may result in a complex and confused syndrome constellation. Many of the features are chronic in evolution but some are acute. In practice, any change in neurological status in a patient with AIDS usually creates a neurological emergency because of the possibility of opportunistic infection. There are excellent accounts of the epidemiology, immunology, and classification of the natural progression of HIV infection available and these matters are not discussed further here.[43-46]

HIV is spread by inoculation of virus by sexual intercourse, by contaminated blood or blood products, or vertically in utero, during birth, or by breast milk. Infection with HIV occurs when the viral glycoprotein, gp 120, binds to the cellular membrane CD4 molecule of T helper lymphocytes (and other cells) and the virus enters the cell cytoplasm. HIV is an RNA virus that encodes for reverse transcriptase, enabling a DNA copy of viral RNA to be produced in an infected cell. This DNA provirus is incorporated into the host genome. Because HIV can infect the neuraxis early and persist in the CNS indefinitely, CSF studies cannot prove that HIV causes a particular neurological syndrome. Some 40% of all HIV patients not receiving antiretroviral drugs have CSF abnormalities, although a large proportion is asymptomatic. There is a lymphocytic pleocytosis, raised protein, and a normal glucose content, and as many as 20% may grow HIV in culture.[47,48] Antibodies, mainly IgG but also IgA and IgM, appear in CSF and p24 antigen is often present in higher concentration than in serum. Unfortunately these levels do not correlate well with clinical status. Viral load can be detected and quantified using PCR.

Primary HIV infection

During the first few weeks after infection with HIV, about 50% of patients develop a self-limiting seroconversion illness.[49,50] The most common symptoms include fever, pharyngitis, malaise, headache, lymphadenopathy, and a maculopapular rash. These coincide with the onset of the immune response and high levels of viraemia. At this time HIV may invade the central nervous system, probably via lymphocytes, monocytes, and as cell free virus. The most common neurological manifestation is an aseptic meningoencephalitis, associated with lymphocytic CSF. Clinical features include headache, confusion, personality change, and retro-orbital pain, exacerbated by eye movements. Although these symptoms settle spontaneously after one to three weeks, primary HIV infection is an important diagnosis to consider both because it is associated with an increased risk of progression to symptomatic disease and also because patients have a high viral load and are thus highly infectious to sexual and needle sharing partners. Diagnosis can be made reliably by positive virological tests (these involve testing for free viral RNA using amplification techniques) in the absence of specific HIV antibodies. The diagnosis should be confirmed by repeat antibody testing, since anti-HIV antibodies appear during the seroconversion illness. Some advocate the use of antiretroviral therapy for symptomatic primary HIV infection,[51] although this is still a contentious matter, without data to confirm any overall benefits. At present, in the UK most patients are monitored and antiretroviral therapy started when their immune dysfunction becomes pronounced.

HIV encephalopathy

A decline in cognitive function is common in advanced HIV infection, although with more subtle neuropsychological and neurophysiological techniques, it is possible to demonstrate mild mentation defects in early infection.[52] Pathological changes found at autopsy include brain atrophy, most prominent in the hippocampus and basal ganglia, with sulcal widening and ventricular dilatation. The usual course is for subjects to become inattentive, clumsy, and to have short term memory loss. In time, the subject becomes withdrawn, apathetic, and mentally slow, with akinetic dementia.[42] The course may, however, be interrupted by acute relapses with confusion and psychosis, when the patient may present as a neurological emergency, when it is necessary to exclude other CNS infections, neoplasia, and systemic illness as a cause.

In HIV encephalopathy, CT is normal or shows cerebral atrophy and MRI demonstrates diffuse white matter abnormalities, which correlate with neuropathological changes. CSF examination is likely to be abnormal as described and it is necessary to exclude complicating infection. In HIV-infected children, 50% develop a similar progressive encephalopathy that is usually fatal within a year.

A decline in the incidence of HIV dementia has been noted following the introduction of highly active antiretroviral therapies (HAART) and there is anecdotal evidence that such treatment improves abnormal brain metabolism associated with HIV dementia.

HIV treatment

There has been extraordinary progress in developing HAART over the past decade and treatment of HIV infection is now an extremely complex and continually evolving subject.[53-55] It is inappropriate to give details here but, in broad terms, modern management involves the use of a combination of at least three antiretroviral drugs. There are a number of classes of drugs including reverse transcriptase inhibitors (either nucleoside analogues, nucleotides, or non-nucleoside drugs), protease inhibitors, and inhibitors of HIV fusion to or entry into cells.[56] If patient compliance with the complex regimens is good then the quantity of HIV in the serum can be suppressed to undetectable levels for many years, leading to prolonged remission.

Opportunistic infections

Although the development of HAART has reduced the incidence of opportunistic infections and tumours they can still complicate and alter the progression of HIV infection and precipitate a neurological emergency. Some patients are unable to take HAART and, in others, antiretroviral regimens have failed: for these prophylaxis against opportunistic infections is needed.[57,58]

A useful way to approach the different cerebral opportunistic infections is to divide them into those that cause focal lesions and those with a more diffuse picture of meningitis or encephalitis. Toxoplasmosis, primary CNS lymphoma, and progressive multifocal leukoencephalopathy (PML) cause over 90% of focal lesions in patients with a CD4 count of less than 50 per microlitre. Tuberculosis, nocardia, and aspergillosis can also present with focal CNS lesions. CMV, HSV, VZV, and syphilis are all frequent pathogens that may cause diffuse disease. Meningitis is usually caused by pathogens such as *Cryptococcus neoformans*, *Mycobacterium tuberculosis*, *Streptococcus pneumoniae* and *Listeria monocytogenes*. More than one syndrome may be present at any given time, confusing the clinical picture.

Toxoplasmosis

Toxoplasmosis is a common cause of focal neurological abnormalities in advanced HIV infection, particularly in those with a CD4 cell count less than 200 per microlitre.[59,60] It almost always results from reactivation of latent cysts of *Toxoplasma gondii*. These rapidly divide, resulting in tissue destruction and progressively enlarging necrotic lesions, mainly in the brain (particularly the basal ganglia), but also in the eye and lung.

The onset of symptoms is usually subacute with the most common abnormalities being a hemiparesis or speech problem. Brain stem involvement may result in cranial nerve abnormalities. Occasionally the onset is more abrupt with seizures or cerebral haemorrhage. Confirming a diagnosis of toxoplasmosis can be difficult. Serology is unhelpful as disease is secondary to reactivation of latent infection and thus detectable IgG to *T. gondii* does not differentiate latent from active infection. If CSF can be safely obtained, PCR for *T. gondii* may be diagnostic.[61] CT or MRI scanning typically demonstrates solitary or multiple, ring-enhancing cerebral lesions, most commonly in the basal ganglia or cerebral hemispheres (Figure 9.1). Whilst ring-enhancing lesions are not diagnostic of cerebral toxoplasmosis, in a patient with AIDS the positive predictive value of detectable toxoplasma IgG and multiple ring-enhancing lesions on CT or MRI is nearly 80%.[60] Thus a presumptive diagnosis may be made if there is a favourable response to treatment. Serial scanning can

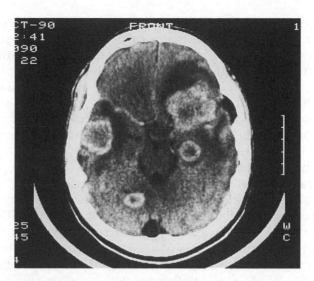

Figure 9.1 CT scan of a patient with AIDS showing multiple ring-enhancing lesions of cerebral toxoplasmosis

be used to monitor lesions. Ninety per cent of patients will have demonstrable clinical and radiological improvement after two to three weeks of appropriate treatment. If improvement does not occur, if there is clinical deterioration, or if diagnostic doubt remains, a cerebral biopsy should take place.

Treatment for cerebral toxoplasmosis is usually with pyrimethamine and sulfadiazine, plus folinic acid to reduce bone marrow suppression.[59] This will result in a clinical response in 68–95% of patients, but 40% will suffer side effects. Pyrimethamine and clindamycin is one of a number of alternative regimens.[62] Steroids are used frequently but there has been no definite benefit described and their use can make the interpretation of the results of empirical therapy difficult. After completion of initial therapy patients should take lifelong suppressive therapy unless immune reconstitution occurs after use of HAART.[57]

Cryptococcosis

Cryptococcus neoformans is an encapsulated yeast-like fungus with a worldwide distribution. It is a common cause of meningitis in AIDS patients with CD4 cell counts of less than 100 per microlitre.[63,64] In many parts of Africa where HIV is very prevalent, it is now the commonest cause of meningitis. Patients present with an acute or insidious onset of non-specific symptoms such as headache, nausea, irritability, confusion, and drowsiness. Signs too are often non-specific with low grade fever and minimal neck stiffness. Focal neurological abnormalities are rare but papilloedema may occur in up to one third of patients.

Diagnosis is made by examination of the CSF. The opening pressure is usually elevated, but microscopy may reveal minimal or no abnormalities or a lymphocytosis with raised protein and low glucose. An India ink stain of the CSF will detect cryptococci in 25–50% of patients with cryptococcal meningitis, whilst tests to detect the cryptococcal polysaccharide capsular antigen (CRAG) in CSF have a sensitivity of 90%. *C. neoformans* will grow in culture. The differential diagnosis of a lymphocytic CSF in the context of HIV infection is wide and includes tuberculous meningitis, other mycoses, viral meningoencephalitis, meningeal metastases, and syphilis.

Treatment of cryptococcal meningitis should probably be with amphotericin B in the initial phase, possibly combined with flucytosine.[65] Some advocate the use of fluconazole in the absence of poor prognostic factors (positive blood culture, CRAG > 128, positive India ink stain of CSF, or an impaired mental status). The continuation phase of treatment should be with fluconazole 400 mg per day for 8 weeks and then maintenance therapy with fluconazole 200 mg per day for life or until there is improvement of CD4 cell count to 100–200 cells/mm^3 with HAART.[57] Even with aggressive management the prognosis associated with cryptococcal meningitis is poor with 25–30% mortality and a relapse rate of 20–25% after initial cure.

Progressive multifocal leukoencephalopathy

Progressive multifocal leukoencephalopathy (PML) is an opportunistic demyelinating infection caused by reactivation of a papovavirus, known as JC virus, and resulting in characteristic unifocal or multifocal white matter lesions.[66] The disorder must be distinguished from AIDS dementia complex and cerebral infarction. JC virus can be detected in

CSF by nucleic acid amplification techniques. There is no specific therapy but marked improvement has been shown following immune reconstitution as a result of HAART.[67]

Tuberculosis

Tuberculosis is an increasing problem in HIV infected persons.[68] It can present in the CNS with a meningitic illness, focal tuberculomas, or combination of the two. The clinical picture is similar to that seen in non-immunosuppressed patients with fever, altered mental status, seizures, and meningism (see below). Where there is diagnostic doubt and focal CNS lesions, the threshold for deciding to perform a biopsy is diminishing, in order to distinguish tuberculosis from toxoplasmosis, cerebral lymphoma, and other causes of focal lesions.

Bacterial meningitis

Meningitis may occur as an isolated illness or as a complication of disease elsewhere and any bacterium is capable of causing meningitis given favourable circumstances (Box 9.2, Table 9.1).[69] In practice, a limited number of

---

Box 9.2 Bacterial meningitis: causal organisms

Neonates
  Gram negative bacilli
  Streptococci (usually group B)
  Listeria monocytogenes

Children
  Meningococci
  Pneumococci

Adults
  Pneumococci
  Meningococci
  Staphylococci
  Listeria monocytogenes
  Streptococci

  Mycobacterium tuberculosis can affect children and adults

Table 9.1 Bacteria linked to underlying causes of meningitis

Cause	Organism
Diabetes mellitus	Pneumococci
	Staphylococci
	Gram negative bacilli
Alcohol	Pneumococci
Sickle cell disease	Pneumococci
Skull fracture	Gram negative bacilli
	Staphylococci
Dural fistula/CSF leak	Pneumococci
	Gram negative bacilli
CNS shunt	*Staphylococcus epidermidis*
Pregnancy/childbirth	*Listeria*
	Streptococci
Cell mediated immune defect	*Listeria*
Humoral immune defect	Pneumococci
	Haemophilus
	Meningococci
Neutropenia	*Pseudomonas*

organisms with particular virulence properties, which allow access to the CNS, cause most cases.

The epidemiology of meningitis is complex and varies with the age of the patient and geography. About 70% of cases are seen in children. The introduction of childhood vaccination against *Haemophilus influenzae* type b has led to a dramatic fall in the incidence of this pathogen, which previously was the most common cause of meningitis in children less than five years old. Now, with the exception of the neonatal period and the elderly, *Neisseria meningitidis* and *Streptococcus pneumoniae* account for about 70% of all cases of bacterial meningitis. Neonatal meningitis may be caused by any organism but the most frequently encountered pathogens are gram negative bacilli, particularly *Escherichia coli*, other enteric bacilli, *Pseudomonas* spp., *Listeria monocytogenes*, and group B streptococci. Neonatal meningitis is not discussed further here. In the elderly there is an increased risk of meningitis caused by gram negative bacilli, staphylococci, and *L. monocytogenes*.

The meningococcus, of which there are a number of serogroups, remains the only significant cause of epidemics.[69–71] In sub-Saharan Africa there are annual epidemics of meningitis due to serogroup A. Serogroup B tends to cause epidemics spread over several years and these have been reported in Europe, Latin America, and New Zealand. Recent years have seen an increased incidence in adolescents and young adults (particularly on college campuses) of meningococcal disease caused by a particularly virulent strain (serotype 2a) of serogroup C organisms. The United Kingdom was the first country to use meningococcal serogroup C conjugate vaccines and their introduction has led to a decline in serogroup C disease in adolescents.[72]

S. pneumoniae meningitis is associated with pneumonia, acute and chronic otitis media, alcoholism, diabetes mellitus, splenectomy, hypogammaglobulinaemia, head trauma, and CSF rhinorrhoea or otorrhoea resulting from dural leaks.

Gram negative bacilli tend to occur in association with head injuries, following neurosurgery, in patients who have compromised immune systems, and in the elderly. One disturbing factor is the increase in the number of cases that have been acquired nosocomially.[73]

Staphylococcal infection may complicate neurosurgical procedures and head trauma and also affects those with immunosuppression or endocarditis. Anaerobic organisms alone or as part of polymicrobial infections cause 1–2% of cases that complicate paranasal sinus and ear infections, skull fractures, neurosurgery, and immunosuppression.[74] Tuberculosis remains a significant cause of meningitis in the United Kingdom and United States.[75] Many other organisms may also cause meningitis, commonly of a more chronic nature, but which may rapidly develop into an acute emergency in those with compromised immune systems.

Advances in the investigation and management of bacterial meningitis over the past 40 years or so, including the continuing development of antibiotics, the introduction of CT and MRI, the application of improved techniques of bacterial culture, and now the widespread use of molecular methods incorporating PCR, have permitted treatment to be given on a more rational basis to a wider range of patients. It is disappointing, therefore, that mortality and morbidity from the main forms of bacterial meningitis have failed to diminish by any substantial degree over the same length of time. Fortunately, in recent years new understanding of the pathophysiology of the changes that occur in bacterial meningitis has become available,[76,77] from which it may be possible to develop new strategies for treatment.

Pathophysiology and clinical presentation

To cause bacterial meningitis, the infecting organism must be able to overcome host defence mechanisms that protect the neuraxis, and their neurotropic qualities derive from their ability to thwart these mechanisms. The upper respiratory tract is the favoured, but not the only, site for colonisation by these organisms which must cross the mucosal epithelium, which secretes IgA. The bacteria render IgA non-functional by secreting IgA proteases and attach to the epithelium by mechanisms that vary between species and await full characterisation. Transient bacteraemia ensues. To enter and survive in the bloodstream, the bacterium must avoid phagocytosis by neutrophils and attack by complement. In this they are often reliant on their polysaccharide capsule. All bacteria commonly causing meningitis have a capsule, the molecular basis of which varies between organisms. Once bacteria are established in the circulation, the blood–brain barrier must be penetrated to enter CSF; this is the least understood element of pathogenesis. The possession of pili to aid binding to surface molecules appears to influence virulence. Once inside the CSF, there is virtually no immunoglobulin, including anticapsular antibodies, or complement activity, so opsonic attack on invading bacteria cannot be mounted.

Host reaction to this bacterial invasion determines the resulting clinical features of meningitis. One of the major features of meningitis is a CSF neutrophil response. The release of bacterial cell wall components into the CSF stimulates the release of inflammatory cytokines, including interleukins 1 and 6, tumour necrosis factor, and prostaglandins, into the CSF and there is strong evidence that their presence induces inflammation and disruption of the blood–brain barrier. The inflammatory response recruits granulocytes to the CSF. By a complex series of interactions, as yet not fully understood, cerebral blood flow increases, inducing vasogenic cerebral oedema and raised intracranial pressure. With the progression of inflammation, cytotoxic oedema develops, cerebral blood flow falls, vasculitis progresses, and intracranial pressure rises further. Interstitial oedema results from obstruction of CSF flow from subarachnoid space to blood. Cerebrovascular autoregulation is disrupted and the brain becomes at risk from either hyper- or hypo-perfusion. Evidence is accumulating that many of these changes occur early in the course of meningitis and treatment regimens that reduce intracranial pressure while maintaining cerebral perfusion and blood flow may be useful.[78,79] The clinical features of a typical case of meningitis are fever, malaise, headache, neck stiffness, irritability, and confusion.[80] Usually these features appear over the space of a day or two, but in some fulminant cases the signs may develop within hours. In as many as 20% of cases, these typical features may be lacking: this is particularly so with the very young, the very old, the very ill, and those with compromised immune systems. The possibility of meningitis should be entertained in every child or adult in the above groups who has lethargy, altered mental status, drowsiness, or pyrexia, especially if neck stiffness is present. It is important to recognise that neck stiffness may *not* be present in the early stages of bacterial meningitis[81,82] and the physician must include meningitis in the differential diagnosis of a very wide range of diseases.

Convulsions occur with meningitis in any age group, are particularly common in young children, affecting up to 40% of cases, and may be the presenting feature. Convulsions associated with pyrexia – "febrile convulsions" – commonly occur in the very young. Each such patient may have meningitis, which poses the question, does each require a lumbar puncture? Evidence suggests that the answer is "no".[83,84] Many febrile convulsions are caused by infection with human herpesvirus type 6.[85] If the convulsion is brief and not associated with continuing neurological deficit or focal feature, if the child rapidly regains consciousness and there are no other signs of meningitis, it is reasonable to observe the child closely for some hours rather than perform a lumbar puncture straight away.

Specific features may suggest the aetiology of meningitis. A diffuse maculopapular eruption, which progresses to include petechiae or frank purpura, accompanies 50–60% of cases of meningococcal meningitis. Other bacteria – *L. monocytogenes*, staphylococci, pneumococci, and *H. influenzae* – and viruses, particularly echovirus 9, may also cause rashes. Rarely, a rash may be due to a reaction to an antibiotic or other drug but this seldom occurs early in the course of the disease. Focal neurological signs, seizures, and cranial nerve palsies resulting from rhomboencephalitis are seen in some patients with listerial infection.[86] Pneumococcal meningitis is associated with otitis media, a history of skull fracture, alcoholism, or sickle cell disease, and up to 50% will have pneumonia. Staphylococci or gram negative bacilli often cause meningitis complicating the implantation of neurosurgical devices such as shunts. In those with immune suppression, including AIDS, simultaneous infection with more than one organism may occur. If there is a history of meningitis, there is probably a dural fistula from previous head injury or, much more rarely, the patient suffers from an inherited complement-deficiency state.

Management

Once the possibility of bacterial meningitis is considered, treatment should be given without delay. Next to the conscious level on admission, the factor that has the most deleterious effect on prognosis is delay in beginning treatment.[87] We recommend that all adult patients in whom a diagnosis of bacterial meningitis is suspected should be given parenteral penicillin or ceftriaxone while urgent transfer to hospital is arranged. If the patient arrives at hospital without having received any prehospital antibiotics then they should be given before any further investigations, other than blood cultures. Pre-admission antibiotics are unlikely to obscure the diagnosis of bacterial meningitis.[88]

Blood cultures and CSF examination are the best ways to confirm the diagnosis of bacterial meningitis and, in established meningitis, there is usually no difficulty in determining the aetiology. In all cases blood cultures and a coagulation screen should be set up immediately, whether or not pre-admission antibiotics have been given.[88] In meningococcal disease organisms may be identified in skin aspirates from areas of rash[89] and meningococci can also be identified from swabs taken perorally from the posterior pharyngeal wall.[90]

The diagnosis of bacterial meningitis is ultimately based on examination of CSF.[80] However, bacterial meningitis raises the intracranial pressure. In most cases physiological mechanisms cope and no long term untoward effects result. Sometimes, however, intracranial pressure may rise to potentially lethal levels, with cerebral oedema and brain herniation: in such circumstances, a lumbar puncture can lead to rapid deterioration and death. To reconcile this with the necessity of reaching an early diagnosis is, in some cases, difficult, the correct decision depending on experience and a degree of luck. It should not be left to junior members of the medical team. Brain imaging, usually with CT, should be undertaken immediately if there are focal neurological signs, papilloedema, the conscious level is reduced, or if there are frequent seizures. One report[91] suggested that CT had little influence on the management of bacterial meningitis in children but it did not address the problem of recognition of raised ICP. Imaging does allow other pathologies that may present like bacterial meningitis to be excluded – subarachnoid haemorrhage, infarction, tumour, and brain abscess. Unfortunately, a normal CT scan does not always mean that it is safe to proceed to lumbar puncture, and cerebral herniation and death do occur as the result of lumbar puncture in cases of suspected meningitis.[92]

Contraindications to lumbar puncture include presence of signs of raised ICP – unless there is a normal CT or MRI scan – severe shock or a coagulation disorder. If, therefore, there is a confident clinical diagnosis of meningococcaemia with a typical rash, then lumbar puncture should *not* be undertaken.[88,93] CSF may be examined later when it is considered to be safe and evidence of bacterial infection can be found by demonstration of bacterial DNA by PCR.[88,94,95] Anxiety that infection may be introduced to CSF by lumbar puncture in patients with bacteraemia is largely unfounded.

CSF findings in bacterial meningitis are of a raised cell count (usually in the range 100–5000) with polymorphs predominating. The protein content is increased and the glucose is reduced. A sample of blood should be taken at the time of lumbar puncture for comparison; a ratio of CSF : blood glucose of less than 0·3 is abnormal and is found in about three quarters of patients.[96] Any one of the following parameters is 99% or more predictive of bacterial rather than viral meningitis: a CSF : blood glucose ratio below 0·23; a protein above 220 mg/dl; more than 1180×10^6/L neutrophils

or more than 2000×10^6/L total white cells.[97] Identification of
the organism under the microscope or on culture should be
possible in up to 90% of patients (less than 50% if antibiotics
have already been given for more than 24 hours).[96,98] If the
CSF findings suggest bacterial meningitis but the gram stain is
negative then latex agglutination tests are available for all the
common meningeal pathogens.[80] However, although these
tests can provide rapid results a negative result does not rule
out bacterial meningitis and they are not widely used in
the United Kingdom. A PCR based test for the detection of
N. meningitidis from both peripheral blood and CSF has been
in routine use since 1996 in the United Kingdom.[94,99] This test
is sensitive and specific and can also provide information on
serogroup to aid serological investigations.[100] PCR tests are also
available for the detection of S. pneumoniae and H. influenzae.
The S. pneumoniae PCR can also provide information on
penicillin sensitivity of the organism.

As stated earlier, once the diagnosis of bacterial meningitis
is suspected, antibiotic treatment should be started on a "best
guess" basis (Box 9.3) and a CSF examination performed as
soon as possible. Precedence is given to maintaining
cardiorespiratory function, adequate oxygenation, and tissue
perfusion while the causal organism is being identified and a
specific antibiotic regimen determined. If no organism is
found on gram stain, the "best guess" antibiotic treatment is
continued (Box 9.3).

To treat meningitis effectively, it is necessary to achieve
adequate bactericidal levels of antibiotic in CSF at least 10-fold
higher than the minimal bactericidal concentration (MIC)
in vitro for the particular organism.[88] Ideally, the antibiotic
should be lipid soluble to facilitate transfer across the
blood–brain barrier but this is not usually a problem in

Box 9.3 Bacterial meningitis: empirical treatment

Neonates: ampicillin and a third generation cephalosporin

Children and adults: a third generation cephalosporin

Adults over age 50 years: ampicillin and a third generation cephalosporin

History of beta-lactam anaphylaxis: chloramphenicol and vancomycin (plus co-trimoxazole if Listeria is thought possible)

practice because meningeal inflammation disrupts the barrier and allows sufficient penetration. It should be active within purulent and acidic CSF and the rate at which it is metabolised and cleared from CSF determines the frequency and dose that should be given. The choice of antibiotic will be modified by knowledge of local drug resistance patterns for pneumococci and *H. influenzae* (penicillin-resistant meningococci do not pose a therapeutic problem).[80] Antibiotics should be given intravenously in high doses. They should not be given intrathecally. It is prudent to discuss the treatment of any but the most straightforward case of meningitis with a microbiologist or a specialist in infectious diseases.

In cases where an organism cannot be identified, children or adults with presumed bacterial meningitis should be treated with a third generation cephalosporin (cefotaxime or ceftriaxone).[88] If cephalosporin-resistant pneumococci are common in the part of world the patient comes from (e.g. Spain or parts of the USA),[101–105] then vancomycin or rifampicin should be added. Patients over 50 years and those with defective cell mediated immunity should have ampicillin added (to cover *Listeria* infection). If there is a clear history of anaphylactic allergy to beta-lactam antibiotics then chloramphenicol and vancomycin should be used (with co-trimoxazole added for the over-50s).[88] For empirical treatment of the neutropenic patient, meropenem and an aminoglycoside (to cover possible *Pseudomonas* infection) are suggested.

Treatment may be modified once pathogens have been identified. For *H. influenzae* type b infections, ampicillin and chloramphenicol are no longer suitable for empirical treatment, owing to widespread antibiotic resistance. The third generation cephalosporins, cefotaxime or ceftriaxone, have been demonstrated to be effective and are the drugs of choice.[80] For meningococcal meningitis, IV benzylpenicillin remains the preferred drug. There have been reports of meningococci resistant to penicillin,[106] but this is not associated with clinical failure if the high doses of penicillin used for meningitis are given. Chloramphenicol or a third generation cephalosporin may be used in people who react adversely to penicillin.

Pneumococcal meningitis caused by fully sensitive organisms can be treated with penicillin but penicillin resistant strains are common and a third generation cephalosporin is now the best choice empirical therapy. Once the sensitivity of the pneumococcus to penicillin is confirmed, benzylpenicillin can be chosen. If the pneumococcus is shown to be penicillin resistant but cephalosporin sensitive then the vancomycin and/or rifampicin can be discontinued.

Third generation cephalosporins and meropenem have been shown to be more effective than aminoglycosides for the treatment of gram negative bacillary meningitis and should now be used.[107,108] Group B streptococcal infection should be treated with penicillin or ampicillin. Listerial infection responds to ampicillin and for those with penicillin allergy, co-trimoxazole is effective. Flucloxacillin or oxacillin in high doses is recommended for *Staphylococcus aureus* meningitis, with vancomycin for those who cannot have penicillin or if the organism is methicillin resistant (MRSA).

Shunt infections are commonly caused by coagulase negative staphylococci, and vancomycin, perhaps with added rifampicin, is effective. In most cases it is necessary to remove the device to eradicate the infection completely.[109] The combination of penicillin with metronidazole is recommended for anaerobic infections.

The length of time for which treatment is given should be tailored to each case: meningococcal meningitis needs five days of parenteral therapy, *H. influenzae* 7–10 days, and other forms a minimum of 14 days. Failure to respond adequately prompts a review of the diagnosis and treatment, search for a continuing source of infection, and repeat brain imaging to demonstrate abscess or subdural fluid accumulation. Repeat CSF examination should be considered in cases where the patient is not responding satisfactorily and no explanation can be found.

As mentioned earlier, the release of bacterial cell wall products into the CSF stimulates inflammation, mediated in part by cytokines. Studies to determine the efficacy of the anti-inflammatory action of corticosteroids in reducing this inflammation have produced encouraging results. There is evidence in children that dexamethasone in a dose of 0·15 mg/kg body weight every six hours for four days reduces the incidence of neurological sequelae,[110,111] and this should be given just before antibiotics are started. There is now evidence that a similar approach (dexamethasone 10 mg given just before or with the first dose of antibiotics and continued every six hours for four days) improves the outcome in most adults with acute bacterial meningitis, particularly that caused by pneumococci.[112] There is some concern that dexamethasone might reduce the penetration of vancomycin into the CSF and hence there is still some doubt about the routine use of dexamethasone in cases where there is suspicion of meningitis caused by pneumococci that are highly resistant to penicillin or cephalosporin.[113]

Several other anti-inflammatory agents which act at different stages have been tried but are unhelpful, including non-steroidal anti-inflammatory drugs, pentoxifylline, naloxone, and monoclonal antibodies targeted specifically against human β-integrin.[114] Encouraging results have been obtained in meningococcal sepsis with recombinant bactericidal/permeability increasing protein[115] and recombinant activated protein C.[116,117]

Adjunctive management of bacterial meningitis includes measures to lower any raised intracranial pressure, appropriate intensive care support of cardiorespiratory, coagulation, and renal problems, and maintenance of electrolyte balance.[88] Details of these measures are beyond the scope of this account.

In the United Kingdom all cases of bacterial meningitis need to be reported to the Public Health Authorities who are charged with the responsibility for ensuring appropriate steps are taken to minimise the risk of secondary cases (particularly of meningococcal disease). These measures include the use of prophylactic antibiotics and, if necessary, vaccination.[118]

Tuberculous meningitis

The time course over which tuberculous meningitis (TBM) develops is usually longer than purulent meningitis, up to three weeks in children and rather longer in adults. In some cases, however, the onset may be acute and exactly similar to purulent meningitis, so TB must be considered in each case.[75] Indeed, given the highly variable clinical presentation of TBM and the frequent absence of fever and/or signs of meningism, a high degree of suspicion of TBM is required in many neurological presentations.

CT and MRI of the brain show changes of meningitis and no specific diagnostic features. Hydrocephalus is common, as is basal meningeal thickening. Tuberculomas may be seen. Low-density changes of infarction are common.[119-121] CSF is typically under increased pressure and is clear or slightly turbid. Rarely, it may look frankly purulent. There is moderate pleocytosis, often in the hundreds, with eventual lymphocyte predominance, but polymorphs may be in the majority at the onset. CSF protein is elevated, sometimes to very high levels, and the glucose content is reduced, although generally not to the levels seen with pyogenic meningitis.[75,122] If tubercle bacilli are seen, the diagnosis is confirmed, but several samples may be required for organisms to be identified, and even then as many as 30–50% of cases are negative. In these cases it may be possible to diagnose TBM by PCR, although the place of this has still not been fully evaluated in TBM.[75]

If TBM is suspected, treatment must be given promptly, as delay worsens morbidity and mortality.[123] Details of treatment regimens may be found elsewhere.[124] Chemotherapy is given for between 6 and 18 months, dependent upon the guidelines followed and the drugs used.[124-126] Even though corticosteroids are often given routinely to those with more severe disease and may be useful for preventing arachnoiditis or other severe residual disability, a Cochrane Review suggested that further large studies were needed to confirm any benefits.[127] Dexamethasone for a short time in high dose is useful to reduce cerebral oedema. Hydrocephalus commonly develops, sometimes acutely, and should be treated early by surgical drainage.

Lyme disease

Lyme disease, caused by the spirochaete *Borrelia burgdorferi*, can present as meningitis, usually of chronic type but sometimes as an acute fulminating illness.[128] Acute meningitis occurs in about 10% of patients as part of the second stage of the disease, one to six months after a bite by the vector, a tick of the genus *Ixodes*. Occasionally the original bite and the skin lesion of erythema chronicum migrans were not noticed or have been forgotten, and acute meningitis may be the presenting illness. Cranial neuritis and radiculopathy may also be present. Treatment of Lyme borrellial meningitis with ceftriaxone for a minimum of two weeks probably hastens symptom resolution.[129] Intravenous cefotaxime or penicillin in high dose are also effective.

Syphilis

Another spirochaete, *Treponema pallidum*, may also cause acute meningitis. Although rare, such cases are occurring more frequently in association with HIV infection.[130,131] It occurs within two years of primary infection and presents acutely with headache, vomiting, pyrexia, and neck stiffness. Cranial nerve palsies and epileptic seizures are not infrequent. CT scan appearances are of non-specific meningeal enhancement and the CSF contains a predominantly mononuclear pleocytosis, raised protein, and normal sugar. The diagnosis is confirmed by finding a positive CSF VDRL test.

Acute syphilitic meningitis is managed with the parenteral administration of large doses of procaine penicillin for 17–21 days,[132] with corticosteroids given for the first 24 hours to diminish the possibility of inducing a Jarisch–Herxheimer reaction. It is necessary to follow up cases closely to ensure that serological changes and CSF revert to normal and to treat any reinfection rapidly.

Rickettsial meningitis

As a consequence of the proliferation of intercontinental air travel, the person arriving from abroad may harbour an infection not usually seen in the United Kingdom and symptoms of some of these infections may not appear until weeks after arrival.[133] It is therefore of prime importance to obtain a full history of recent travel, places visited (including stopovers), and activities undertaken from any person who presents with an acute meningoencephalitis. Such an illness may be caused by rickettsial diseases, which are transmitted to humans by the bites of ticks or mites and are prevalent in every continent except Antarctica. Rocky Mountain spotted fever caused by *Rickettsia rickettsii* may be contracted in the Americas; Mediterranean spotted fever (*R. conorii*) in Africa, Asia, and the Mediterranean basin; scrub typhus (*R. tsutsugamushi*) in Asia, the Pacific, and Australia. Typhus

(*R. prowazekii*) and Q fever (*Coxiella burnetii*) are ubiquitous.[133] Rickettsiae invade small blood vessels throughout the body and multiply, causing endothelial wall proliferation, thrombosis, and perivascular inflammation, and when this affects the brain, meningoencephalitis results.

The incubation period, clinical features, and progression of the illness vary between organisms, but all share the triad of high fever, skin rash, and headache, with meningoencephalitis developing during the second week of the illness in a significant proportion of cases. Rocky Mountain spotted fever may occur without a rash; a rash does not usually accompany Q fever; and Mediterranean spotted fever is characterised by a distinctive eschar at the site of the bite.

Neurological features are typically non-focal, with headache, neck stiffness, photophobia, and, in more severe cases, confusion and reduction in conscious level. Convulsions may occur. CSF examination reveals no specific features; there may be a slight pleocytosis, the protein content may be raised, and glucose is normal. Diagnosis is confirmed by serological tests (PCR based tests for rickettsial DNA are not widely available as yet), but treatment must be started on the basis of clinical suspicion and not delayed for test results to become positive. The treatment of choice is tetracycline or doxycycline in adults.

Malaria

Involvement of the brain occurs in patients who are infected with *Plasmodium falciparum* and results in cerebral malaria. *P. vivax*, *P. ovale*, and *P. malariae* do not cause cerebral malaria.

Falciparum malaria is found in large parts of Asia, sub-Saharan Africa, the Middle East, and Central and South America. People who live in endemic areas may acquire a degree of immunity that diminishes with time. Those most at risk of developing severe malaria are the traveller who has no immunity and is being exposed for the first time, the emigrant returning home from a long spell abroad whose immunity has lapsed, pregnant women, and those who have immune suppression. It is not always necessary to stay in an endemic country to contract the disease; "runway malaria" occurs when an infected mosquito that has travelled on an aeroplane from an endemic country bites a person.[134]

Cerebral malaria is an acute diffuse encephalopathy with fever, which can kill within 72 hours if not recognised and treated, and even then carries a mortality of 25–50%.[135] Delay in making the diagnosis and initiating treatment is a major factor contributing to this mortality.

Female *Anopheles* mosquitoes spread falciparum malaria. When they feed on humans they inject sporozoites, which circulate in the blood and are rapidly cleared by the liver, where they enter hepatocytes and reproduce asexually. One to three weeks later they rupture into the bloodstream as motile merozoites, which rapidly invade erythrocytes, where they can be seen microscopically on blood films. There they feed on haemoglobin and further asexual reproduction occurs (schizogeny). The progeny mature through the stage of trophozoite to merozoite, multiplying approximately 10–fold, to rupture out of the red cell and invade other uninfected red cells. This dispersal occurs every 48 hours and induces fever. A proportion of merozoites develop into the sexual gametocyte stage of the parasite and it is these that are ingested by a feeding mosquito to continue the cycle.

The clinical manifestations of cerebral malaria are the end result of a complex and not fully understood series of interactions mediated by humoral, vascular, and haematological factors within the cerebral capillaries. There is evidence of immune mediated inflammatory reactions that release vasoactive products and produce endothelial damage.[135] The presence of trophozoites within erythrocytes induces changes, which renders the cells capable of adhering to vascular endothelium. These red cells packed with mature trophozoites are to be found sequestrated in small cerebral vessels, resulting in microvascular congestion and tissue hypoxia.

Other organ systems are vulnerable to similar changes. Acute tubular necrosis and the adult respiratory distress syndrome may need simultaneous treatment. Disseminated intravascular coagulation occurs in severe cases. Whether cerebral oedema contributes significantly to the pathogenesis of cerebral malaria is debatable. It would be surprising if a disease which causes intracranial vasculitis and microthrombosis did not raise intracranial pressure, but it is clear that administration of dexamethasone does not improve the outcome.[136]

Hypoglycaemia is an important and frequent complication of cerebral malaria and undoubtedly contributes to depression of consciousness and the appearance of neurological signs. It results from a complex series of interactions, which include malabsorption of glucose from the gut, hyperinsulinaemia (which may be induced by treatment using intravenous quinine), the metabolic demands of infection, and increased metabolism of available glucose by a large biomass of parasites. Pregnant women are particularly susceptible.

Definitions of the clinical criteria required to justify a diagnosis of cerebral malaria have been drawn up to standardise parameters for research.[135] For the purposes of this discussion, any person from an endemic area with cerebral symptoms or signs should be suspected of suffering from cerebral malaria and demands immediate monitoring, investigation, and treatment. Such a patient will usually have been ill for days and have a high temperature. Exceptions occur: the onset of neurological symptoms may be abrupt and very ill patients may be hypothermic. Commonly there are convulsions, more so in the young, and in 45% of adults coma follows the convulsion. Young children have convulsions associated with many varieties of infection and with those, consciousness is rapidly regained. Coma lasting more than an hour or two in such circumstances should raise the suspicion of cerebral malaria.

Symptoms before the onset of the cerebral state are diverse and non-specific and the most common misdiagnosis is of flu. The level of consciousness is invariably impaired and there is evidence of an organic brain syndrome that manifests as confusion, hallucinations, delirium, and psychosis, complicated in some by motor signs and movement disorders. Meningism and opisthotonus may be found and it is important to remember that bacterial and other forms of meningitis may coexist with malaria. Furthermore, severely ill patients are susceptible to gram negative septicaemia. There may be signs of damage to other organ systems: anaemia is common and may be severe, jaundice complicates severe infection in adults, hepatosplenomegaly of mild to moderate degree is frequent, and haemorrhages may be found in the retina. Prolonged coma and frequent convulsions should trigger a search for hypoglycaemia and pyogenic meningitis.

Confirmation of the diagnosis of a case of suspected malaria must be obtained forthwith but if this cannot be done and suspicion is high, treatment should be given straight away. The best way to confirm the diagnosis is to have thick and thin smears of blood examined by an experienced microscopist after appropriate staining. If no parasites are seen and the diagnosis seems likely, treatment should be given and the blood re-examined every six to eight hours for the next 48 hours. Blood sugar should be estimated and monitored frequently and hypoglycaemia corrected if found. A full blood count, urea, electrolytes, and blood gases must be checked and monitored as treatment progresses. All such patients should be nursed in intensive care.

Because of widespread resistance of *P. falciparum* to chloroquine, this should not be used; quinoline compounds or artemisinin derivatives are the treatments of choice. Quinine is the most widely used. In severe malaria, when there is intensive care support the World Health Organization recommends it should be given in an initial dose of 7 mg/kg over 30 minutes, followed immediately by 10 mg/kg over four hours.[135] Infusions of 10 mg/kg over four hours are repeated eight to twelve hourly. Use of quinine loading doses reduces the fever resolution in severe malaria but has not been clearly shown to reduce the risk of death or convulsions.[136] Quinine should not be given by bolus injection. Plasma glucose and ECG should be monitored. After the patient regains consciousness, oral quinine (600 mg) may be given. Quinine therapy should be followed by either pyrimethamine-sulfadoxine (Fansidar, three tablets as a single dose) and/or doxycycline for one week. In situations where quinine is not available, quinidine may be used but there is still discussion about the correct dosage regimens.[135] Various artemisinin derivatives are as effective as quinine in preventing death in severe or complicated malaria.[137] If the parasite load is very high and the patient very ill, exchange transfusion may be beneficial.[135] The utility of the routine use of anticonvulsants in cerebral malaria is still unclear.[138] Full intensive care support is required for patients with cerebral malaria,[135] but there is no evidence of benefit from corticosteroids.[139]

Features that adversely affect the outcome are failure to make the diagnosis or delay in starting treatment, not recognising concurrent infection, deep and prolonged coma, and continuing seizures.

Primary amoebic encephalitis

This condition is caused by free living amoebae of the species *Naegleria fowleri*. They live in moist soil and most cases have been reported in children who have been swimming or playing in stagnant water. Amoebae enter the nasal cavity, cross the nasal epithelium, and ascend to the brain along olfactory nerves and blood vessels to frontal and basal meninges and spread, causing a florid necrotising inflammation.

Clinically the presentation is of a sudden onset of severe meningitis indistinguishable from bacterial meningitis.[140] The clue to diagnosis is the history of exposure to warm, stagnant water. CSF examination reveals pleocytosis in which polymorphs predominate, raised protein, and reduced glucose. No organisms are seen on the gram stain and special examination of fresh, warm specimens of CSF will show motile trophozoites. Most patients die rapidly despite treatment, but survival following treatment with amphotericin B has been described,[141] and this should be given in the highest tolerated dose parenterally, reinforced by intracisternal injection and by rifampicin and tetracycline, which have some activity against *Naegleriae*.[142]

Acanthamoeba spp. tend to cause a subacute granulomatous meningoencephalitis.

Brain abscess and subdural empyema

Intracranial abscesses remain a diagnostic and therapeutic challenge despite the considerable advances that have taken place in recent decades in imaging techniques, neurosurgical practice, bacteriological isolation of causal organisms, and the introduction of more potent antibiotics.[143,144] They frequently present as emergencies and, as with all forms of cerebral infection, delay in diagnosis and implementation of treatment, and inappropriate investigation, adversely affect the outcome.[145]

The incidence of brain abscess is 1·3 per 100 000 person-years and this has fallen in recent years. Brain abscesses account for approximately 1 in 10 000 admissions in the United States.[144] Both brain abscesses and subdural empyemas are more common in young men.[145,146]

Pathogenesis

Bacteria reach the brain parenchyma via the bloodstream, by direct extension from an adjacent focus of infection or by implantation through wounds as a result of trauma or neurosurgery. In about 15% of cases the source of infection cannot be identified. Haematogenous spread has been implicated in approximately 25% of cases. The most common primary foci are endocarditis and pulmonary infections. Brain abscesses resulting from haematogenous spread are often multifocal and more frequently involve middle cerebral artery territory. Congenital cyanotic heart disease and pulmonary suppuration (for example, bronchiectasis or lung abscess) are associated with an increased frequency of brain abscess. Sinusitis, otitis, and dental abscess are the most commonly implicated foci of infection that result in direct spread of infection to the brain parenchyma and subdural space. With improved treatment of these conditions the incidence of suppurative complications has declined. Spread of infection beyond the dural barrier is unusual in bacterial meningitis, but when it occurs is often secondary to gram negative organisms. Penetrating head injuries, particularly those secondary to gunshot wounds or associated with bone fragments, are occasionally associated with brain abscess. There is also a small risk following neurosurgical procedures.

The risk of brain abscess increases with immunosuppression, particularly that associated with the use of high dose corticosteroids, repeated episodes of rejection, and prolonged neutropenia in bone marrow/stem cell and solid organ transplant patients.

Experimental data indicate that bacteria cannot set up a nidus of infection in normal, undamaged brain and an area of devitalised or ischaemic tissue is a prerequisite. Generally it is believed that either a thrombophlebitis spreads from contiguous infection or that microinfarction from emboli or hypoxaemia produces a microscopic area of necrosis in which infection can become established. This is followed by cerebritis, with surrounding oedema of white matter; next the centre of cerebritis becomes necrotic and enlarges, capsule formation begins with the appearance of fibroblasts and neovascular change at the periphery, reactive astrocytosis, and surrounding oedema. Thereafter capsular development and thickening occurs.[147] The time course is variable and may be as short as three weeks.

Causative organisms

In the non-immunocompromised host, most brain abscesses are bacterial in origin and are frequently polymicrobial. A wide spectrum of organisms, both aerobic and anaerobic, has been isolated from brain abscesses. Streptococcal species, particularly *Streptococcus milleri*, are the most commonly identified and are found in up to 70% of abscesses. Suppurative infections complicating ear and sinus infections commonly have a mixed flora, which includes Enterobacteriaceae, streptococci (aerobic and anaerobic), *Staphylococcus aureus*, and *Bacteroides* spp. Dental sepsis causes infections with a mixed bag of streptococci, *Bacteroides* spp., and *Fusobacterium* spp.; pulmonary disease is associated with fusobacteria, other anaerobes, streptococci, and actinomycetes. Patients with congenital heart disease are likely to have anaerobic and microaerophilic streptococci. Staphylococci are found with penetrating head trauma, as are streptococci and *Clostridium* spp.

The organism implicated in abscesses associated with immunocompromised individuals depends on the type of defect. In those suffering from neutropenia and defects in neutrophil function, gram negative rods and fungi (*Aspergillus* spp., *Candida* spp., and Mucoraceae) are most commonly involved. T cell dysfunction predisposes to infection with *Listeria monocytogenes*, *Nocardia asteroides*, mycobacteria, *Cryptococcus neoformans*, and *Toxoplasma gondii*. In recipients of bone marrow transplants and solid organ transplants 92% of brain abscesses are associated with a single fungal pathogen.[148] *Aspergillus* is most commonly identified followed by *Candida*. Other fungi are occasionally found.

Diagnosis

The clinical features of brain abscesses and other focal CNS suppuration are largely caused by the presence of a space occupying lesion. They are usually described as headache, fever, and focal neurological signs, but this triad is only found in half of all patients.[144] Other common clinical features are focal signs pointing to the site of the lesion, convulsions, which are usually generalised but may be focal, nausea and vomiting, raised intracranial pressure even to the point of coning, and neck stiffness to suggest meningitis. There may be pyrexia and symptoms relating to the source of infection, such as otitis or sinusitis. Cerebral abscesses, therefore, must be included in the differential diagnosis of patients who present acutely with a wide range of neurological features.

Faced with a patient in whom intracranial abscess is a possible diagnosis, the priority is to confirm the diagnosis and identify the source of infection and the responsible organism or organisms. Once vital functions have been stabilised, a full examination should be made for a focus of infection, such as otitis media or pelvic sepsis, and if found, cultures should be made and steps taken to eradicate the source. Blood cultures should be set up. Contrast-enhanced CT or MRI should be done as soon as possible. In addition to visualising the intracranial contents, note should be made of the state of the paranasal sinuses and the mastoid air cells. Skull fractures and cranial defects should be looked for.

CT classically shows ring-enhancing lesions, although in the early stages ring enhancement may be absent. There may be surrounding oedema. Unfortunately, such appearances are not specific and may be seen with brain tumours, granulomas, necrotising encephalitis, and infarction. MRI is more sensitive than CT in demonstrating early cerebritis, cerebral oedema, and the contents of abscess cavities.[144]

Lumbar puncture should *never* be carried out on patients suspected of having a brain abscess.

Treatment

When the diagnosis of brain abscess is confirmed, the therapeutic strategy will be influenced by several factors. Most patients require surgical drainage: reasons for surgery are relief of space occupation, confirmation of the diagnosis, and obtaining specimens of pus for culture. It is seldom necessary to resort to complete surgical excision of an abscess. Simple aspiration of the contents of an abscess is the most frequently advocated technique; when carried out under stereotactic CT-guided control[149] diagnostic material is obtained in more than 90% of cases. If the abscess is a consequence of head trauma, then surgery is mandatory to perform appropriate toilet, debridement, removal of fragments, and closure of dural defects. If the abscesses are small or in the cerebritis stage, then surgery may not be needed and it is appropriate to treat with antibiotics on the basis of organism identification from other sources or, if that is not possible, on a "best guess" principle governed by the likely source of infection. Close monitoring of the lesions with serial CT or MRI is necessary; if they do not diminish in size, aspiration should be undertaken. In people with immunosuppression, including those with AIDS, the threshold for aspiration of pus to identify the offending organism is substantially lowered.

Choice of antibiotics

In the immunocompetent patient, empirical treatment should be with a combination of a third generation cephalosporin (for example, cefotaxime) and metronidazole.[150] Vancomycin is added to this regimen if staphylococci are suspected. Treatment should be given for no less than six weeks but must be determined for each case by clinical response and improvement of CT scan appearances. In the immunosuppressed the choice of treatment will depend on the immune defect, as outlined above. For neutropenic patients and those post transplantation, empirical therapy should include amphotericin B because of the high frequency of fungal infections that occur. In HIV positive patients with multiple lesions, pyrimethamine and sulfadiazine are used to treat toxoplasmosis. If there is not a rapid clinical and radiological response then other pathologies need to be considered.

Dexamethasone is commonly used to treat cerebral oedema and, in practice, the benefit obtained in reducing intracranial pressure outweighs the potential hazard of diminishing the host inflammatory response. The risk of developing epileptic seizures is not insubstantial and prophylactic anticonvulsants are recommended. Mortality is about 25–30% and another third of individuals will have long-term sequelae.

Spinal subdural empyema and epidural abscess

The presenting features of spinal epidural and subdural suppuration are back pain that may progress rapidly to limb paralysis and bowel or bladder dysfunction. The management of these uncommon conditions is very similar to their intracranial counterparts. The key to a successful outcome is clinical awareness, prompt diagnosis with MRI, and urgent surgical decompression and drainage. A six to eight week course of intravenous antibiotics is generally advised.[151]

Management of cerebral infection

- Cerebral infection may be due to meningitis, encephalitis, or focal space occupation.
- Viral meningitis must be distinguished from partly treated bacterial and other causes of aseptic meningitis.
- Viral encephalitis in the UK and Europe is usually due to herpes simplex which must be treated quickly with intravenous acyclovir. However other causes must be considered including, especially in other parts of the world, rabies and arborviruses.
- At seroconversion HIV infection may cause aseptic meningoencephalitis and later it may cause HIV encephalopathy. AIDS is associated with cytomegalovirus, toxoplasmosis, progressive multifocal leukoencephalopathy, and tuberculosis.
- Bacterial meningitis is a serious neurological emergency. The commonest causative organisms, except in neonates and the elderly, are Neisseria meningitidis and Streptococcus pneumoniae. Immediate treatment should be given to adult patients with ceftriaxone. Advice about other antibiotic treatment is contained in this chapter.
- Cerebral malaria is fatal in 25–50% of cases. Patients with febrile illnesses returning from malarial areas should be suspected of having malaria. Quinine is the drug of choice for severe malaria.
- Cerebral abscess may be caused by a wide variety of organisms but Streptococci are the commonest in non-immunocompromised hosts. Most patients require surgical drainage and empirical treatment with antibiotics. These usually include a third generation cephalosporin, metranidazole, and, if Staphylococci are suspected, vancomycin.

References

1 Wallgren A. Une nouvelle maladie infectieuse du systeme nerveux central? (Meningite septique aigue). *Acta Paediatr Scand* 1925;**4**:158–82.
2 Johnson RT, Mims CA. Pathogenesis of viral infections of the nervous system. *N Engl J Med* 1968;**278**:23–30.
3 Dropulic B, Masters GL. Entry of neurotropic arboviruses into the central nervous system. *J Infect Dis* 1990;**161**:691.

4   Rotbart H. Enteroviral infections of the central nervous system. *Clin Infect Dis* 1995;**20**:971–81.
5   Feigin RD, Shackelford PG. Value of repeat lumbar puncture in the differential diagnosis of meningitis. *N Engl J Med* 1973;**289**:571–4.
6   Jeffery KJM, Bangham CRM. Recent advances in the laboratory diagnosis of central nervous system infections. *Curr Opin Infect Dis* 1996;**9**:132–7.
7   Jeffery KJM, Read SJ, Peto TEA, Mayon-White RT, Bangham CRM. Diagnosis of viral infections of the central nervous system: clinical interpretation of PCR results. *Lancet* 1997;**349**:313–17.
8   Schiff GM, Sherwood JR. Clinical activity of pleconaril in an experimentally induced coxsackievirus A21 respiratory infection. *J Infect Dis* 2000;**181**:20–6.
9   Rotbart HA, Webster AD, for the Pleconaril Treatment Registry Group. Treatment of potentially life-threatening enterovirus infections with pleconaril. *Clin Infect Dis* 2001;**32**:228–35.
10 Johnson RT. The pathogenesis of acute viral encephalitis and postinfectious encephalomyelitis. *J Infect Dis* 1987;**155**:359–64.
11 Whitley RJ, Gnann JW. Viral encephalitis: familiar infections and emerging pathogens. *Lancet* 2002;**359**:507–14.
12 Plotkin SA. Rabies. *Clin Infect Dis* 2000;**30**:4–12.
13 Whitley RJ. Viral encephalitis. *N Engl J Med* 1990;**323**:242–50.
14 Smith RR, Caldemeyer KS. Neurologic review of intracranial infection. *Curr Prob Diagn Radiol* 1999;**28**:1–26.
15 Rowley AH, Whitley RJ, Lakeman FD, Wolinsky SM. Rapid detection of herpes-simplex-virus DNA in cerebrospinal fluid of patients with herpes simplex encephalitis. *Lancet* 2001;**335**:440–1.
16 Lakeman FD, Whitley RJ, the National Institute of Allergy and Infectious Diseases Collaborative Antiviral Study Group. Diagnosis of herpes simplex encephalitis: application of polymerase chain reaction to cerebrospinal fluid from brain-biopsied patients and correlation with disease. *J Infect Dis* 1995;**171**:857–63.
17 Lipkin WI. European consensus on viral encephalitis. *Lancet* 1997;**349**:299–300.
18 Pickard JD, Czosnyka M. Management of raised intracranial pressure. *J Neurol Neurosurg Psychiatry* 1993;**56**:845–55.
19 Whitley RJ, Lakeman F. Herpes simplex virus infections of the central nervous system: therapeutic and diagnostic considerations. *Clin Infect Dis* 1995;**20**:414–20.
20 Whitley RJ. Herpes simplex virus. In: Scheld WM, Whitley RJ, Durack DT, eds. *Infections of the central nervous system*. Philadelphia: Lippencott-Raven, 1996.
21 Whitley RJ, Cobbs CG, Alford CA, *et al.* Diseases that mimic herpes simplex encephalitis. Diagnosis, presentation, and outcome. *JAMA* 1989;**262**:234–9.
22 Whitley RJ, Alford CA, Hirsch MS, *et al.* Vidarabine versus acyclovir therapy in herpes simplex encephalitis. *N Engl J Med* 1986;**314**:144–9.
23 McGrath N, Anderson NE, Croxson MC, Powell KF. Herpes simplex encephalitis treated with acyclovir: diagnosis and long term outcome. *J Neurol Neurosurg Psychiatry* 1997;**63**:321–6.
24 Kennedy C. Acute viral encephalitis in childhood. *Br Med J* 1995;**310**:139–40.
25 Kennedy PGE. Neurological complications of varicella-zoster virus. In: Kennedy PGE, Johnson RT, eds. *Infections of the nervous system*. London: Butterworths, 1987.
26 Johnson R, Milbourn PE. Central nervous system manifestations of chickenpox. *Can Med Assoc J* 1970;**102**:831–4.

27   Peterslund NA. Herpes zoster associated encephalitis: clinical findings and acyclovir treatment. *Scand J Infect Dis* 1988;**20**:583–92.

28   Whitley RJ, Schlitt M. Encephalitis caused by herpesviruses, including B virus. In: Scheld WM, Whitley RJ, Durack DT, eds. *Infections of the central nervous system*. New York: Raven Press, 1991.

29   Whitley RJ, Cloud G, Gruber W, *et al*. Ganciclovir treatment of symptomatic congenital cytomegalovirus infection: results of a phase II study. *J Infect Dis* 1997;**175**:1080–6.

30   Gautier-Smith PC. Neurological complications of glandular fever (infectious mononucleosis). *Brain* 1965;**88**:323–34.

31   Tsutsumi H, Kamazaki H, Nakata S, *et al*. Sequential development of acute meningoencephalitis and transverse myelitis caused by Epstein–Barr virus during infectious mononucleosis. *Pediatr Infect Dis J* 1994;**13**:665–7.

32   Johnson RT, Griffin DE, Hirsch RL, *et al*. Measles encephalomyelitis – clinical and immunologic studies. *N Engl J Med* 1984;**310**:137–41.

33   Gnann JW Jr. Meningitis and encephalitis caused by mumps virus. In: Scheld WM, Whitley RJ, Durack DT, eds. *Infections of the central nervous system*. New York: Raven Press, 1991.

34   Tsai TF, Popovici F, Cernescu C, Campbell GL, Nedelcu NI. West Nile encephalitis epidemic in southeastern Romania. *Lancet* 1998;**352**: 767–71.

35   Tyler KL. West Nile virus encephalitis in America. *N Engl J Med* 2001;**344**: 1858–9.

36   Chua KB, Goh KJ, Wong KT, *et al*. Fatal encephalitis due to Nipah virus among pig-farmers in Malaysia. *Lancet* 1999;**354**:1257–9.

37   Cunha BA. Acute encephalitis. *Infect Dis Pract* 1989;**12**:1–12.

38   McJunkin JE, de los Reyes EC, Irazuzta JE, *et al*. La Crosse encephalitis in children. *N Engl J Med* 2001;**344**:801–7.

39   Monath TP. Japanese encephalitis – a plague of the Orient. *N Engl J Med* 1988;**319**:641–3.

40   Dickerson RB, Newton JR, Hausen JE. Diagnosis and immediate prognosis of Japanese B encephalitis. *Am J Med* 1952;**12**:277–90.

41   Price RW. Neurological complications of HIV infection. *Lancet* 1996;**348**:445–52.

42   Price RW, Brew B, Sidtis J, Rosenblum M, Scheck AC, Cleary P. The brain and AIDS: central nervous system HIV-1 infection and AIDS dementia complex. *Science* 1988;**239**:586–92.

43   Piot P, Bartos M, Ghys PD, Walker N, Schwartlander B. The global impact of HIV/AIDS. *Nature* 2001;**410**:968–73.

44   McCune JM. The dynamics of CD4+ T-cell depletion in HIV disease. *Nature* 2001;**410**:974–9.

45   McMichael AJ, Rowland-Jones SL. Cellular immune responses to HIV. *Nature* 2001;**410**:980–7.

46   Harrington M, Carpenter CCJ. Hit HIV-1 hard, but only when necessary. *Lancet* 2000;**35**:2147–52.

47   Hollander H, Levy JA. Neurologic abnormalities and recovery of human immunodeficiency virus from cerebrospinal fluid. *Ann Intern Med* 1987;**106**:692–5.

48   Levy JA, Shimabukuro J, Hollander H, Mills J, Kaminsky L. Isolation of AIDS associated retroviruses from cerebrospinal fluid and brain of patients with neurological symptoms. *Lancet* 1985;**ii**:586–8.

49   Apoola A, Ahmad S, Radcliffe K. Primary HIV infection. *Int J STD AIDS* 2002;**13**:71–8.

50   Jolles S, Kinloch de Loës S, Johnson MA, Janossy G. Primary HIV-1 infection: a new medical emergency? *Br Med J* 1996;**312**:1243–4.

51   Ho DD. Time to hit HIV, early and hard. *N Engl J Med* 1995;**333**:450–1.

52 Lipton SA, Gendelman HE. Dementia associated with the acquired immunodeficiency syndrome. *N Engl J Med* 1995;**332**:934–40.
53 Richman DD. HIV chemotherapy. *Nature* 2001;**410**:995–1001.
54 Omrani AS, Pillay D. Multi-drug resistant HIV-1. *J Infect* 2000;**41**:5–11.
55 Carr A, Cooper DA. Adverse events of antiretroviral therapy. *Lancet* 2000;**356**:1423–30.
56 D'Souza MP, Cairns JS, Plaeger SF. Current evidence and future directions for targeting HIV entry. Therapeutic and prophylactic strategies. *JAMA* 2000;**284**:215–22.
57 Centers for Disease Control and Prevention. Guidelines for preventing opportunistic infections among HIV-infected persons – 2002 recommendations of the US Public Health Service and the Infectious Diseases Society of America. *MMWR* 2002;**51**(No. RR-8):1–52.
58 Kovacs JA, Masur H. Prophylaxis against opportunistic infections in patients with human immunodeficiency virus infection. *N Engl J Med* 2000;**342**:1416.
59 Luft BJ, Hafner R, Korzun AH, *et al.* Toxoplasmic encephalitis in patients with the acquired immunodeficiency syndrome. *N Engl J Med* 1993;**329**: 995–1000.
60 Porter SB, Sande MA. Toxoplasmosis of the central nervous system in the acquired immunodeficiency syndrome. *N Engl J Med* 1992;**327**:1643–8.
61 Østergaard L, Nielsen AK, Black FT. DNA amplification on cerebrospinal fluid for diagnosis of cerebral toxoplasmosis among HIV-positive patients with signs or symptoms of neurological disease. *Scand J Infect Dis* 1993;**25**:227–37.
62 Katlama C, De Wit S, O'Doherty E, Van Glabeke M, Clumeck N, the European Network for Treatment of AIDS (ENTA) Toxoplasmosis Study Group. Pyrimethamine-clindamycin vs. pyrimethamine-sulfadiazine as acute and long-term therapy for toxoplasmic encephalitis in patients with AIDS. *Clin Infect Dis* 1996;**22**:268–75.
63 Sepkowitz KA. Opportunistic infections in patients with and patients without acquired immunodeficiency syndrome. *Clin Infect Dis* 2002;**34**:1098–107.
64 Dismukes WE. Cryptococcal meningitis in AIDS. *J Infect Dis* 1988;**157**: 624–7.
65 Saag MS, Graybill RJ, Larsen RA, *et al.* Practice guidelines for the management of cryptococcal disease. *Clin Infect Dis* 2000;**30**:710–18.
66 Greenlee JE. Progressive multifocal leukoencephalopathy progress made and lessons relearned. *N Engl J Med* 1998;**338**:1378–80.
67 Giudici B, Vaz B, Bossolasco S, *et al.* Highly active antiretroviral therapy and progressive multifocal leukoencephalopathy: effects on cerebrospinal fluid markers of JC virus replication and immune response. *Clin Infect Dis* 2000;**30**:95–9.
68 Colebunders R, Lambert ML. Management of co-infection with HIV and TB. *Br Med J* 2002;**324**:802–3.
69 Roos KL, Tunkel AR, Scheld WM. Acute bacterial meningitis in children and adults. In: Scheld WM, Whitley RJ, Durack DT, eds. *Infections of the nervous system*. Philadelphia: Lippencott-Raven, 1997.
70 Achtman M. Clonal properties of meningococci from epidemic meningitis. *Trans R Soc Trop Med Hyg* 1991;**85**(Suppl 1):24–31.
71 Schwartz B, Moore PS, Broome CV. Global epidemiology of meningococcal disease. *Clin Microbiol Rev* 1989;**2**(Suppl):S118–24 [review].
72 Ramsay ME, Andrews N, Kaczmarski EB, Miller E. Efficacy of meningococcal serogroup C conjugate vaccine in teenagers and toddlers in England. *Lancet* 2001;**357**:195–6.

73   Durand ML, Calderwood SB, Weber DJ, et al. Acute bacterial meningitis in adults: a review of 493 episodes. N Engl J Med 1993;328:21–8.
74   Law DA, Aronoff SC. Anaerobic meningitis in children: case report and review of the literature. Pediatr Infect Dis J 1992;11:968–71 [review].
75   Thwaites G, Chau TTH, Mai NTH, Drobniewski F, McAdam K, Farrar J. Tuberculous meningitis. J Neurol Neurosurg Psychiatry 2000;68:289–99.
76   Quagliarello V, Scheld WM. Bacterial meningitis: pathogenesis, pathophysiology, and progress. N Engl J Med 1992;327:864–72.
77   Tunkel AR, Scheld WM. Pathogenesis and pathophysiology of bacterial meningitis. Clin Microbiol Rev 1993;6:118–36.
78   Ashwal S, Perkin RM, Thompson JR, Schneider S, Tomasi LG. Bacterial meningitis in children: current concepts of neurologic management. Adv Pediatr 1993;40:185–215.
79   Schaad UB. Management of bacterial meningitis in childhood. Rev Med Microbiol 1997;8:171–8.
80   Tunkel AR, Scheld WM. Acute bacterial meningitis. Lancet 1995;346: 1675–80.
81   Thomas KE, Hasbun R, Jekel J, Quagliarello VJ. The diagnostic accuracy of Kernig's sign, Brudzinski's sign and nuchal rigidity in adults with suspected meningitis. Clin Infect Dis 2002;35:46–52.
82   Attia J, Hatala R, Cook DJ, Wong JG. Does this adult patient have acute meningitis? JAMA 1999;282:175–81.
83   Rutter N, Smales OR. Role of routine investigations in children presenting with their first febrile convulsion. Arch Dis Child 1977;52:188–91.
84   Lorber J, Sunderland R. Lumbar puncture in children with convulsions associated with fever. Lancet 1980;i:786.
85   Osman H. Human herpesvirus 6 and febrile convulsions. Herpes 2000;7:33–7.
86   Uldry PA, Kuntzer T, Bogousslavsky J, et al. Early symptoms and outcome of Listeria monocytogenes rhomboencephalitis: 14 adult cases. J Neurol 1993;240:235–42.
87   Aronin SI, Peduzzi P, Quagliarello VJ. Community-acquired bacterial meningitis: risk stratification for adverse clinical outcome and effect of antibiotic timing. Ann Intern Med 1998;129:862–9.
88   Begg N, Cartwright KAV, Cohen J, et al. Consensus statement on diagnosis, investigation, treatment and prevention of acute bacterial meningitis in immunocompetent adults. J Infect 1999;39:1–15.
89   Taylor MRH, Keane CT, Periappuran M. Skin scraping is a useful investigation in meningococcal disease. Br Med J 1997;314:831–2.
90   Cartwright K, Reilly S, White D, Stuart J. Early treatment with parenteral penicillin in meningococcal disease. Br Med J 1992;305:143–7.
91   Friedland IR, Paris MM, Rinderknecht S, McCracken GH. Cranial computed tomographic scans have little impact on management of bacterial meningitis. Am J Dis Child 1992;146:1484–7.
92   Rennick G, Shann F, de Campo J. Cerebral herniation during bacterial meningitis in children. Br Med J 1993;306:953–5.
93   Nadel S, Levin M, Habibi P. Treatment of meningococcal disease in childhood. In: Cartwright K, eds. Meningococcal Disease. Chichester: Wiley, 1995.
94   Kaczmarski EB, Ragunatha PL, Marsh J, Gray SJ, Guiver M. Creating a national service for the diagnosis of meningococcal disease by polymerase chain reaction. Commun Dis Public Health 1998;1:54–6.
95   Urwin R, Kaczmarski EB, Guiver M, Fox AJ, Maiden MC. Amplification of the meningococcal porB gene for non-culture serotype characterisation. Epidemiol Infect 1998;120:257–62.

96   Marton KI, Gean AD. The spinal tap: a new look at an old test. *Ann Intern Med* 1986;**104**:840–8.

97   Spanos A, Harrell FE Jr, Durack DT. Differential diagnosis of acute meningitis: an analysis of the predictive value of initial observation. *JAMA* 1989;**262**:2700–7.

98   Bonadio WA. The cerebrospinal fluid: physiologic aspects and alterations associated with bacterial meningitis. *Pediat Infect Dis J* 1992;**11**:423–32.

99   Newcombe J, Cartwright K, Palmer WH, McFadden J. PCR of peripheral blood for the diagnosis of meningococcal disease. *J Clin Microbiol* 1996;**34**:1637–40.

100 Borrow R, Claus H, Guiver M. Non-culture diagnosis and serogroup determination of meningococcal B and C by a sialyltransferase (siaD) PCR ELISA. *Epidemiol Infect* 1997;**118**:111–17.

101 Klugman KP, Saunders J. Pneumococci resistant to extended-spectrum cephalosporins in South Africa. *Lancet* 1993;**341**:1164.

102 Whitney CG, Farley MM, Hadler J, *et al*. Increasing prevalence of multidrug-resistant *Streptococcus pneumoniae* in the United States. *N Engl J Med* 2000;**343**:1917–24.

103 Song JH, Lee NY, Ichiyama S, *et al*. Spread of drug-resistant *Streptococcus pneumoniae* in Asian countries: Asian Network for Surveillance of Resistant Pathogens (ANSORP) Study. *Clin Infect Dis* 1999;**28**:1206–11.

104 Leggiadro RJ. Penicillin- and cephalosporin-resistant *Streptococcus pneumoniae*: an emerging microbial threat. *Pediatrics* 1994;**93**:500–3.

105 McCracken GH. Emergence of resistant *Streptococcus pneumoniae*: a problem in pediatrics. *Pediatr Infect Dis J* 1995;**14**:424–8.

106 Saez-Nieto JA, Lujan R, Berron S, *et al*. Epidemiology and molecular basis of penicillin-resistant *Neisseria meningitidis* in Spain: a 5-year history (1985–1989). *Clin Infect Dis* 1992;**14**:394–402.

107 Landesman SH, Corrado ML, Shah PM, Armengaud M, Barza M, Cherubin CE. Past and current roles for cephalosporin antibiotics in treatment of meningitis: emphasis on use in gram-negative bacillary meningitis. *Am J Med* 1981;**71**:693–703.

108 Bradley JS, Garau J, Lode H, Rolston KVI, Wilson SE, Quinn JP. Carbapenems in clinical practice: a guide to their use in serious infection. *Int J Antimicrob Agents* 1999;**11**:93–100.

109 Infection in Neurosurgery Working Party of the British Society for Antimicrobial Chemotherapy. The management of neurosurgical patients with postoperative bacterial or aseptic meningitis or external ventricular drain-associated ventriculitis. *Br J Neurosurg* 2000;**14**:7–12.

110 Lauritsen A, Oberg B. Adjunctive corticosteroid therapy in bacterial meningitis. *Scand J Infect Dis* 1995;**27**:431–4.

111 McIntyre PB, Berkey CS, King SM, *et al*. Dexamethasone as adjunctive therapy in bacterial meningitis: a meta-analysis of randomized clinical trials since 1988. *JAMA* 1997;**278**:925–31.

112 de Gans J, van de Beek D, for the European Dexamethasone in Adulthood Bacterial Meningitis Study Investigators. Dexamethasone in adults with bacterial meningitis. *N Engl J Med* 2002;**347**:1549–56.

113 Tunkel AR, Scheld WM. Corticosteroids for everyone with meningitis? *N Engl J Med* 2002;**347**:1613–15.

114 Lynn WA, Cohen J. Adjunctive therapy for septic shock: a review of experimental approaches. *Clin Infect Dis* 1995;**20**:143–58.

115 Levin M, Quint PA, Goldstein B, *et al*. Recombinant bactericidal/permeability-increasing protein (rBPI$_{21}$) as adjunctive treatment for children with severe meningococcal sepsis: a randomised trial. *Lancet* 2000;**356**:961–7.

116 Smith OP, White B, Vaughan D, *et al.* Use of protein-C concentrate, heparin, and haemofiltration in meningococcus-induced purpura fulminans. *Lancet* 1997;**350**:1590–3.

117 White B, Livingstone W, Murphy C, Hodgson A, Rafferty M, Smith OP. An open-label study of the role of adjuvant hemostatic support with protein C replacement therapy in purpura fulminans-associated meningococcemia. *Blood* 2000;**96**:3719–24.

118 PHLS Meningococcal Infections Working Group and Public Health Medicine Environmental Group. Control of meningococcal disease: guidance for consultants in communicable disease control. *CDR Rev* 1995;**5**:R189–95.

119 Bullock MRR, Welchman JM. Diagnostic and prognostic features of tuberculous meningitis on CT scanning. *J Neurol Neurosurg Psychiatry* 1982;**45**:1098–101.

120 Bhargava S, Gupta AK, Tandon PN. Tuberculous meningitis: a CT study. *Br J Radiol* 1982;**55**:189–96.

121 Jamieson DH. Imaging intracranial tuberculosis in childhood. *Pediatr Radiol* 1995;**25**:165–70.

122 Thwaites GE, Chau TTH, Stepniewska K, *et al.* Diagnosis of adult tuberculous meningitis by use of clinical and laboratory features. *Lancet* 2002;**360**:1287–92.

123 Kent SJ, Crowe SM, Yung A, Lucas CR, Mijch AM. Tuberculous meningitis: a 30-year review. *Clin Infect Dis* 1993;**17**:994.

124 Joint Tuberculosis Committee of the British Thoracic Society. Chemotherapy and management of tuberculosis in the United Kingdom: recommendations 1998. *Thorax* 1998;**53**:536–48.

125 Donald PR, Schoeman JF, Van Zyl LE, De Villiers JN, Pretorius M, Springer P. Intensive short-course chemotherapy in the management of tuberculous meningitis. *Int J Tuberc Lung Dis* 1998;**2**:704–11.

126 Phuapradit P, Vejjajiva A. Treatment of tuberculous meningitis: role of short-course chemotherapy. *Q J Med* 1987;**62**:249–58.

127 Prasad K, Volmink J, Menon GR. Steroids for treating tuberculous meningitis. In: Cochrane Collaboration. *Cochrane Library*. Issue 4. Oxford: Update Software, 2002.

128 Nadelman RB, Wormser GP. Lyme borreliosis. *Lancet* 1998;**352**:557–65.

129 Wormser GP, Nadelman RB, Dattwyler RJ, *et al.* Practice guidelines for the treatment of Lyme disease. *Clin Infect Dis* 2000;**31**(suppl 1):S1–14.

130 Musher DM, Baughn RE. Neurosyphilis in HIV-infected persons. *N Engl J Med* 1994;**331**:1516–7.

131 Hook EWI. Syphilis and HIV infection. *J Infect Dis* 1989;**160**:530–4.

132 Clinical Effectiveness Group (Association of Genitourinary Medicine and the Society for the Study of Venereal Diseases). National guideline for the management of late syphilis. *Sex Transm Inf* 1999;**75**(Suppl1): S34–7.

133 Parola P, Raoult D. Ticks and tickborne bacterial diseases in humans: an emerging infectious threat. *Clin Infect Dis* 2001;**32**:897–928.

134 Conlon CP, Berendt AR, Dawson K, Peto TEA. "Runway malaria". *Lancet* 1990;**335**:472.

135 World Health Organization. Severe falciparum malaria. *Trans R Soc Trop Med Hyg* 2000;**94**(suppl 1):51–90.

136 Lesi A, Meremikwu M. High first dose quinine regimen for treating severe malaria. In: Cochrane Collaboration. *Cochrane Library*, Issue 4. Oxford: Update Software, 2002.

137 McIntosh HM, Olliaro P. Artemisinin derivatives for treating severe malaria. In: Cochrane Collaboration. *Cochrane Library*, Issue 4. Oxford: Update Software, 2002.

138 Meremikwu M, Marson AG. Routine anticonvulsants for treating cerebral malaria. In: Cochrane Collaboration. *Cochrane Library*, Issue 4. Oxford: Update Software, 2002.

139 Prasad K, Garner P. Steroids for treating cerebral malaria. In Cochrane Collaboration. *Cochrane Library*, Issue 4. Oxford: Update Software, 2002.

140 Davies AH. Metronidazole in human infections with syphilis. *Br J Venereol* 1967;**43**:197–200.

141 Thong YH. Chemotherapy for primary amebic meningoencephalitis. *N Engl J Med* 1982;**306**:1295–6.

142 Seidel J. Chemotherapy for primary amebic meningoencephalitis. *N Engl J Med* 1982;**306**:1296.

143 Colli BO, Carlotti CG, Machado HR, Assirati JA. Intracranial bacterial infections. *Neurosurg Q* 1999;**9**:258–84.

144 Townsend GC. Brain abscess and other focal pyogenic infections. In: Armstrong D, Cohen J, eds. *Infectious diseases*. London: Mosby, 1999.

145 Nathoo N, Nadvi SS, Van Dellen JR, *et al.* Intracranial subdural empyemas in the era of computed tomography: a review of 699 cases. *Neurosurgery* 1999;**44**:529–36.

146 Yen PT, Chan ST, Huang TS. Brain abscess: with special reference to otolaryngologic sources of infection. *Otolaryngol Head Neck Surg* 1995; **113**:15–22.

147 Britt R, Enzmann D, Yeager A. Neuropathological and computed tomographic findings in experimental brain abscess. *J Neurosurg* 1981;**55**:590–603.

148 Hagensee ME, Bauwens JE, Kjos B, Bowden RA. Brain abscess following marrow transplantation: experience at the Fred Hutchinson Cancer Research Center, 1984–1992. *Clin Infect Dis* 1994;**19**:408.

149 Shahzadi S, Lozano AM, Bernstein M, Guha A, Tasker RR. Sterotaxic management of bacterial brain abscesses. *Can J Neurol Sci* 1996;**23**:34–9.

150 Townsend GC, Scheld WM. Infections of the central nervous system. *Adv Intern Med* 1998;**43**:403–47.

151 Kim KD, Johnson JP, Masciopinto JE. Management of spinal epidural abscess and subdural empyema. *Tech Neurosurg* 1999;**5**:293–302.

10: Acute spinal cord compression

J BROWN, RA JOHNSTON

Introduction

A wide variety of pathological lesions may cause spinal cord compression. The clinical presentation sometimes indicates the nature of the causal lesion and usually indicates its anatomical location. With modern imaging techniques, the relevance of making a clinical diagnosis of pathology has diminished but the importance of the anatomical diagnosis to guide the choice of imaging site and modality remains fundamental to management. The important diagnostic aspect of acute spinal cord compression is that it should be recognised as early as possible and be referred with the urgency that the particular case merits. Prompt referral enhances the likelihood of reversing neurological deficits by appropriate decompressive surgery. The prognosis for recovery depends mainly on the severity of the deficit before decompression, but the duration of the deficit and rapidity of its onset may also play a role. Trauma results in a virtually instantaneous onset of compression and in this setting, the benefit of urgent decompressive surgery has not been demonstrated. By contrast, compression of a more gradual onset, for example in infectious or neoplastic cord compression, allows an opportunity for intervention before spinal cord function is lost completely. This window of opportunity may be brief and so deteriorating spinal cord function on serial neurological examinations demands immediate consultation with a specialist unit.

Successful spinal cord decompression means return of normal function in affected limbs and a stable, painless spine.

Generally, this means restoring independent walking, although both patient and surgeon may have to settle for lesser degrees of functional recovery.

Spinal cord compression implies a "structural" lesion of the vertebral column compromising the spinal canal and producing a myelopathy. The signs and symptoms of any spinal cord dysfunction are motor and sensory deficit and reflex changes, but a common feature of "structural" lesions is pain. Spinal pain or nerve root pain, occurring in the presence of myelopathic symptoms, strongly implies a surgically remediable aetiology. Most patients presenting with spinal cord compression reach hospital by referral through their general practitioner or through an accident and emergency department and are usually admitted to general medical or surgical wards. In the early stages abnormal neurological signs may be difficult to detect, especially if these are subtle and the pain is severe. For a variety of reasons, including late self-referral to any medical practitioner, delays can and do occur in the transfer of such a patient to a specialist spinal unit. This was the subject of a candid and disturbing report by Maurice-Williams and Richardson illustrating the diverse causes for delayed referral and its consequences.[1]

Any surgeon who carries out spinal decompression has experience of patients who are referred having been paraplegic for several days. Surgical treatment is very unlikely to result in a functional recovery when motor power has deteriorated below MRC grade 3 (active movement against gravity). Recognition of signs and symptoms of spinal cord compression may be difficult outside a neuroscience environment and it is important that neurosurgeons, spinal orthopaedic surgeons, and neurologists take the trouble to facilitate referral from physicians and general surgeons at an early stage. This includes an ongoing educational element, of which a most important aspect is to encourage colleagues to recognise the early signs of myelopathy. Easier access to spinal imaging should help.

Diverse factors are taken into consideration when planning surgical management of spinal cord compression including general fitness, life expectancy, tumour pathology, and the extent of any metastatic spread if the lesion is neoplastic. Details of past medical history are thus important information to relay to the specialist unit.

Trauma

The most acute form of spinal cord compression is caused by trauma, of which 50% occurs in the cervical spine and most of the remainder at the thoracolumbar junction or in the lumbar spine. Patients are usually young males involved in road traffic accidents, falls, and occasionally sport related activities.[2] The forces involved can be resolved into flexion, extension, compression, and rotation, although most patterns of fracture and subluxation seen in practice result from a combination of these forces. In approximately 10% of cases, two non-contiguous levels of the cervical spine are damaged, separated by normal segments.[3]

The management of acute spinal cord injury can be intimidating to those unfamiliar with this clinical problem. In fact, the major components of management of spine trauma are analogous to the management of a fracture of a long bone. The steps involved are recognition, immobilisation, investigation, reduction, fixation, and rehabilitation.

In most cases, the combination of neurological deficit and a painful, tender cervical region leads to recognition of the injury. Where the patient is unable to provide a history, for example, in the presence of an associated head injury with a decreased conscious level, it is best to presume that a spinal injury is present until proven otherwise.

The cervical spine can be immobilised easily by holding the head firmly between two hands and maintaining the cervical spine in a neutral position until better facilities are available. If the patient needs to be moved, to examine the back for example, a strict "logrolling" technique with an adequate number of personnel should be observed. Depending on the circumstances, the patient may be fitted with an appropriate sized Philadelphia style collar or be placed in cervical traction. Soft cervical collars are not adequate as they barely restrict flexion and extension movements of the cervical spine. A Philadelphia style collar supports the occiput, spreads over the shoulders, rises over the chin, and provides more effective immobilisation (Figure 10.1). Cervical tongs such as the Gardner–Wells variety may be applied in the casualty department within a matter of seconds. These require local anaesthetic and are placed 4 cm above the external auditory meatus. The pins are hand-screwed through the anaesthetised

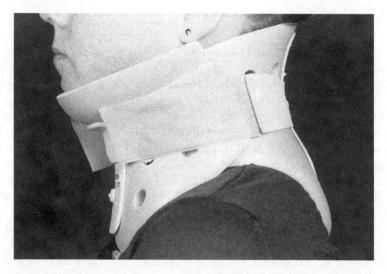

Figure 10.1 The main points of support for a Philadelphia style collar are the occiput, shoulders, and chin

scalp into the outer skull cortex to a preset tension. The clinician then has full control of the patient's cervical spine.

Definitive investigations at an early stage must include a lateral plain radiograph of all cervical vertebrae. Some cases of missed fracture in the cervical spine are the result of inadequate radiographs that omit the lower vertebrae. Flexion/extension views can be particularly revealing and, if carried out carefully, the patient will come to no harm even should the films show abnormal movement. These dynamic views should only be carried out under supervised conditions and after senior or specialised consultation. Cervical spine radiographs are difficult to read, especially for inexperienced junior staff, and experienced staff should be consulted before management decisions are made. More definitive investigation is carried out by CT, which almost always reveals more damage than was initially expected from plain radiographs. If C7 is not seen on ordinary radiographs it is always accessible by CT. MRI may show damage to ligaments, discs, and prevertebral tissues which have a clearly altered signal with this form of scanning, but which may not be recognised using plain radiographs[4] (Figure 10.2).

At or before this stage in management, referral should be made to a specialised spinal unit, preferably an acute spinal

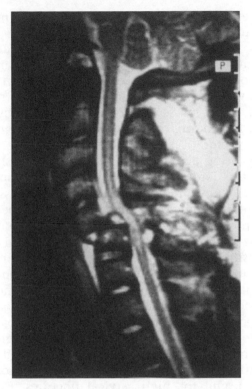

Figure 10.2 MRI (1·5T Siemens Magnetom, T2 weighted scan). Discoligamentous injury at C5/6 with anterior subluxation of C5 on C6. *Note the altered cord signal at the level of the injury and the high signal in the interspinous ligaments posteriorly*

cord injury unit. The Queen Elizabeth National Spinal Injuries Unit for Scotland receives patients with spine trauma, with and without cord injury, usually within 24 hours of injury. The pathophysiological consequences of acute spinal cord injury on cardiovascular and respiratory function and the intensive nursing requirements make early referral of these patients to an appropriate unit imperative. Spinal cord damage results in attenuated sympathetic neural control causing hypotension and bradycardia. These are "normal" for a patient who has functional cord transection and attempts at "volume loading" to elevate blood pressure are misplaced. Loss of intercostal innervation due to cervical cord trauma produces ventilatory insufficiency that is best managed in specialised units.[5]

Fractures, subluxations, or dislocations usually require reduction into normal alignment. This may be relatively easily brought about using simple cervical traction. In the 1970s there was a vogue for using high weight cervical traction, but this carries a risk of secondary cord damage by excessive distraction. Depending on the type and displacement of the injury, the vector of traction may need to be varied, for example by using a rolled up sheet under the shoulders to exaggerate the lordotic curve of the cervical spine. These techniques require frequent radiographic assessment and management experience and are best left to the specialist unit. Should appropriate cervical traction be unsuccessful in reducing the fracture-dislocation, the options are manipulation under anaesthesia, rarely used now, or open reduction and internal fixation. Those patients who have vertebral damage but no spinal cord injury are vulnerable to secondary injury through inadvertent or accidental mishandling of the spine and have potentially more to lose than those patients who sustain major spinal cord damage at the time of impact.

Fixation of the cervical spine may be carried out using external orthotic supports such as a halo fixator which is particularly useful for high cervical fractures. Even in this device a small range of flexion and extension can still occur. Methods of internal fixation have evolved and improved, especially in recent years. In the cervical spine, plate or rod and screw constructs are increasingly replacing sublaminar wires and laminar clamp devices. Internal fixation enables the patient to begin mobilisation and rehabilitation at an earlier stage.[6] For thoracic and lumbar fractures the use of pedicle screw fixation reduces the number of vertebral levels permanently immobilised and allows intraoperative fracture reduction and restoration of alignment.[7] Malalignment of the spinal column is reduced using internal fixation, but long term stability only comes through bone union. There is continued debate among specialists over the merits, demerits, and appropriate timing of surgical intervention in spinal injury. It is clear that in selected circumstances internal fixation and fusion does have a role to play and does impart advantages to patients, allowing earlier mobilisation for rehabilitation and conferring better long term stability. There is no evidence, however, that surgical intervention improves neurological outcome. Despite anecdotal reports, there is no recognised causal association between surgical decompression and fixation and neurological recovery in patients with acute spinal trauma.[8]

Enthusiasm for the use of high dose methylprednisolone in acute spinal trauma, especially in North America, followed the publication of the second national acute spinal cord injury study (NASCIS 11).[9] This prospective, randomised trial showed statistical improvement in limb function where the steroid was administered as a bolus infusion of 30 mg/kg given over 15 minutes and, after a 45 minute pause, followed by an infusion of 5·4 mg/kg per hour over 23 hours. This statistical improvement, however, was mainly sensory so that it did not result in any clear functional or clinical gain by the patient. The steroid treated group had a higher rate of infectious complications. For these reasons, this practice has not become established in the United Kingdom. Methylprednisolone is not given routinely at the Queen Elizabeth National Spinal Injuries Unit for Scotland.

More recently, substantial concern has been raised about the methodology of the study and of the subsequent NASCIS III trial.[10] Coleman *et al.* questioned the appropriateness of generalising results from a trial population that included individuals with minor cord injury to the more severely injured population and pointed out a concern that the positive result of the trial could be a statistical artefact. The placebo group treated before eight hours did poorly not only when compared to the group that received steroids but also when compared to the second placebo group, treated after eight hours, suggesting that the early placebo group was perhaps more severely injured than either of the other two groups. Finally, a concern that the primary data from NASCIS were not publicly available even nine years after completion of the trial means that reporting of these studies does not meet standards required for FDA approval.[11]

Hurlbert called the use of methylprednisolone in spinal cord injury "an inappropriate standard of care" and raised further concerns that half of the data from the trials (all observations on the left side of all patients) were excluded from analysis.[12] The primary outcome analysis was negative and despite more than 60 *post hoc* tests, no correction for multiple comparisons was provided. He analysed six other studies of steroids in spinal cord injury demonstrating that the results are not reproducible, and offered compelling arguments and an analysis of the available data supporting the view that methylprednisolone should be considered an investigational agent with an unproven role in spinal cord injury. The handicap posed to future studies in neuroprotection if this status is not recognised is also highlighted.[13] Although the NASCIS trials were prospective and randomised, well designed, and well executed, they do not provide compelling data, appropriate analysis, or evidence of clinically meaningful outcomes. The results are not reproducible and thus they fall well short of criteria for Level I evidence (evidence sufficient to support a standard of care). The use of steroids in spinal cord trauma should be considered unproven and experimental.

As in severe head injury, the primary traumatic event in spinal cord injury is followed by microvascular and biochemical changes that compound the original injury. It may be possible to block or attenuate some of these changes pharmacologically. For example, the action of the excitotoxin glutamate, released following trauma to central neural tissue, can be modified using N-methyl-D-aspartate receptor blockade in experimental models. Although considerable attention has been focused on biochemical methods of preventing or modifying the secondary damage produced following brain and spinal cord injury,[14] none are yet proven in clinical trials. A randomised controlled trial of ganglioside GMI (Syngen) failed to show a benefit of the drug in a primary efficacy analysis. It did suggest, however, an earlier recovery in the treated group and that further studies of the drug in incomplete injuries should be undertaken, as these patients showed a trend to improvement that did not reach significance due to small numbers of patients. The hope that effective pharmacological neuroprotective agents may be found thus persists though it is as yet unrealised.[15]

Inflammatory conditions

The most common inflammatory condition leading to spinal cord compression is rheumatoid disease, which affects approximately 1% of the population in Western Europe. The cervical spine is involved in a substantial percentage of patients with rheumatoid disease and the incidence and severity increase directly with the duration of the disease. The most common site of involvement is at the occipito–Cl/C2 level, although all levels of the cervical spine may be involved.[16]

The fluctuating progress of the condition gradually destroys the joint tissues and articular surfaces and leads to subluxation or even dislocation. This is frequently seen in the fingers and wrist joints of patients with rheumatoid disease, but also occurs at the occipito–CI/C2 level.

The most common form of dislocation is anterior subluxation of Cl on C2, and this may be fixed or mobile depending on the activity of the inflammatory process[17–19] (Figure 10.3). Eventually the condition "burns out" and the joints may become ankylosed in an abnormal position. Loss of height of the lateral masses of C1 results in vertical translocation of the odontoid process and this occurs in about 10% of the affected population. Less frequently occurring abnormalities include posterior subluxation of C1 on C2 where the odontoid is totally eroded and the atlas can move posteriorly relative to the body of C2. Asymmetrical involvement of the lateral mass joints may lead to rotational deformities or lateral subluxations.[20] The demonstration of these different types of atlantoaxial abnormality was enormously enhanced by the advent of CT myelography, including sagittal plane reconstruction. Magnetic resonance scanning is now more commonly used. Either type of study may be carried out in flexion and extension to demonstrate instability.[21,22]

With any subluxation in this region or in the subaxial region, spinal canal compromise may occur, causing a myelopathy (Figure 10.4). Although pain and radiographic abnormalities are common in rheumatoid disease, extensive epidemiological and clinical studies have shown no sure method of predicting which patients will deteriorate neurologically and which patients, even with relatively severe radiological involvement, will never develop neurological signs and symptoms. More recent work suggests that measurement of cord diameter or area may prove to be a better predictor of the requirement for surgical intervention and of surgical outcome than clinical markers.[23,24]

(a)

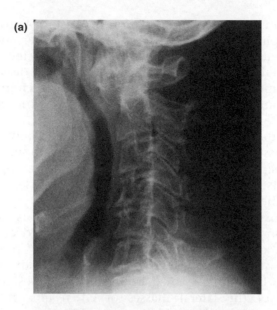

(b)

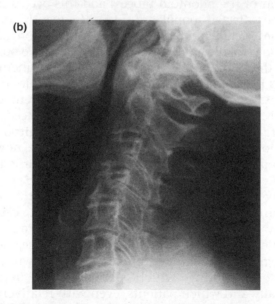

Figure 10.3 Plain lateral cervical spine radiograph performed in flexion (a) and extension (b). This patient with rheumatoid arthritis has anterior subluxation of C1 on C2 in flexion with complete reduction in extension. Note the compromise of the spinal canal between the posterior surface of the odontoid process and the posterior arch of C1 in the flexion film

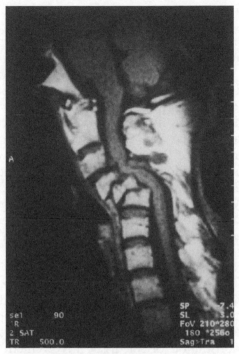

Figure 10.4 MRI (1·5T Siemens Magnetom, T1 weighted scan). Subaxial spinal cord compression presenting as gait disturbance and loss of coordination over a period of weeks

Acute spinal cord compression is not common in rheumatoid disease although there are anecdotal cases of patients suddenly collapsing with paralysis and succumbing due to gross odontoid subluxation. Usually neurological symptoms develop over a period of weeks or even months, but a few patients do develop neurological signs and deteriorate with progressive myelopathy over a period of days. They present with deterioration in gait quality and complain of sensory alteration or sensory loss, including loss of manual dexterity. A clear clinical history is of paramount importance in confirming the myelopathy, since severe widespread synovial joint involvement frequently precludes accurate assessment of deep tendon reflexes and muscle power.

Patients can often distinguish between new symptoms such as loss of strength, paraesthesia, or significant gait deterioration and identify these separately from the symptoms of multiple joint involvement with which they are already very familiar. Isolated tendon reflexes may be elicited, although plantar responses are almost never obtainable because of local joint involvement or previous surgery. Vertical subluxation of the odontoid process may occasionally give rise to lower cranial nerve signs and symptoms. Formation of a fibrous inflammatory mass (often erroneously referred to as pannus) around the odontoid process can also cause compression of the high spinal cord or lower medulla. The differential diagnosis of speech difficulty and dysphonia includes rheumatoid involvement in the temporomandibular and cricoarytenoid joints.[25,26] In one of the largest series of rheumatoid patients that has been studied neurologically, nystagmus only occurred in those patients with a pre-existing Chiari I malformation.[23]

When a cervical myelopathy is confirmed in a patient with rheumatoid disease, the most common cause is anterior atlantoaxial subluxation. This can be confirmed easily and rapidly by a plain lateral radiograph of the cervical spine taken in flexion and extension. This shows bone movement and position, whereas demonstration of soft tissue involvement requires the use of CT myelography or MRI. The purpose of management in this situation is to reduce compression on the cervical cord and in most cases this can be achieved by extending the upper cervical spine and bringing the C1 and C2 vertebrae into more normal alignment. It cannot be assumed, however, that because vertebral alignment has been restored, spinal cord compression has been reduced. This becomes apparent once scanning of the region has been carried out. A spine surgeon should be consulted at this point for decisions concerning continued immobilisation or surgical decompression, fixation, and fusion.

There are a variety of surgical approaches to the craniocervical junction. The odontoid region can be approached directly by the transpharyngeal route in order to decompress the anterior cervicomedullary region directly. It is recommended that this should be followed by a posterior stabilising operation to generate fusion of C1 and C2 or occipital bone to C2.[27–29] If the spinal cord compression is primarily posterior, a standard posterior approach and decompression with or without stabilisation may be preferable. For many patients a posterior

C1–C2 fixation and fusion is sufficient.[30-35] Subaxial spinal cord compression is less common than at C1–C2, but also may require a combination of anterior and posterior surgery. A careful history sometimes elicits an episode of trauma that was initially thought to be trivial. Extreme caution must be exercised in reducing deformities at this level. Overzealous attempts at reduction may result in cord injury in the setting of chronic spinal deformity secondary to rheumatoid disease or other inflammatory conditions such as ankylosing spondylitis. At all levels the aim is to directly decompress the spinal cord, to restore vertebral alignment, and to prevent further malalignment.

The postoperative mortality and morbidity rates are greatest in those patients who are severely neurologically affected, that is, tetraparetic and unable to walk.[24] The systemic effects of rheumatoid disease, especially interstitial pulmonary involvement, may adversely affect postsurgical recovery. In those patients in whom the myelopathy is recognised and treated in the early stages the outlook for recovery is good and postoperative mortality is low.[17]

Infective lesions

Infections of the spine are uncommon, but can usefully be classified as either vertebral osteomyelitis or intraspinal infection. Vertebral osteomyelitis is the more common variety of infection and can lead to intraspinal infection. "Pure" intraspinal infection implies no associated infection of the vertebral column and includes extradural, subdural, or intramedullary abscess in descending order of frequency.[36,37] Intraspinal infections occur at a frequency of approximately one per million per year in United Kingdom neurosurgical units and are predominantly caused by pyogenic organisms, usually *Staphylococcus* sp., whereas in Asia or Africa *Mycobacterium tuberculosis* is the common infecting organism.[38]

An abscess may be found anywhere within the spinal epidural space but the most common location is posterior where the epidural space is most prominent and thoracic and lumbar levels are most commonly affected (Figure 10.5). The spinal epidural space does not communicate with the

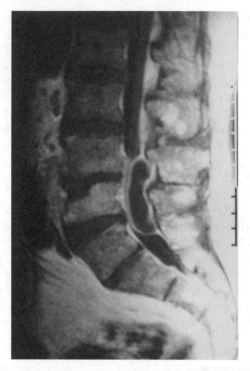

Figure 10.5 MRI (1·5T Siemens Magnetom, T1 weighted scan with gadolinium enhancement). Spinal epidural abscess in the lumbar spine presenting as a complete cauda equina syndrome

intracranial extradural space and has no true intracranial analogue because at the foramen magnum the outer, endosteal layer of the intracranial dura adheres to bone and becomes continuous with the pericranium. The spinal dura is a single layer continuous with the inner, meningeal layer of the intracranial dura. Cervical epidural abscess is uncommon and is usually associated with vertebral osteomyelitis. The abscess may extend over few or many vertebral levels, and it is well recognised that non-contiguous abscesses may occur.[39,40]

A spinal epidural abscess is a neurosurgical emergency and is one of the few instances where the history and clinical examination may provide the pathological diagnosis. The patient may or may not present with systemic infective illness, but as the abscess enlarges and compression of the spinal cord occurs then myelopathic symptoms gradually develop, usually over the course of a small number of days.[41–43] The outstanding clinical feature is spinal pain and the marked local tenderness of the spine that may be elicited by lightly tapping the spinous processes with a tendon hammer. Several studies have reported the frequent misdiagnosis of this condition in its early stages. A complaint of spinal pain, particularly in younger patients, and of thoracic pain in all patients should be regarded seriously and not be attributed to minor "mechanical dysfunction". The presence of neurological symptoms may occur before neurological signs and it is at this stage that the chance of surgical cure without residual disability is highest. The patient presenting with paraplegia should be regarded as a failure of diagnosis, as symptoms are frequently present for several days before this end stage.

The most valuable investigation is high grade MRI.[44] This confirms the diagnosis of epidural abscess, indicates its upper and lower limits, demonstrates whether or not there is an associated primary osteomyelitis, and in most cases differentiates between epidural abscess and subdural abscess. Myelography with CT is the next best diagnostic investigation, although the distinction between abscess, haematoma or even in some cases metastatic tumour is not always possible.

Investigations should be carried out without delay and managed by immediate surgical decompression. As abscesses are very commonly located in the posterior extradural space, albeit extending laterally on either side, a decompressive laminectomy is the operation of choice. Attention should be paid to the upper and lower limits of the abscess, although the laminectomy may not need to be taken to these extremes should the pus be liquid. The laminectomy may need to be taken to the limits if the compressive material is semisolid, infected granulation tissue.

The poor results of surgery in severely affected or paraplegic patients underline the urgency of timely referral. The mortality rate for this condition has diminished over the years with improving diagnosis, but nevertheless remains substantial for a spinal condition and is reported at between 17% and 36%.[38,45]

Vertebral osteomyelitis is a relatively uncommon condition, but familiar to spine surgeons in the United Kingdom. The commonest organisms involved are staphylococci, streptococci, *Escherichia coli*, and occasionally an unusual organism such as *Salmonella* or *Brucella* sp. For the most part the spinal cord is not affected and the problem is one of structural integrity in

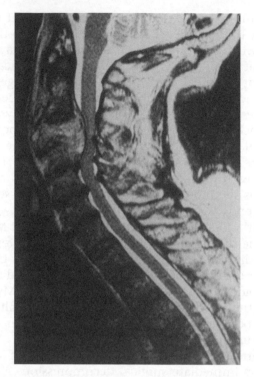

Figure 10.6 MRI (1·5T Siemens Magnetom, T2 weighted scan). Vertebral osteomyelitis secondary to tuberculosis and associated with anterior cord compression at C3 and C4

the vertebral column.[46] Both pyogenic and tuberculous osteomyelitis may lead to the formation of an extradural abscess lying anterior to the spinal cord, which may cause acute spinal cord compression in fashion not dissimilar to a "pure" epidural abscess. The gradual and progressive nature of bone infection produces a more protracted clinical history, including spinal pain, aches, malaise, discomfort, and systemic signs of infection culminating in neurological deterioration (Figure 10.6).

Plain radiographs of the spine may give the diagnosis by revealing bone erosion and loss of height in contiguous vertebrae with destruction of the intervertebral disc. The diagnosis of coexisting extradural abscess is made by MRI or by CT myelography done as a matter of some urgency. It requires only a few millilitres of localised liquefied pus in the anterior cervical spinal canal to cause tetraparesis. Recovery is entirely possible with expeditious diagnosis and decompression. Scanning also reveals the extent of vertebral and paravertebral infection and can usually distinguish infection from metastatic disease.[47]

For pyogenic osteomyelitis, which predominates in the United Kingdom, direct ventral spinal canal decompression is often required. In the cervical spine this involves an anterior cervical decompression procedure carried out through an intervertebral disc space or by a vertebrectomy. Division of the posterior longitudinal ligament usually results in the egress of a small volume of liquefied pus that is sometimes less than impressive considering the degree of paralysis that it has produced. In these acute situations the surgeon is best advised not to incorporate spinal reconstruction, but rather to return the patient to a period of external spinal stabilisation, usually by cervical traction, accompanied by appropriate intravenous antibiotic therapy. Once the infection has been treated in such a way for a period of several days, more definitive spinal stabilisation can be established. Once the pyogenic infection is under control, bone grafting almost always results in a solid fusion. In selected cases it is accepted practice to use internal metal fixation while continuing antibiotic treatment. As in osteomyelitis at any location, a prolonged course of antibiotics is required. The erythrocite sedimentation rate (ESR) and C-reactive protein (CRP) are useful parameters to follow during the course of treatment.

In the thoracic and lumbar spine surgical decompression involves more difficult access, either by costotransversectomy or posterior thoracotomy in the thoracic region or the extraperitoneal route in the lumbar region. In tuberculous osteomyelitis a limited posterolateral decompression by costotransversectomy to release indolent purulent material is a satisfactory means of decompression, with reconstruction and stabilising surgery reserved for later if necessary.[48]

Degenerative pathology

Degenerative change within the spine causes acute spinal cord compression rarely, usually having a more prolonged course of progressive neurological symptoms.[49] Protrusion of an intervertebral disc into the spinal canal, whether in the presence of existing osteophytic compression or not, can produce a rapidly developing myelopathy. Acute disc protrusions most commonly occur in the lumbar spine with 90% being located either at the L4–L5 or L5–S1 level. Central compression of the thecal sac at this level causes an acute cauda equina syndrome, which is a spinal emergency. Isolated or "pure" cervical intervertebral disc protrusion is much less common than compression due to osteophyte formation, although it is common to find a combination of both. "Pure" cervical disc prolapse can occur at any age, and in some cases a pre-existing mild myelopathy rapidly becomes much worse because of protrusion of cervical disc a few millimetres further into the spinal canal. Acute myelopathy may present in older patients who have degenerative changes superimposed on a developmentally narrow cervical spinal canal (< 10 mm anteroposterior diameter). In these patients the usual mechanism is violent extension of the neck.[50] "Pure" thoracic disc protrusion is uncommon and these patients present to neurosurgical units at a frequency of one per million population per year.[51] It is common to find that the so-called thoracic "disc" is in fact a combination of osteophyte and calcified disc material, rather than degenerate nucleus pulposus that has prolapsed into the spinal canal.

Acute disc protrusion at any level commonly presents with spinal pain, usually accompanied by nerve root pain. The level of root pain provides a good indication of which intervertebral disc is the culprit. When the disc protrudes sufficiently into the spinal canal to cause spinal (or cauda equina) compression, neurological symptoms and signs accompany the pain. The sensory level gives a good indication of the level of thoracic disc prolapse and the distribution of pain, numbness, or "dropped" reflexes in the upper limbs provides a good clinical indicator of the level of cervical disc disease. When the patient presents with loss of manual dexterity the compression is often at the level of the C3–C4 intervertebral disc. In the lumbar spine, compression of the cauda equina produces loss of sensation across the sacral dermotomes, either unilaterally or bilaterally, associated with nerve root pain in both legs and loss of bladder sensation and sphincter function. The clinical diagnosis of an acute disc

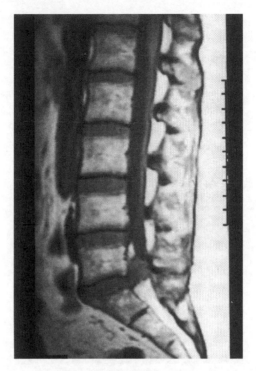

Figure 10.7 MRI (1·5T Siemens Magnetom, T1 weighted sagittal image). Acute L5–S1 disc herniation presenting as an acute cauda equina syndrome.
The image shows severe compression of the thecal sac by soft disc

prolapse in the cervical and lumbar spine is relatively straightforward, but misdiagnosis often occurs in the thoracic region. A background history of thoracic spine pain should raise suspicion, but several studies have confirmed that, probably because of the rarity of thoracic disc disease, other pathological diagnoses are often given prior consideration.

The diagnosis of disc prolapse is confirmed radiologically by MRI of the appropriate spinal region (Figures 10.7, 10.8). CT myelography may also be used though with modern CT scanners contrast is usually not required to confirm lumbar disc prolapse.[52]

Acute myelopathy or cauda equina syndrome secondary to disc prolapse requires urgent surgical decompression. In the

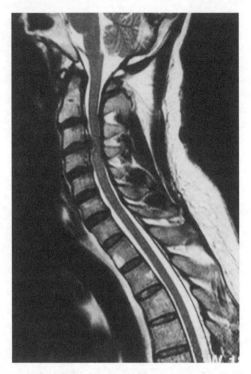

Figure 10.8 MRI (1·5T Philips T2 weighted scan). Anterior spinal cord compression by a degenerative disc at C3/4 presenting as a rapidly progressive myelopathy

lumbar spine this may be carried out through a posterior approach as for elective microdiscectomy because the thecal sac will tolerate some retraction to reach the disc space. Occasionally the access has to be increased by either a hemilaminectomy or, on rare occasions, a full laminectomy, especially in the presence of coexisting lumbar canal stenosis. The risk of a postsurgical cauda equina syndrome is about one in 500 lumbar disc operations.[53]

In the cervical spine, the disc must be approached anteriorly as the spinal cord cannot be retracted at this level. The standard approach to the anterior subaxial spine is the plane between the carotid sheath laterally and the pharynx/larynx medially. When the compression is due to disc prolapse alone, a simple disc excision may be sufficient. This is carried out using an operating microscope with excision of the disc material and the cartilaginous endplates down to the level of the posterior longitudinal ligament and laterally to the medial part of the uncovertebral joints. It is necessary to open the posterior longitudinal ligament to directly visualise and explore the extradural space for disc material that can find its way through the longitudinally orientated fibres of this ligament. Fusion may be carried out either by a variety of techniques using iliac crest graft or specially designed implants but is not always necessary. The use of a bone fusion does not confer additional neurological recovery, although it may be required (or preferred) if spinal stability is significantly degraded.

For those patients who develop an acute myelopathy due to a hyperextension injury superimposed on a narrow spinal canal, there is little, if any, convincing evidence that surgical decompression improves neurological recovery. About 60% of these patients improve neurologically in the natural course of the condition. A few patients who have a narrow cervical spinal canal develop an acute non-traumatic myelopathy. Laminectomy or multiple level anterior decompression and fusion are the surgical alternatives, although the presumed ischaemic pathogenesis does not incline to the favourable outcome associated with slowly developing spondylotic myelopathy.[49]

For a thoracic disc protrusion the surgical access must be either lateral or anterior or a combination of both. The recommended approaches to the thoracic spinal canal give access to the disc prolapse without requiring retraction of the spinal cord and allow the disc material to be removed in a direction away from the spinal dura. They are pediculectomy, costotransversectomy, or transthoracic partial vertebrectomy.[51,54,55] A laminectomy is *only* indicated for thoracic disc prolapse if the disc material is entirely free and is located lateral to the spinal cord. This does happen, but rarely. A laminectomy approach to an anteriorly placed thoracic disc prolapse invites major neurological deterioration.

For patients who present with an acute disc prolapse causing cauda equina syndrome, prognosis for recovery is primarily based on the severity of the preoperative neurological deficit rather than the duration of neurological symptoms, although it is difficult to separate these two components entirely.[56] The

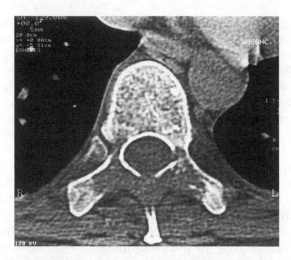

Figure 10.9 Axial CT scan. Bone windows through a metastatic breast tumour in the thoracic spine. Destruction of the posterior elements and pedicles is demonstrated

same is likely to apply to prognosis for recovery from myelopathy secondary to cervical or thoracic discs. Good recovery can only be expected for expeditiously diagnosed and optimally managed patients.

Neoplastic cord compression

By far the commonest type of neoplastic spinal cord compression is that caused by secondary tumour deposits. Up to one third of patients with malignant disease have deposits in the spine.[57,58] These are most commonly found in the vertebral body and pedicles with direct spread into the spinal canal (Figure 10.9). Metastatic tumour is confined to the spinal extradural space in only about 5% of cases.[59] The most common primary tumours are bronchus, breast, gastrointestinal tract, prostate, kidney, myeloma, and lymphoma. Most secondary deposits are found in the thoracic spine, and where there are multiple lesions they may not be contiguous. Secondary deposits are less common in the lumbar and cervical spine and they are uncommon or rare in the sacral spine. This distribution may be explained by the venous drainage of affected primary organs through the spinal extradural venous plexus and the relatively larger size of the thoracic spine.

As the tumour enlarges and encroaches on the spinal cord, the signs and symptoms of myelopathy develop progressively. This is associated with spinal pain in over 90% of patients and in retrospect these patients are often found to have complained of pain in the affected region for many weeks before the development of clinical myelopathy.[60] In most cases the myelopathy progresses gradually, usually over a period of days or weeks. As the compression increases, the ability of the spinal canal to accommodate the extra volume is exhausted and the rate of neurological deterioration increases rapidly. The typical patient has complained of thoracic spinal pain for perhaps four to six weeks with gradual development of fatigue in the lower limbs followed by decreased gait quality and finally rapid development of weakness and loss of sensation. The apparent acute presentation is therefore usually only the final stage of a more gradual process.[61] Spinal pain in a patient with a known malignancy demands investigation even in the absence of neurological symptoms and signs. Once these occur the need for imaging becomes emergent.

Acute spinal cord compression due to secondary tumour does occur when the tumour enlarges very rapidly as a result of haemorrhage or where a vertebral body suddenly collapses because of extensive neoplastic infiltration.

The clinical features of acute neoplastic cord compression are not sufficiently characteristic to permit an accurate pathological diagnosis. Other causes of acute cord compression may present in a similar clinical fashion. The diagnosis must be confirmed by appropriate spinal imaging. Initially plain radiographs of the relevant spinal region should be obtained, although the whole spine needs to be imaged as up to 17% of patients have multiple lesions.[60] The typical features of metastatic involvement include loss of vertebral height, an irregular lucent appearance within the fine architecture of the bone, preservation of the intervertebral disc space, and the possibility of multiple lesions (Figure 10.10). Spinal radiographs

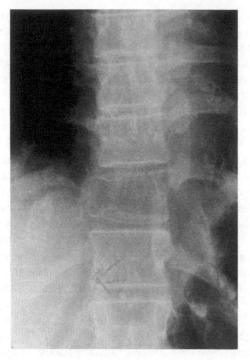

Figure 10.10 Plain AP thoracic film of the same patient shown in Figure 10.9.
Loss of vertebral height, irregular lucency within the vertebral body and right pedicle, and preservation of the adjacent disc spaces are shown

should be taken in combination with chest radiographs and a clinical examination, either or both of which may reveal evidence of a primary lesion. Definitive spinal imaging is MRI or CT myelography.[62] All the relevant information can be obtained from MRI including the number of levels affected, the extent of local extravertebral infiltration, and soft tissue involvement. CT gives a clear indication of the extent of bone involvement and makes surgical planning of the route of access and the achievable extent of excision easier.

If the primary tumour is known or can be identified, the pathological nature of the secondary tumour can be inferred. When no primary can be found a histological diagnosis is required. In the spine between about T8 and L5 this can be achieved through percutaneous vertebral body biopsy carried out under biplanar imaging intensifier control.[63] CT guided needle biopsy may be performed at almost any level, although this technique does not readily provide samples of bone tissue but rather of infiltrated soft tissue immediately adjacent to the vertebra. Either technique is safe in experienced hands and yields a high rate of positive diagnosis.

The subsequent management takes account of a number of factors.[64] The histopathology of the tumour must be considered primarily, with the overall tumour load, that is, the number of secondary deposits, and the best estimate of the patient's life expectancy. The severity of the neurological deficit has the major influence on neurological and functional recovery following decompressive surgery. The most severely affected patients and those who are paraplegic have the lowest chance of regaining the ability to walk independently. Levels of recovery which do not permit the patient either to transfer, stand, or walk are of little practical benefit, although return of sensation is of great importance to someone who is confined to a wheelchair.

The first surgical decision to be made is whether or not a surgical procedure is indicated. Surgery provides the most rapid method of cord decompression. By contrast, radiotherapy may take several days to have its optimum decompressive effect. Even patients with highly radiosensitive tumours such as myeloma or lymphoma occasionally require urgent surgery where the compression is due to a collapsed vertebra rather than to tumour tissue surrounding the spinal cord.

The route of access should then be decided and at all spinal levels the surgeon has a choice of posterior, lateral, or anterior routes. In general, where the compression and major disease lie anterior to the spinal cord this should be the preferred route to decompression. This may be transoral, transcervical, transthoracic, or retroperitoneal depending on the level of the spine affected. Lateral access can be achieved through a laminectomy extended laterally to include the pedicle and facet joint, a true costotransversectomy, or a lateral extracavity approach which is the equivalent of an extended multiple level costotransversectomy. Where the spinal cord is primarily compressed posteriorly, laminectomy still has a role to play, but studies from the late 1970s and early 1980s clearly showed how ineffective a laminectomy is in the presence of vertebral body disease. In this situation about 20% of patients are made neurologically worse and a similar number are made unstable by the posterior approach. The decompression may entail removal of a considerable amount of bone from the spine and necessitate stabilisation using internal metallic fixation, bone graft, or in some cases methyl methacrylate in combination with metal fixation.

Surgical decision making in these situations is complex. The overriding aims are to provide the most effective form of decompression of the spinal cord and to leave the patient with a pain free stable spine in order to facilitate return of spinal cord function. In some situations, such as a patient with widespread metastatic bronchogenic tumour, it is inappropriate to carry out a transthoracic spinal decompression. In a patient who has multiple non-contiguous spinal lesions, major surgery on any one of these is likely to be followed by further cord compression at a different level. In selected patients, however, even relatively major surgery, to access and decompress the spinal cord and stabilise the spine, is indicated before further treatment with radiotherapy or chemotherapy.

Haemorrhagic spinal cord compression

Extradural and subdural haematomas are common and well known conditions in cranial neurosurgery, but are uncommon in the spine.[65] Subdural haematomas in particular are rare, with few cases being reported. Epidural haematomas, although uncommon, are a recognised cause of cord compression and about a third are associated with patients receiving anticoagulant therapy. Lumbar puncture may lead to the formation of a spinal epidural haematoma, but a substantial proportion have no apparent reason although in the literature they are coincidentally associated with or even causally related to what might be described as minor trauma of everyday living.[66,67] It seems more likely that these are coincidental rather than causal factors. There is little evidence that arteriovenous abnormalities in the vertebra or other forms of angiomatous malformation are causally related to more than a very small number of spinal epidural haematomas.[68,69]

The clinical presentation of spinal haematomas is similar to several other forms of structural spinal cord compression. They produce a combination of spinal pain and root pain, followed by a progressive myelopathy, whose features will depend on the level of compression. Occasionally the process develops over several days and there are documented cases in whom the myelopathy has developed over several weeks.[70] Most present relatively rapidly, within one or two days, and the diagnosis is confirmed by MRI or CT myelography.[71] The appearances are those of an extradural compressive lesion, although with MRI it is possible to distinguish haematoma from pus or extradural tumour in some cases. Treatment is by laminectomy across the level of compression.[72]

Management of acute spinal cord compression: the role of the non-specialist

- The importance of the non-specialist in prompt recognition and specialist referral of cases of spinal cord compression has been emphasised. It is better to err on the side of "false alarm" than to make a late diagnosis and referral when function is no longer salvageable.
- The history should include the site and duration of spine and root pain, sensory or motor loss, and sphincter disturbance, any history of trauma, malignancy, or rheumatoid disease, relevant medications such as anticoagulants and coincident symptoms of systemic illness such as fever, night sweats, or weight loss. Spinal pain in patients under about 25 years of age or with a history of malignancy and thoracic or radicular pain in any patient should raise suspicion of an organic lesion and should not be attributed to non-specific or degenerative conditions. "Hysterical paralysis" is a diagnosis of exclusion and should not be made by junior staff without consultation with senior colleagues or spinal specialists.
- Examination should note whether the patient is ambulatory and whether the power in the lower limbs is MRC grade 3 or better. Motor power in the proximal arm muscles and the hands should be noted separately. The distribution of sensory loss should be recorded. The presence of a sensory level helps to target imaging studies. Careful examination may reveal that reflexes are depressed at the level of compression and exaggerated below, although this pattern may take some days to develop. A detailed

neurological examination is not necessary and can be left to the specialist unit, but early clinical information can be useful in monitoring change.

- Investigation is dependent on the urgency for transfer and the resources available to the referring clinician. Plain radiographs of the symptomatic level of the spine are invaluable in trauma, neoplastic cord compression, rheumatoid arthritis, and vertebral osteomyelitis. Cervical flexion/extension films may be appropriate but only after discussion with a specialist or senior clinician. If CT or MRI scanning facilities are available at the referring hospital, obtaining these studies prior to transfer may expedite the patient's management. Other imaging studies may include a chest radiograph, bone scan, and abdominal ultrasound to suggest an origin and define the extent of neoplastic disease. Further investigations that may aid pathological diagnosis are serum prostate specific antigen, urine Bence Jones protein, ESR, and CRP. Depending on the severity and duration of cord compression, it is not always practical to obtain all or even any of these investigations prior to transfer to the specialist unit and each case should be assessed and discussed individually.

- In preparation for transfer, an unstable spine should be immobilised using traction, a cervical collar, and/or a spinal backboard as appropriate. Trauma patients should be stabilised according to principles of trauma management: establish an airway, respiration, and haemodynamic stability, manage life threatening head and torso injuries, and reduce and splint long bone fractures. A medical escort should accompany patients who remain at risk of recurrent circulatory or respiratory instability after initial resuscitation. All radiographic studies and not just a report should accompany the patient if they have not been sent to the specialist unit prior to transfer.

- Early recognition of acute cord compression by the non-specialist along with a thorough history, physical examination, and investigations with appropriate arrangements for transfer to a specialist unit provide the patient with the greatest chance of functional recovery following spinal cord compression.

References

1   Maurice-Williams RS, Richardson PL. Spinal cord compression: delay in the diagnosis and referral of a common neurosurgical emergency. *Br J Neurosurg* 1988;2:55–60.
2   Meyers PR. Acute injury retrieval and splinting. In: Meyer PR, ed. *Surgery of spine trauma*. New York: Churchill Livingstone, 1989;1–21.
3   Vaccaro AR, An HS, Lin S *et al.* Noncontiguous injuries of the spine. *J Spinal Dis* 1992;5:320–9.

4 Schaefer DM, Flanders AE, Osterholm JL, Northrup B. Prognostic significance of magnetic resonance imaging in the acute phase of cervical spine injury. *J Neurosurg* 1992;**76**:218–23.

5 Cane RD, Shapiro BA. Pulmonary effects of acute spinal cord injury: assessment and management. In: Meyer PR, ed. *Surgery of spine trauma*. New York: Churchill Livingstone, 1989;173–83.

6 Aldrich EF, Weber PB, Crow WN. Halifax interlaminar clamp for posterior cervical fusion: a long term follow up review. *J Neurosurg* 1993;**78**: 702–8.

7 McNamara MJ, Stephens GC, Spengler DM. Transpedicular short segment fusions for treatment of lumbar burst fractures. *J Spinal Dis* 1993;**5**: 183–7.

8 Fehlings MG, Lali S, Tator CH. The role and timing of decompression in acute spinal cord injury: what do we know? What should we do? *Spine* 2001;**26**(24S):S101–10.

9 Bracken MB, Shepard MJ, Collins EF, *et al.* Methylprednisolone or naloxone treatment after acute spinal cord injury: 1 year follow up data. Results of the second national acute spinal cord injury study. *J Neurosurg* 1992;**76**:23–31.

10 Bracken MB, Shepard MJ, Holford TR, *et al.* Administration of methylprednisolone for 24 or 48 hours or tirilazad mesylate for 48 hours in the treatment of acute spinal cord injury: results of the third National Acute Spinal Injury randomized controlled trial. *JAMA* 1997;**277**:1597–604.

11 Coleman WP, Benzel E, Cahill DW, *et al.* A critical appraisal of the reporting of the National Acute Spinal Cord Injury Studies (II and III) of methylprednisolone in acute spinal cord injury. *J Spinal Dis* 2000;**13**: 185–99.

12 Hurlbert RJ. Methylprednisolone for acute spinal cord injury: an inappropriate standard of care. *J Neurosurg* 2000;**93**(1 suppl):1–7.

13 Hurlbert RJ. The role of steroids in acute spinal cord injury: an evidence-based analysis. *Spine* 2001;**26**(24S):S39–46.

14 Tator CH, Fehlings MG. Review of the secondary injury theory of acute spinal cord trauma with emphasis on vascular mechanism. *J Neurosurg* 1991;**75**:15–26.

15 Geisler FH, Coleman WP, Grieco G, *et al.* The Syngen® multicentre acute spinal cord study. *Spine* 2001;**26**:S87–98.

16 Johnston RA. Review of the spinal complication of rheumatoid disease. *Neurosurg Q* 1998;**8**:206–15.

17 Santavirta S, Kottinen YT, Laasonen E, Honkanen V, Antti-Poika l, Kauppi M. Ten year results of operation for rheumatoid cervical spine disorders. *J Bone Joint Surg* 1991;**73B**:116–20.

18 Mathews JA. Atlanto-axial subluxation in rheumatoid arthritis. *Ann Rheum Dis* 1974;**33**:526–31.

19 Pellicci PM, Ranawat CS, Tsairis P, Bryan WJ. A prospective study of the progression of rheumatoid arthritis of the cervical spine. *J Bone Surg* 1981;**63A**:342–50.

20 Santavirta S, Kankaanpaa U, Sandelin J, Laasonen E, Kottinen Y, Slatis P. Evaluation of patients with rheumatoid cervical spine. *Scand J Rheumatol* 1987;**16**:9–16.

21 Bell GR, Stearns KL. Flexion-extension MRI of the upper rheumatoid cervical spine. *Orthopaedics* 1991;**14**:969–74.

22 Krodel A, Refior HJ, Westermann S. The importance of functional magnetic resonance imaging in the planning of stabilizing operations on the cervical spine in rheumatoid patients. *Arch Orthop Trauma Surg* 1989;**109**:30–3.

23   Dvorak J, Grob D, Baumgartner H, Gschwent N, Graver W, Larsson S. Functional evaluation of the spinal cord by magnetic resonance imaging in patients with rheumatoid arthritis and instability of the upper cervical spine. *Spine* 1989;**14**:1057–64.

24   Casey ATH, Crockard HA, Bland JM, *et al*. Predictors of outcome in the quadriparetic, non ambulatory myelopathic patient with rheumatoid arthritis: a prospective study of 55 surgically treated Ranawat Class IIIb patients. *J Neurosurg* 1996;**85**:574–81.

25   Rogers MA, Crockard HA. Nystagmus and joint position sensation: their importance in posterior occipito-cervical fusion in rheumatoid arthritis. *Spine* 1994;**19**:16–20.

26   Toolaner G. Cutaneous sensory impairment in rheumatoid atlanto-axial subluxation assessed quantitatively by electrical stimulation. *Scand J Rheumatol* 1987;**16**:27–32.

27   Dickman CA, Lacantro J, Fessler RG. The influence of transoral odontoid resection on stability of the craniovertebral junction. *J Neurosurg* 1992;**77**:525–30.

28   Crockard HA, Calder I, Ransford AO. One stage transoral decompression and posterior fixation in rheumatoid atlanto-axial subluxation. *J Bone Joint Surg* 1990;**72B**:682–5.

29   Hadley MN, Spetzler RF, Sonntag VKH. The transoral approach to the superior cervical spine. *J Neurosurg* 1989;**71**:16–23.

30   Wertheim SB, Bohlman HH. Occipitocervical fusion. *J Bone Joint Surg* 1987;**69A**:833–6.

31   Ranawat CS, O'Leary P, Pellicci P, Tsairis P, Marchisollo P, Dorr L. Cervical spine fusion in rheumatoid arthritis. *J Bone Joint Surg* 1979;**61A**:1003–10.

32   Chan CP, Ngian KS, Cohen L. Posterior upper cervical fusion in rheumatoid arthritis. *Spine* 1992;**17**:268–72.

33   Ferlie DC, Clayton ML, Leidholt JD, Gamble WE. Surgical treatment of the symptomatic unstable cervical spine in rheumatoid arthritis. *J Bone Joint Surg* 1975;**57A**:349–54.

34   Brattstöm H, Granholm L. Atlanto-axial fusion in rheumatoid arthritis. *Acta Orthop Scand* 1976;**47**:619–28.

35   Grob D, Dvorak J, Gschwent N, Froehlich M. Posterior occipito-cervical fusion in rheumatoid arthritis. *Arch Orthop Trauma Surg* 1990;**110**:38–44.

36   Dutton JEM, Alexander GL. Intramedullary spinal abscess. *J Neurol Neurosurg Psychiatry* 1954;**17**:303–7.

37   Fraser RAR, Ratzan K, Wolpert SM, *et al*. Spinal subdura empyema. *Arch Neurol* 1973;**28**:235–8.

38   Johnston RA. Intraspinal infection. In: Findlay G, Owen R, eds. *Surgery of the spine*. London: Blackwell, 1992;621–8.

39   Dandy WE. Abscesses and inflammatory tumors in the spinal epidural space (so called pachymeningitis externa). *Arch Surg Chicago* 1926;**13**: 477–94.

40   Heusner AP. Non tuberculous spinal epidural infections. *N Engl J Med* 1948;**239**:845–54.

41   Statham P, Gentleman D. Importance of early diagnosis of acute spinal extradural abscess. *J R Soc Med* 1989;**82**:584–7.

42   Baker AS, Ojemann RG, Swartz MN, *et al*. Spinal epidural abscess. *N Engl J Med* 1975;**293**:463–8.

43   Hakin RN, Burt AA, Cook JB. Acute epidural abscess. *Paraplegia* 1979; **17**:330–6.

44   Ross J. Inflammatory disease. In: Modic M, Masaryk T, Ross J, eds. *Magnetic resonance imaging of the spine*. Chicago; Year Book Medical, 1989;167–82.

45 Holme A, Dott DM. Spinal epidural abscess. *Br Med J* 1954;**64**:64–8.
46 Ho EKW, Leong JCY. Spinal osteomyelitis. In: Findlay G, Owen R, eds. *Surgery of the spine*. London: Blackwell, 1992;621–8.
47 Modic MT, Feiglin DH, Piraino DW, *et al*. Vertebral osteomyelitis: assessment using MR. *Radiology* 1985;**157**:157–63.
48 Johnston RA, Hadley DM. Tuberculous infection of the thoracic spine. In: Tarlov EC, ed. *Neurosurgical treatment of disorders of the thoracic spine*. Illinois: American Association of Neurological Surgeons, 1991;95–101.
49 Ferguson RJL, Kaplan LR. Cervical spondylitic myelopathy. *Neurol Clin* 1985;**3**:373–82.
50 Epstein N, Epstein J, Benjamin V, *et al*. Traumatic myelopathy in patients with cervical spinal stenosis without fracture or dislocation. *Spine* 1980;**5**:489–96.
51 Russell T. Thoracic intervertebral disc protrusion: experience of 67 cases and review of the literature. *Br J Neurosurg* 1989;**3**:153–60.
52 Wesolowski DP, Wang AM. Radiologic evaluation. In: Rothman RH, Simeone FA, eds. *The spine*. Philadelphia: WB Saunders, 1992;570–6.
53 McLaren AC, Bailey SI. Cauda equina syndrome: a complication of lumbar discectomy. *Clin Orthop* 1986;**204**:143–9.
54 Fidler MW, Goedhart ZD. Excision of prolapse of thoracic intervertebral disc. *J Bone Joint Surg* 1984;**66B**:518–22.
55 Russell T. Thoracic intervertebral disc protrusion. In: Findlay G, Owen R, eds. *Surgery of the spine*. London: Blackwell, 1992;813–20.
56 O'Laoire SA, Crockard HA, Thomas DG. Prognosis for sphincter recovery after operation for cauda equina compression owing to lumbar disc prolapse. *Br Med J* 1981;**282**:1852–4.
57 Schabert J, Gainor B. A profile of metastatic carcinoma of the spine. *Spine* 1985;**10**:19–20.
58 Wong D, Fornaisier V, MacNab I. Spinal metastases: the obvious, the occult and the impostors. *Spine* 1990;**15**:1–4.
59 Constans J, de Divitus E, Donzelli R, *et al*. Spinal metastases with neurological manifestations: review of 600 cases. *J Neurosurg* 1983;**59**:111–18.
60 Gilbert R, Kim J, Posner J. Epidural spinal cord compression from metastatic tumor: diagnosis and treatment. *Ann Neurol* 1978;**3**:40–51.
61 Shapiro W, Posner J. Medical versus surgical treatment of metastatic spinal cord tumour. In: Thompson R, Green J, eds. *Controversies in neurology*. New York: Raven Press, 1983;57–65.
62 Godersky J, Smoker W, Knutzon R. Use of magnetic resonance imaging in the evaluation of metastatic spinal disease. *Neurosurgery* 1987;**21**:676–80.
63 Findlay G, Sandeman D, Buxton P. The role of needle biopsy in the management of malignant spinal compression. *Br J Neurosurg* 1988;**2**:479–84.
64 Findlay GFG. Metastatic spinal disease. In: Findlay G, Owen H, eds. *Surgery of the spine*. London: Blackwell, 1992;557–72.
65 Reisen TE, Goldberg E, Cranato DB, *et al*. Spinal subdural haematoma: a rare cause of recurrent postoperative radiculopathy. *J Spinal Dis* 1993;**6**:62–7.
66 Cowie RA. Acute spinal haematoma. In: Findlay G, Owen R, eds. *Surgery of the spine*. London: Blackwell, 1992;621–8.
67 Bruyn GW, Bosma NJ. Spinal extradural haematoma. In: Vilken PJ, Bruyn GW, eds. *Handbook of clinical neurology*. Amsterdam: Elsevier, 1976;1–30.
68 Harris DJ, Fornasier VL, Livingstone KE. Haemangiopericytoma of the spinal canal. Report of three cases. *J Neurosurg* 1978;**49**:914–20.

69 Stuart Lee K, McWhorter JM, Angelo IV. Spinal epidural haematoma associated with Pagets disease. *Surg Neurol* 1988;**30**:131–4.
70 Boyd HR, Pear BL. Chronic spontaneous spinal epidural haematoma: report of two cases. *J Neurosurg* 1972;**36**:239–42.
71 Larsson EM, Holtas S, Cronqvist S. Emergency magnetic resonance examination of patients with spinal cord symptoms. *Acta Radiol* 1988;**29**:69–75.
72 Johnston RA, Bailey IC. Spinal extradural haematoma: report on two cases. *Ulster Med J* 1983;**52**:157–61.

11: Acute neuromuscular respiratory paralysis

RAC HUGHES, A McLUCKIE

This chapter reviews the recognition, diagnosis, and management of respiratory failure in acute neuromuscular disease. Respiratory failure requiring artificial ventilation occurs in about 20% of patients with Guillain–Barré syndrome (GBS), a small percentage of patients with myasthenia gravis and polymyositis, and also in acute rhabdomyolysis and a wide range of other less common disorders. Neuromuscular disorders are responsible for only a tiny proportion of admissions to most intensive care units, 10 (0·4%) of 2506 consecutive admissions to our own unit in the last two years. Of those patients, 75% required mechanical ventilation and 20% died in hospital. These figures exclude those patients who were admitted to the intensive care unit because of operation or systemic disease and then developed neuromuscular disease that caused respiratory failure or delayed weaning from mechanical ventilation.

Respiratory failure in the setting of chronic progressive neuromuscular disease, such as Duchenne muscular dystrophy and motor neuron disease, presents a challenging management problem beyond the scope of this chapter.

Pathophysiology

Respiratory failure is particularly dangerous when it is caused by neuromuscular rather than lung disease because its development may be insidious and unrecognised until sudden decompensation causes life threatening hypoxia. The arterial hypoxaemia of these patients is the result of both hypoventilation and also microatelectasis arising from the retention of secretions.[1] Hypercapnia occurs only as a late feature in this form of respiratory failure, usually when respiratory muscle strength has fallen to approximately 25% of predicted, and often heralds an impending respiratory arrest. Bulbar involvement from the primary disease process may prevent clearing of secretions and cause upper airway obstruction and significant pulmonary aspiration. Infection of the lower respiratory tract may supervene at any stage and contribute to a further deterioration in pulmonary gas exchange. Underlying these changes is the profound respiratory muscle dysfunction which interferes with the usual process of spontaneous breathing.[2]

The severity of respiratory failure is related primarily to the number and nature of the muscle groups disabled by the primary disease. Weakness of the diaphragm has different effects from weakness of the intercostal and abdominal muscles. The diaphragm is inserted at an acute angle into the lower border of the ribcage, pulls the ribcage upwards, and enlarges the cross-sectional area of the thorax. At the same time the dome of the diaphragm moves caudally and elongates the thoracic cavity. As the diaphragm descends the anterior abdominal wall is forced anteriorly. Thus the action of the diaphragm is to move both the ribcage and the abdomen outwards. During quiet breathing and sleep the diaphragm performs nearly all the work of breathing.

When the diaphragm is paralysed, the accessory muscles of respiration perform expansion of the ribcage. When the ribcage expands, the fall in intrapleural pressure moves the flaccid diaphragm cephalad into the thorax, and the anterior abdominal wall, being coupled to the diaphragm movement through the abdominal contents, moves passively inwards during inspiration. This "paradoxical abdominal movement" is most marked in the supine posture as gravity assists the cephalad movement of the abdominal contents. The change in volume of the ribcage is partly absorbed by the cephalad movement of the abdominal contents and the volume of air inspired is reduced. In the upright posture gravity partially counteracts the upward movement of the abdominal contents and improves the efficiency of the accessory muscles producing inspiration. Consequently, in diaphragmatic paralysis, patients use the accessory muscles of respiration, become distressed when supine, and have smaller supine than erect vital capacities. Furthermore, the majority of neural drive to the respiratory muscles during sleep is directed to the phrenic nerves, so that patients with diaphragm paralysis are particularly prone to hypoventilation during sleep.

Patients with intact diaphragms but impaired intercostal and abdominal muscle function show paradoxical ribcage movement. As the diaphragm lowers intrapleural pressure during inspiration, the intercostal spaces and the upper ribcage move inwards because of the lack of intercostal muscle tone. In the upright posture, gravity pulls the abdominal contents caudally and the flaccid anterior abdominal wall bulges anteriorly. The diaphragm is thus flattened and shortened and is inefficient in lifting the ribcage and elongating the thorax. In this situation respiratory distress may be experienced in the upright position. The resultant poor vital capacity and inability to cough contribute to ventilatory failure.

Clinical diagnosis of neuromuscular respiratory failure

The danger of respiratory failure should be considered in every patient with progressive weakness, especially if the upper limbs and bulbar muscles are involved. The patient complains of weakness and fatigue but, unlike a patient with parenchymal lung disease or airway obstruction, does not appear wheezy or cyanosed. Instead, the patient prefers to sit or lie still in bed, becomes breathless on talking or swallowing, and uses the accessory muscles of respiration (pectoral, scalene, sternocleidomastoid, and levators of the nostrils). Diaphragm weakness may be detected by indrawing of the abdominal wall during inspiration, that is, paradoxical abdominal movement. Although the respiratory rate may be rapid and shallow, and the observation chart may show an increase in heart and respiratory rate over the previous few hours, this is not invariable and some patients present with ventilatory failure and a normal or reduced respiratory rate. All such patients should be monitored from the outset, especially during sleep, by pulse oximetry for the early detection of arterial desaturation. Clinical assessment, however, is better than blood gas analysis in assessing the need for ventilatory support. As respiratory failure worsens, the patient becomes increasingly anxious and, though exhausted, may be unable to sleep. Additional bulbar weakness or insensitivity with the attendant danger of inhalation is particularly hazardous.

Although the decision to intubate and start artificial ventilation depends primarily on the overall clinical assessment, measurement of vital capacity provides a useful quantitative assessment of respiratory muscle strength and helps to determine when intubation is necessary. In general, a steady fall in vital capacity over several consecutive hours usually predicts the need for ventilation. Impaired clearance of secretions occurs at values below 30 ml/kg and frank respiratory failure at less than 10 ml/kg. In practice, mechanical ventilation is usually instituted when vital capacity is approximately 15 ml/kg.[3] Whilst measurement of vital capacity is a useful guide to the timing of intubation in patients with GBS, it is less so in patients with myasthenia gravis, perhaps due to the fluctuating nature of this disease.[4] Respiratory rate should also be monitored closely, since the development of rapid shallow breathing indicates that the patient is likely to require intubation within the next eight hours.[3] Arterial $P\mathrm{co}_2$ measurements are not a reliable guide to the timing of intubation, and indeed bulbar function may have deteriorated to the point of frank pulmonary aspiration before any rise in $Pa\mathrm{co}_2$ is observed.

Maximal static respiratory pressures (maximum inspiratory pressure, PI_{max}, measured at residual volume; maximum expiratory pressure, PE_{max}, measured at total lung capacity) obtained while breathing against an occluded mouthpiece are said to be more sensitive indicators of respiratory muscle weakness.[5] A PE_{max} of less than 40 cmH$_2$O (adult normal = 100 cmH$_2$O) is associated with an inability to cough and clear secretions adequately, whereas a PI_{max} of less than -20 cmH$_2$0 (adult normal of more than -70 cmH$_2$O) precludes effective ventilation and maintenance of a normal arterial CO$_2$ tension. In patients who find this manoeuvre difficult to perform, measurement of sniff nasal pressure (SNIP) is an alternative. This is done by placing a tight plug, connected to a pressure transducer, into one nostril and asking the patient to inhale deeply through the unobstructed nostril.[6]

Respiratory muscle strength may also be assessed by recording transdiaphragmatic pressure during tidal breathing

> **Box 11.1 Central nervous system disorders causing respiratory failure**
>
> Sedative drugs
> Secondary effects of metabolic disorders
> Central transtentorial herniation
> Brain stem lesions
>   Infarction
>   Haemorrhage
>   Extrinsic compression
>   Intrinsic tumour
>   Encephalitis
>   Multiple sclerosis
>   Motor neuron disease
>   Central pontine myelinolysis
> Spinal cord lesions
>   Cord compression
>   Motor neuron disease
>   Intrinsic tumour
>   Multiple sclerosis
>   Transverse myelitis
>   Poliomyelitis
>   Rabies

and on maximal inspiration (± measurement of the diaphragmatic EMG). Alternatively magnetic stimulation of the phrenic nerves may be used to assess diaphragmatic contractility. However, neither of these tests is routinely performed outside research centres.

Diagnosis of the cause

Central nervous system causes

Diseases of the nervous system can cause respiratory failure by damaging the respiratory centre in the medulla or its connections with the cervical and thoracic spinal cord (Box 11.1). In practice the commonest causes are the secondary consequences of CNS depression by drugs, metabolic abnormalities, or primary cerebral or brain stem disease. These are important in differential diagnosis but this review is confined to disorders affecting the lower motor neuron, peripheral nerves, neuromuscular junction, and muscles. The localisation of the disease process to the brain stem or spinal cord does not usually present the neurologist with any difficulty because of the presence of symptoms and signs at the level of the lesion and involvement of the long tracts.

Wild type poliomyelitis remains a common problem in the Indian subcontinent and south east Asia. Rare vaccine-associated cases still occur throughout the world. Poliomyelitis should still be considered in the differential diagnosis of acute flaccid paralysis when sensory deficit is absent, the onset is asymmetrical, and the CSF shows a pleocytosis especially in recent vaccine recipients or their contacts.[7,8] Enteroviruses other than polio and flaviviruses which cause tick-borne encephalitis can also produce a poliomyelitis-like illness.[9] The diagnosis of polio may be confirmed by culturing the stool, and sometimes a throat swab or CSF, and by finding a rising titre of neutralising antibody in the serum.

Peripheral neuropathy

Peripheral neuropathy causing respiratory failure can usually be identified clinically from the gradual evolution of ascending, or sometimes descending, weakness associated with paraesthesiae, sensory deficit, and reduced or absent tendon reflexes. Difficulties in diagnosis arise in rapidly evolving pure motor neuropathies, especially in the earliest stages when the tendon reflexes may be preserved. Also paraesthesiae occur in occasional cases of toxic neuromuscular conduction block, including botulism.[10]

Guillain–Barré syndrome is so much more common than any of the other causes of neuromuscular respiratory failure that there is a danger that other causes, including other causes of neuropathy, will be overlooked. The diagnosis of GBS cannot be made by any diagnostic test but requires the exclusion of other conditions (Table 11.1). The diagnosis of GBS itself is no longer sufficient since it is now recognised to be a syndrome with several underlying pathological processes.[11] In Europe and North America over 90% of cases are due to acute inflammatory demyelinating polyradiculoneuropathy and the remainder to acute motor or motor and sensory axonal neuropathy.[12] In northern China, Japan, India, and Central America the axonal forms of the disease are more common, accounting for up to 40% of cases. The distinction during life is difficult and depends on careful neurophysiological studies. In acute inflammatory demyelinating polyradiculoneuropathy there is multifocal partial conduction block or slowing of motor nerve conduction. In the axonal forms there is a reduction of compound muscle action potential amplitude with relative preservation of motor nerve conduction velocity.[11-13] In very severe cases the action potentials may be unrecordable in which case the diagnosis can only be made by biopsy of an affected nerve. This is not worth performing except in a specialist centre.

The other causes of neuropathy (Table 11.1) can be ruled out by a careful history. Critical illness polyneuropathy occurs in the setting of an extremely ill patient who is being ventilated, has had sepsis and multiorgan failure, and cannot be weaned from the ventilator. It is due to an axonal neuropathy. The aetiology of critical illness polyneuropathy is not known but probably multifactorial.[14] Careful enquiry about possible toxin exposure as a cause of polyneuropathy is always necessary. Acute ingestion of organophosphorus compounds is often due to attempted suicide and usually causes vomiting. After one to five days, as survivors emerge from coma, some develop acute paralysis with respiratory failure. This is called the "intermediate syndrome" to distinguish it from the later organophosphate induced delayed sensory and motor polyneuropathy which organophosphates may also cause. Electromyography shows pre- and postsynaptic impairment and the intermediate syndrome is probably due to necrosis of the neuromuscular junctions.[15] The majority of patients with the intermediate syndrome recover spontaneously provided they do not suffer hypoxic brain injury. Inadequate pralidoxime therapy is proposed but not established as contributory. Poisoning with heavy metals severe enough to cause a neuropathy with respiratory failure has usually been preceded by an acute illness with vomiting and an altered level of consciousness often misdiagnosed as viral illness. Prominent cutaneous and muscular pain, especially in the soles of the feet, and preservation of the reflexes in the early stages should raise the suspicion of thallium poisoning.[16] Painful tingling and weakness begin within one to five days from ingestion of thallium, before the characteristic hairfall. In arsenic poisoning, sensory symptoms such as pins and needles predominate early, and weakness may then develop.

Table 11.1 Peripheral neuropathies that cause respiratory failure

Condition	Specific test	Specific treatment
GBS (demyelinating from)	Nerve conduction block	IVIg PE
GBS (axonal form)	Small CMAPs	IVIg PE
	Relatively normal MCV	
CIDP	Nerve conduction block	IVIg PE S
	Nerve biopsy	
Critical illness polyneuropathy[14]		
Toxins		
Organophosphorus compounds[94]	Red cell cholinesterase*	Atropine
	Blood OP	Pralidoxime
	Urine OP	
Thallium[95]	Dystrophic anagen hairs with dark bands	
	95% sensitive and specific for thallium poisoning	
	Whole blood thallium	Prussian blue
	24 hour urine thallium	
Arsenic[17,96–98]	24 hour urine arsenic	Dimercaprol
	Whole blood arsenic†	DMSA
Lead	Whole blood lead	Sodium calcium edetate DMSA
Gold[99]		Dimercaprol
Lithium[100,101]	Plasma lithium	Haemodialysis
Drugs:		
Vincristine[21,102]		Withdrawal
Lymphoma[103]	Nerve biopsy	Cytotoxics
Vasculitis: systemic lupus erythematosus[104]	Nerve biopsy	S cyclophosphamide IVIg?
Metabolic: acute intermittent porphyria[23]	Urine porphobilinogen Urine d-ALA	Avoidance of precipitants Intravenous haematin
Hereditary tyrosinaemia[25]		High calorie intake Liver transplant
Diphtheria[105]	Throat swab culture	Antitoxin
Buckthorn neuropathy (central America)[20,106]		

GBS = Guillain–Barré syndrome; PE = plasma exchange; IVIg = intravenous immunoglobulin; CIDP = chronic idiopathic demyelinating polyradiculoneuropathy; S = steroids; CMAPs = compound muscle action potentials; MCV = maximum conduction velocity; OP = organophosphorus d-ALA = d-aminolaevulinic acid; Prussian blue = potassium ferric hexacyanoferrate; DMSA = 2,3-dimercaptosuccinic acid.

*An isolated cholinesterase level may neither confirm nor exclude exposure because a normal cholinesterase level is based on population estimates. Ideally the diagnosis is based on a drop of 50% from baseline cholinesterase determinations. Animal studies have suggested in intermediate syndrome that AchE must be 20% or lower before muscle activity is affected.
† An elevated arsenic level verifies the diagnosis whereas a low level does not exclude arsenic toxicity. Seafood ingestion may transiently increase arsenic levels too.

The early clinical picture sometimes closely resembles GBS and neurophysiological changes may initially show partial conduction block and slowing of conduction before giving way to changes suggestive of axonal degeneration.[17]

Diphtheria is now extremely rare in Europe and North America but cases were recently reported from Estonia[18] and the diagnosis should be considered in patients with a recent upper respiratory infection, especially if there is prominent palatal involvement.[19] Buckthorn neuropathy need only be suspected in those who have consumed berries from this bush in Mexico.[20] Drugs usually cause an insidiously progressive distal axonopathy without respiratory involvement, but acute paralysis with respiratory failure occurred in a patient being treated with vincristine, possibly due to coincidental GBS.[21] Both T and B cell lymphomas may cause acute neoplastic infiltration of the peripheral nervous system which can resemble GBS.[22] Sometimes acute neuropathy is the presenting feature of the lymphoma. Vasculitic neuropathy rarely causes respiratory failure and usually only does so in the setting of a systemic illness with cutaneous, renal, and lung involvement. Acute neuropathy occurs in acute intermittent porphyria, usually after abdominal pain and vomiting, but sometimes as the presenting feature.[23] It may be diagnosed during attacks by detecting increased urine porphobilinogen excretion, a test which should be considered in every case of undiagnosed acute neuromuscular paralysis.[24] Recurrent neuropathy in infants is a feature of hereditary tyrosinaemia.[25]

Neuromuscular junction disorders

Respiratory failure can herald disorders of the neuromuscular junction (Table 11.2), which can be distinguished from neuropathic causes by the absence of sensory deficit and preservation of tendon reflexes. In myasthenia gravis respiratory failure usually occurs in the setting of established disease that has failed to respond to conventional treatment. Even in an acute case the diagnosis is usually evident because of ptosis, facial weakness, and bulbar palsy with muscle fatigue. The diagnosis can be confirmed by showing a decrement in the compound muscle action potentials elicited by a train of stimuli, neurophysiological tests, or detecting variable conduction block (jitter) in terminal motor nerve fibres in

Table 11.2   Disorders of neuromuscular transmission that cause respiratory failure

Condition	Specific test	Specific treatment
Myasthenia gravis	Single fibre EMG for jitter Anti AChR antibody Edrophonium test[*]	IVIg, PE, S
Anticholinesterase overdose	Negative edrophonium test	Drug withdrawal
Antibiotic induced paralysis[107]		Drug withdrawal
Hypermagnesaemia[28]	Plasma magnesium EMG increment on 50 Hz stimulation	Intravenous calcium
Botulism[27]	Injection of serum into mice	Antitoxin
Snake, scorpions, and spider bite[108]	Identifying the snake or its venom[†]	Antivenin
Fish, shellfish, crab poisoning[31,32,108]	Identifying the fish	Varies
Tick paralysis[33]	Finding the tick	Removal/antitoxin depending on tick species
Eaton–Lambert syndrome[34]	EMG increment on repetitive stimulation	PE, S Anti VGCC antibody

PE = plasma exchange; S = steroids; AChR = acetylcholine esterase receptor; VGCC = voltage gated calcium channel.
[*]This runs the risk of fatal bradycardia and should only be performed by an experienced clinician after giving atropine and in an intensive care setting.
[†]Kits are now available to detect some snake venoms (especially in Australia) and allow the most appropriate antivenin to be chosen.

almost all cases. Acetylcholine receptor antibodies are present in 90% of patients and in about half of the remainder there are antibodies to the muscle specific kinase, which is closely apposed to the acetylcholine receptor.[26] The rare occurrence of asystole following intravenous edrophonium has led some experts to stop using it. If it is used, atropine should be given first and resuscitation facilities should be available. In treated myasthenia, weakness can be caused by overdose of anticholinesterase drugs causing depolarisation of motor nerve terminal in a cholinergic crisis. This will be accompanied by diarrhoea, colic, excessive salivation, and small pupils, and will be worsened rather than improved by intravenous edrophonium.

Other causes of neuromuscular junction blockade are rare and the diagnosis is usually obvious from the clinical setting. Suspect botulism when autonomic features, dry mouth, constipation, poorly reactive pupils, ptosis, and bulbar palsy have heralded acute descending paralysis. In the early stages the symptoms and signs are entirely anticholinergic and the reflexes are normal. These symptoms have usually been immediately preceded by nausea, vomiting, abdominal pain, and diarrhoea from eating foul smelling food contaminated by *Clostridium botulinum*.[27] Magnesium-containing antacids and aperients in patients with impaired renal function can produce severe hypermagnesaemia. The increased magnesium interferes with the release of acetylcholine so as to cause weakness, which may develop into respiratory failure.[28] The aminoglycoside and polymyxin antibiotics and some other drugs also cause neuromuscular blockade by interfering with the release of acetylcholine.[29] This is usually only significant when weaning infected patients off ventilation.[30] Physicians practising in the tropics have to cope with a much wider range of toxic causes of neuromuscular conduction blockade whose diagnosis will be obvious from the history (Table 11.2).[31] Fish or shellfish toxin poisoning (usually Caribbean or Pacific fish) causes a gastrointestinal upset before the development of weakness.[32] In North America paralysis is sometimes caused by the bite of a female tick, *Dermacentor* spp., whose saliva contains an unidentified toxin which interferes with terminal motor nerve conduction perhaps by inhibiting sodium flux across the axolemma. The tick may be difficult to find but its removal is curative.[33] In Australia tick paralysis caused by *Ixodes holocyclus* is due to a toxin which inhibits acetylcholine release and causes neuromuscular conduction block. Respiratory failure occurs in the Lambert–Eaton myasthenic syndrome, but only rarely and then usually in the setting of gradually progressive weakness.[34] The diagnosis may be suggested clinically by autonomic symptoms, including a dry mouth, the finding of depressed reflexes that are enhanced after exercise, and confirmed by electrophysiological tests showing an increment in muscle action potential amplitude following repetitive nerve stimulation. It may be associated with a small cell lung carcinoma or autoimmune disease.

Myopathy

Respiratory failure in muscle disease usually occurs insidiously following progressive proximal weakness, which has evolved over months or years, and presents with nocturnal hypoventilation causing morning headache and daytime sleepiness. This form of respiratory failure may develop in the advanced stages of severe muscular dystrophy and also in polymyositis. Sometimes, especially in myotonic dystrophy, the respiratory failure is worsened by depression of central respiratory drive. When the ventilatory reserve has fallen so far that the vital capacity is less than 55% of its predicted normal, there is a grave danger that an intercurrent lung infection will precipitate respiratory failure.[35] In acid maltase deficiency the diaphragm is particularly severely affected and the patient may present with respiratory failure before consulting a neurologist about weakness.[36] Acid maltase deficiency should be suspected if there is proximal upper limb weakness and marked wasting of the paraspinal muscles, and confirmed by seeking glycogen containing granules in the lymphocytes which stain red with periodic anti-Schiff reagent applied to a blood film.[37]

Although rare, some muscle diseases may present with acute respiratory failure (Table 11.3). When a patient presents with flaccid paralysis and respiratory failure over a few hours or days, a correctable electrolyte disturbance should be sought immediately. The feature that distinguishes muscle disease from neuropathy is the preservation of the reflexes and the absence of sensory symptoms or signs. Hypokalaemia induced by potassium loss from the gut or kidneys is the commonest cause and is probably responsible for the muscle fibre necrosis in acute rhabdomyolysis, which occurs following some drugs, such as carbenoxolone.[38] Severe hypophosphataemia can also cause paralysis requiring respiratory failure. It is often precipitated by parenteral glucose infusions in alcoholic patients.[39]

Acute rhabdomyolysis is a rare condition in which acute muscle necrosis causes the very rapid onset of muscle pain, tenderness, swelling, and weakness, sometimes severe enough

Table 11.3   Disorders of muscle that cause acute respiratory failure

Condition	Specific test	Specific treatment
Hypokalaemia[38,109]	Plasma K[+]	K[+]
Polymyositis[110]	Plasma CK EMG Muscle biopsy	S, IVIg
Acute rhabdomyolysis[87]	EMG Muscle biopsy	Urine alkalinisation
Hypophosphataemia[39]	Plasma phosphate	Phosphate
Acid maltase deficiency[36,37]	PAS stain of blood film	
Combined neuromuscular blockade and steroids[111]	Muscle biopsy	Withdrawal
Barium intoxication[112]	Plasma K[+]	Intravenous K[+] Oral magnesium sulphate haemodialysis
Critical illness thick filament myopathy	Muscle electron microscopy	

CK = creatine kinase; PAS = periodic acid-Schiff reagent.

to cause respiratory failure. The muscle enzyme concentrations, including creatine kinase, are markedly increased in the plasma, and the electromyogram (EMG) shows myopathic changes and spontaneous fibrillation. A muscle biopsy is necessary to confirm the diagnosis and will show massive muscle fibre necrosis and often numerous regenerating fibres but relatively little inflammation. The neurological picture is overshadowed by the development of myoglobinuria and acute renal failure. Causes of acute rhabdomyolysis are alcohol abuse, viruses (influenza, Coxsackie B5, echo 9, adenovirus 21, Epstein–Barr), *Mycoplasma*,[40] and a wide variety of drugs, especially potassium-lowering drugs, amphetamine-like agents including Ecstasy (MDMA) and Speed (amphetamine sulphate), barbiturates, and the combination of the muscle relaxant pancuronium and corticosteroids.[41] If the causative agent is withdrawn and the patient can be nursed through the period of respiratory and renal failure, regeneration of the necrotic muscle and full recovery are usual.

In critically ill patients weakness and failure to wean from the ventilator may be due to either acute neuropathy (see above) or acute myopathy due to dissolution of the thick filaments that are composed of myosin.[42] A favoured hypothesis is that steroids given to patients with paralysed muscles cause loss of the thick filaments.

Respiratory muscle involvement was a presenting feature in 4% of 118 patients with polymyositis. More commonly it developed later, contributing to death in 14%.[43] Neuromuscular respiratory failure may be worsened by simultaneous interstitial infiltration and fibrosis of the lungs.[43] Inflammatory changes in muscle are usually so extensive that the diagnosis can be readily confirmed by the increased plasma creatine kinase concentration, myopathic EMG with additional spontaneous discharges, and inflammatory changes in a muscle biopsy. Antibodies to nuclear and cytoplasmic antigens, especially cytoplasmic ribonucleoproteins, are present in up to 20% of patients with different forms of myositis. The commonest antibody, anti-Jo1, is associated with interstitial lung disease and also occurs with interstitial lung disease in the absence of myositis.[44]

Institution of mechanical ventilation

The decision to institute respiratory support depends much more on the clinical state of the patient than on any physiological measurement. Arterial blood gas analysis is not particularly helpful. Intervention is required to prevent the development of arterial hypoxaemia and carbon dioxide retention before they become life threatening. As a rule of thumb, mechanical ventilation should be instituted once the vital capacity has fallen to 15 ml/kg, or sooner if there is evidence of bulbar dysfunction and pulmonary aspiration. Continuous positive airway pressure (CPAP) or non-invasive positive pressure ventilation via a facemask (NPPV) may temporarily improve hypoxaemia and hypercarbia. However, these techniques should be used with caution since they confer no protection against pulmonary aspiration, and usually only delay rather than avoid the need for intubation. On the whole, it is safer to proceed rapidly to tracheal intubation to ensure control of the airway, adequate oxygenation, ventilation and tracheal toilet (especially in patients with an inadequate cough reflex), and the prevention of pulmonary aspiration.

Intubation should be performed by a skilled operator in the setting of an intensive care unit. This requires referral and involvement of the intensive care medical staff at an early stage to avoid the need for emergency intervention on a general medical ward. Intubation is best achieved via the oral route following adequate intravenous sedation in combination with muscle relaxation. Although it is often said that nasotracheal tubes are a well tolerated alternative, we have found them to be unsuitable because they carry a high risk of sinusitis,[45] and their extra length with the narrow internal diameter makes them more difficult to aspirate adequately and increases the resistance of the ventilatory circuit. Any increase in work of breathing associated with nasotracheal intubation is especially harmful during the weaning period when a weak patient is asked to make some effort while receiving graded reductions in ventilatory support. Following pre-oxygenation, etomidate, propofol, or a benzodiazepine (midazolam) may be used to render the patient unconscious and this on its own – in the presence of cricoid pressure – may be sufficient for the experienced operator to perform the necessary laryngoscopy and intubation. A non-depolarising muscle relaxant, such as rocuronium, in adequate doses will abolish all remaining muscular tone and can improve the inexperienced operator's ability to visualise the larynx. Suxamethonium should never be used in this setting because of reports of ventricular tachycardia and asystole caused by a sudden rise in serum potassium in patients with denervated muscles.[46] Cricoid pressure should always be used because, although patients may not have eaten for some time before the induction of anaesthesia, gastric stasis and ileus are common particularly in the early stages of GBS. Following successful tracheal intubation, a nasogastric tube should be placed to facilitate the initiation of enteral nutrition. When etomidate is used to induce anaesthesia, it is our practice to administer hydrocortisone 100 mg eight hourly for 24 hours, to compensate for the effect of etomidate on steroid synthesis.[47]

Management during mechanical ventilation

General principles

The principles that govern management during mechanical ventilation centre upon three primary concerns – access to the airway with the provision of adequate pulmonary gas exchange, the maintenance of nutrition, and the prevention of nosocomial infection. Other issues, very often taken for granted but which require special attention, include: the need for scrupulous nursing care to avoid nerve compression syndromes and bed sores; physiotherapy with the provision of adequate analgesia and splints, to prevent irreversible contractures and joint immobilisation; subcutaneous heparin for the prophylaxis of deep venous thrombosis; and finally extensive psychological support during the period when patients are entirely dependent upon their attendants and the mechanical ventilator. Keeping a paralysed but conscious patient comfortable requires careful positioning and frequent gentle repositioning: sitting up, especially out of bed, may help and is good for morale. A particular problem in patients with GBS is the management of autonomic dysfunction, which can result in wide fluctuations in pulse and blood pressure as well as a wide variety of atrial and ventricular arrhythmias.[48-50]

Airway access and mechanical ventilation

Most patients who develop respiratory failure as a consequence of neuromuscular dysfunction will require a tracheostomy. This is usually performed at a relatively early stage, in our unit five to seven days after the institution of mechanical ventilation. It simplifies the management of the patient considerably and allows the withdrawal of all sedation. The tracheostomy tube is well tolerated, gives excellent access for tracheal toilet and chest physiotherapy, and facilitates weaning by virtue of allowing the patient to be placed on and off different modes of respiratory support at will. Percutaneous dilatational tracheostomy is now the technique of choice for the majority of intensive care patients. It can be performed at the bedside, takes less time than a surgical tracheostomy, and is associated with a lower incidence of the most important complications, which are bleeding and infection.[51,52] Long term follow up of patients undergoing this procedure has also identified a rate of subglottic stenosis which compares favourably with that of the surgical technique.[51,53] It is our impression that the long term cosmetic result is also superior.

In the absence of severe pulmonary aspiration or infection, it is not difficult to achieve adequate pulmonary gas exchange in these patients. Initially, most patients are too weak to generate an adequate negative pressure to "trigger" the ventilator and so require "controlled ventilation". During this phase, tidal volume should be limited to 6–8 ml/kg, plateau pressure to less than 30 cmH$_2$O, and the level of positive end expiratory pressure (PEEP) titrated according to the inspired oxygen concentration (Fio$_2$) in order to prevent ventilator induced lung injury.[54] Many modern ventilators, for example the Siemens Servo 300, have a triggering mechanism that requires the patient to change a baseline flow within the machine rather than to reduce a pressure. These machines are much more sensitive to the respiratory efforts of a patient and should theoretically be beneficial in management. In fact, no particular kind of ventilation or ventilator has been shown to be superior in supporting these patients. Most intensivists rely on pressure support or some combination of intermittent mandatory ventilation with pressure support to provide an adequate tidal volume and minute ventilation. Humidification of the inspired gases is essential to avoid the development of mucus plugs. The application of positive end expiratory pressure (with a pressure of 5–15 cmH$_2$O), together with physiotherapy, is used in the often vain attempt to prevent atelectasis.

Provision of nutrition

Every effort should be made to feed these patients early via the enteral route.[55] Although it is impossible to prevent muscle wasting related to denervation, loss of muscle bulk will only be more exaggerated if an external source of calories and nitrogen is not forthcoming.[56] Muscle wasting is particularly marked in those cases who develop nosocomial sepsis and may contribute to a prolongation of the period of dependence on mechanical ventilation.[57] Use of the enteral route ensures that the gastrointestinal mucosa does not atrophy and the integrity of the gut barrier is maintained. Theoretically this should contribute to the prevention of nosocomial infection by reducing the likelihood of translocation of bacteria and endotoxin from the lumen of the gut into the portal venous circulation and lymphatic system.[58] Parenteral nutrition on the other hand, especially that containing large amounts of intravenous fat, may contribute to an increased risk of sepsis and is best avoided.[59,60]

During the first few days, enteral feed is usually delivered via a standard gauge nasogastric tube. Once the target rate of feeding (25 non-protein calories/kg/day) has been reached and is tolerated, this tube may be replaced with a fine bore one. In cases where tube feeding is likely to be required for longer than two to three weeks, it is our practice to perform a percutaneous gastrostomy, which is more comfortable for the patient and avoids the risk of sinusitis associated with a nasogastric tube.[61] In some patients, the presence of an ileus makes the establishment of enteral nutrition difficult, and in our experience this is often related to the excessive use of opiates. Early tracheostomy and the subsequent withdrawal of all sedation (other than simple night sedation to ensure an appropriate sleep pattern) will often resolve the problem. A prokinetic agent, such as erythromycin,[62] or insertion of a nasojejunal tube may be required in more difficult cases.[63] Diarrhoea usually reflects the administration of broad spectrum antibiotics, or the development of *Clostridium difficile* colitis secondary to antibiotic administration, rather than any effect of the feed itself. The stool should be examined for *Cl. difficile* toxin. If toxin is present the patient should be treated with a course of enteral metronidazole or vancomycin. Symptomatic treatment is usually all that is required in cases of non-infective diarrhoea, with every effort being made to withdraw the offending antibiotics.

The specific composition of the enteral feed preparation deserves consideration, with the incidence of nosocomial infection, duration of ventilation and hospital stay all being reduced in patients who receive a feed whose composition has been modified to enhance immune function by adding arginine, yeast RNA, and ω-3 polyunsaturated fatty acids.[64] Tight control of blood sugar levels (target range 4·5–6 mmol/L) has also been shown to play an important part in reducing morbidity, including nosocomial infection rates, and mortality in critically ill patients. An intravenous infusion of insulin is usually required to maintain blood sugar at the desired level.[65]

Patients being ventilated for acute illness are at increased risk of peptic ulceration. This has led to the use of prophylactic H_2-receptor antagonists to increase gastric pH. Unfortunately this increases bacterial colonisation and risks causing nosocomial infection. A randomised trial was undertaken in 1200 ventilated patients to compare ranitidine with sucralfate, a cytoprotective agent which does not alter gastric pH. Only 1·7% of the ranitidine compared with 3·8% of the sucralfate recipients had clinically important gastrointestinal bleeding (relative risk 0·44, 95% CI 0·21–0·92).[66] A trend towards increased risk of ventilator associated pneumonia with ranitidine was present but not significant. Consequently many authorities recommend the use of stress ulcer prophylaxis in ventilated patients.[67]

Prevention of nosocomial infection

The prevention of hospital acquired infection is at the heart of good intensive care practice. It is especially important in patients who are intubated and ventilated, since this is the most important risk factor for the development of nosocomial pneumonia. The actuarial risk of developing pneumonia increases by 12% with each day of ventilation, reaching 28% by day 30,[68] whilst the cumulative incidence rises from 8·5% during the first three days of ventilation to 45% in those ventilated for more than 14 days.[69] Every unit should have a written infection control policy developed in conjunction with local microbiological experts. Central issues are local practices of hand washing, nursing numbers, strict intravenous line/urinary catheter and antimicrobial policies, and an infection surveillance programme.

Autonomic dysfunction

In respiratory paralysis due to acute neuropathy and especially in GBS, autonomic dysfunction is common.[48–50,70] Tachycardia and loss of sinus arrhythmia are usual. Rapid fluctuations of pulse and blood pressure and sweating may occur and are sometimes the harbingers of asystole, especially during tracheal toilet. This can usually be prevented by hyperoxygenation before tracheal suction, but if it persists it may be necessary to use atropine and even an endocardial pacemaker. Serious arrhythmias usually only occur in patients who need ventilation, but we have had a patient with early GBS who developed asystole before needing ventilation. We monitor the ECG from the time of admission in all patients with GBS who have any sign of respiratory or bulbar involvement and continue until improvement has begun and the endotracheal tube has been removed. Although the bladder is spared in the early stages of GBS, it may be affected in severe cases and bladder catheterisation is often needed as part of the intensive care of the ventilated patient. Postural hypotension is common when the patient is being mobilised so that the blood pressure should be monitored. This is best done with the aid of a tilt table.

Pain control

Achieving good pain control presents a considerable challenge in caring for patients with GBS. Musculoskeletal pain often responds well to a combination of non-steroidal anti-inflammatory drugs, such as diclofenac, and opiates. Neuropathic pain related to injury or dysfunction of the nerves is more difficult to manage, and tricyclic antidepressants or antiepileptic drugs are usually more efficacious.[71,72] If the side effects of carbamazepine (liver dysfunction, hyponatraemia, and blood dyscrasias) are problematical, gabapentin and ketamine are useful second-line agents.

Specific interventions

Guillain–Barré syndrome

Plasma exchange (PE) was the first treatment to be shown to be effective in GBS.[73] Subsequent trials confirmed its efficacy so that it became accepted as the gold standard[74] before being superseded by intravenous immunoglobulin (IVIg). A Dutch trial showed that the rate of recovery was similar or possibly slightly faster in patients treated with IVIg 0·4 g/kg daily for five days compared with those treated with PE.[75] A large international trial compared PE alone with IVIg alone and PE followed by IVIg.[76] A Cochrane review including these and other smaller trials concluded that there is no significant difference in outcome between the treatments.[77] Although IVIg is expensive, it is not much more expensive than PE and it is more widely available and simpler to give. Although there was a trend towards more rapid recovery in the patients who received combined treatment with PE followed by IVIg, this was not significant, and not sufficient to justify the extra inconvenience, risk, and cost.[76] The usual regimen is 0·4 g/kg of intravenous immunoglobulin by intravenous infusion daily for five consecutive days. There is a small risk of anaphylaxis which is greatest during the first 20 minutes of each infusion. There is also a concern about exacerbating pre-existing renal failure. Side effects include headache, myalgia, flushing, hypotensive reactions, and skin rashes including eczema on the hands.

Although steroids might have been expected to be beneficial in GBS, neither a small trial of oral prednisolone nor a large double-blind trial of intravenous methylprednisolone 500 mg daily for five days demonstrated any benefit. A Cochrane systematic review concluded that corticosteroids should not be used in GBS.[78] This conclusion may need to be revised when the results of another large trial comparing combined IVIg and intravenous methylprednisolone 500 mg daily for five days with IVIg and placebo is published. The abstract reports slightly faster recovery with the combined treatment but no difference in the long term outcome.[79] It is unlikely that the meta-analysis of all the high quality evidence will show benefit from steroids. Physicians will have to decide whether to draw conclusions from the overall analysis or only from the most recent trial, which might be considered more relevant since the patients all received IVIg which is now almost universally used as the first-line treatment.

Myasthenia gravis

After establishing that a patient has respiratory failure due to myasthenia gravis the dose of anticholinesterase drugs should be optimised. The vital capacity should be monitored before and after small (2 mg) doses of intravenous edrophonium. Swallowing is usually impaired and a nasogastric tube is often needed. Pyridostigmine should be given orally or via the nasogastric tube. Doses more than 90 mg three hourly are rarely necessary. When enteral fluids cannot be absorbed, neostigmine should be given intramuscularly, substituting each 60 mg of oral pyridostigmine with 1 mg of parenteral neostigmine.

Patients with myasthenia gravis respond so dramatically in the short term to PE that a controlled trial has never been undertaken. We used to use 50 ml/kg exchanges on alternate days until an adequate response has been achieved, in most cases after two to five exchanges. Improvement was usually noticeable after the second exchange and lasts for about four to six weeks. However similar clinical benefit and fall in anti-acetylcholine receptor antibody titre have been reported followed IVIg, and we now use IVIg as our treatment of choice for myasthenic crises. This practice has now been endorsed by a randomised trial which showed similar benefit from PE and IVIg.[80,81] Cosi et al.[82] reported clinical improvement 12 days after a standard course of 0·4 g/kg in 70% of 37 patients treated and the improvement lasted for 60 days in 57%. Arsura et al.[83] reported improvement in 11 of 12 patients commencing 3·6 days after IVIg treatment began, reaching a maximum after 8·6 days, and lasting an average of 52 days. Sustained improvement has been maintained with repeated courses in a small number of cases.[84]

As IVIg or PE provide only temporary relief, immunosuppressive treatment should be started, or increased, at the same time. We use oral prednisolone 1·5 mg/kg on alternate days initially, bring the disease under control, and then taper the dose. In patients with early respiratory failure steroids should be introduced slowly and cautiously because of the danger of a transient worsening during the first week or two of the course. In patients with established respiratory failure on artificial ventilation, this cautious approach is superfluous and a full dose of steroids can be started immediately. Very large doses of steroids, including boluses of intravenous methylprednisolone, should be avoided because of the danger of inducing acute myopathy.[42,85] For patients who are inadequately controlled with steroids we add azathioprine. The addition of azathioprine to steroids has been shown to achieve better control of chronic myasthenia.[86] If azathioprine is not tolerated, other immunosuppressive agents, such as cyclophosphamide or methotrexate, can be tried. When the respiratory failure due to a myasthenic crisis has been controlled, younger patients and those with thymoma should be assessed for thymectomy.

Polymyositis

Treatment of polymyositis with large doses of steroids is universally recommended and so clearly helpful, at least in the short term, that a controlled trial has never been considered necessary. A typical regimen[87] is prednisolone 1 mg/kg daily for four to six weeks followed by gradual withdrawal at the rate of 5 mg of the daily dose per week. After the dose has reached 25–35 mg daily further reductions should be made more slowly, perhaps at 5 mg every two weeks. A wide range of doses are used and we prefer an alternate day dose, but others feel that this is not so effective.[87] It is important to bring the disease under control before beginning the reduction and then to monitor the course of the disease closely with serial measurements of muscle strength and plasma creatine kinase concentrations. Although PE combined with cyclophosphamide has been reported to be beneficial in polymyositis,[88,89] the usefulness of PE alone was not confirmed in a controlled trial in which three groups of 13 patients were treated with leucopheresis, PE, or sham PE.[90] The authors of that trial claim an 80% power of detecting a minimal improvement in functional capacity. The trial did not answer the question whether PE followed by immunosuppression would provide a more rapid response than immunosuppression alone. Further exploration of this possibility would be worthwhile, as the PE group had a highly significant fall in plasma creatine kinase concentration compared with the sham PE group. Intravenous immunoglobulin was dramatically effective in two cases resistant to steroids and immunosuppressive drugs.[91] Its use has been endorsed in dermatomyositis by the demonstration of benefit in a randomised trial.[92] Immunosuppressive treatment with azathioprine, cyclophosphamide, or methotrexate has often been tried when steroids have failed. However standard oral immunosuppression does not have the rapid effect necessary to prevent or reverse the acute onset of respiratory failure. In desperation, total body low dose irradiation has sometimes been used and remissions have occurred in those cases that have been published.[87]

Withdrawal of mechanical ventilation

The course of respiratory failure related to neuromuscular disease is extremely variable. Numerous factors such as the primary diagnosis, chronic health status, treatment, and the presence or absence of supervening complications dictate the rate of recovery. Attempts to wean the patient from mechanical ventilation are unlikely to be successful until the vital capacity is greater than 7 ml/kg, and should only proceed if the patient is stable in other respects. The most commonly used weaning techniques are to place the patient on slowly decreasing levels of pressure support, or to allow them to breathe through a T-piece for increasing periods of time, returning them to the pressure support mode in between the periods. Irrespective of the strategy chosen, a low level of pressure support (10 cmH$_2$O) is maintained overnight to allow the patient to rest and avoid nocturnal hypoxaemia. Synchronised intermittent mandatory ventilation (SIMV) should not be used once the patient is able to trigger the ventilator, as it prolongs the duration of mechanical ventilation.[93]

Many patients find that this period of ventilator withdrawal provokes extreme anxiety because of psychological dependence on the presence and the sound of the ventilator. Careful assessment of respiratory function and extensive psychological support are required to meet the physical and emotional needs of the patient at this stage.

Aftermath

Prevention of death from respiratory failure is merely the first stage in treatment of an illness such as GBS. Maintenance of morale and recognition and treatment of depression are important and difficult tasks that call on all the resources of the intensive care team. For some conditions, patient support groups exist which offer counselling services (for example,

Guillain–Barré Syndrome Support Group International, PO Box 262, Wynnewood, PA 19096, United States, www.guillain-barre.com; Guillain–Barré Syndrome Support Group, Foxley, Holdingham, Sleaford, Lincs NG34 8NR, United Kingdom, www.gbs.org.uk). There are no easy guidelines. The patient and the family need clear information about what is happening and what may be expected. Overoptimistic prognoses may be greeted eagerly at first but reap a grim harvest of dashed hopes later. Above all, a conscious patient festooned with monitoring equipment in a modern intensive care unit needs a sympathetic caring approach tailored to his or her own needs.

Management of acute neuromuscular paralysis

- Respiratory paralysis occurs in a small percentage of patients with acute neuromuscular disease and accounts for less than 1% of admissions to general intensive care units. Its development may be insidious so that patients with acute neuromuscular disease should have their vital capacity monitored. Orotracheal intubation and ventilatory support should be instituted prophylactically when the vital capacity is falling towards 15 ml/kg. Earlier intervention is necessary in the presence of bulbar palsy.
- The cause of the respiratory paralysis can usually be deduced from the clinical history and examination. It is necessary to distinguish disease affecting the respiratory centre and its CNS connections to the cervical and thoracic spinal cord (Box 11.1), peripheral neuropathy, disorders of neuromuscular conduction, and muscle disease. In practice the commonest cause is Guillain–Barré syndrome, but the possibility of metabolic, vasculitic, and toxic neuropathies should not be ignored (Table 11.1). If the reflexes are preserved and there is no sensory deficit, the possibility of myasthenia, botulism, other rare causes of neuromuscular conduction block (Table 11.2), and muscle disease (Table 11.3) should be considered.
- If artificial ventilation is likely to be required for more than about seven days, a tracheostomy should be created and is more comfortable for the patient than continued orotracheal intubation. Nutrition should be provided early via a nasogastric tube. Strenuous efforts should be made to reduce the incidence of nosocomial infection. Patients with neuropathy should be monitored for autonomic dysfunction causing cardiac arrhythmia or fluctuating blood pressure. Deep vein thrombosis should be avoided by regular passive limb movements and low dose subcutaneous heparin (for example enoxaparin 40 mg daily).
- Specific interventions to shorten the duration of artificial ventilation should be applied appropriate to the nature of the

underlying condition. Metabolic disturbances such as hypokalaemia or hypermagnesaemia should always be sought and corrected first. In Guillain–Barré syndrome we recommend intravenous immunoglobulin as being equally effective to plasma exchange, safer, and more convenient. We do not recommend steroids but will review this advice when the results of the latest trial have been published and included in the Cochrane review. In myasthenia gravis we recommend intravenous immunoglobulin followed by thymectomy or, where thymectomy is inappropriate or has been unsuccessful, intravenous immunoglobulin combined with steroids and azathioprine. In polymyositis and dermatomyositis steroids are the mainstay of treatment but intravenous immunoglobulin is also effective.

Acknowledgements

We thank Dr L Loh, Radcliffe Infirmary, Oxford, for advice and Dr D Bihari who co-authored the first two editions of this chapter.

References

1 Kelly BJ. The diagnosis and management of neuromuscular diseases causing respiratory failure. *Chest* 1991;**99**:1485–94.
2 Roussos C. The respiratory muscles. *New Engl J Med* 1982;**307**:786–97.
3 Chevrolet JC, Deleamont P. Repeated vital capacity measurements as predictive parameters for mechanical ventilation need and weaning success in the Guillain–Barré Syndrome. *Am Rev Respir Dis* 1991;**144**:814–18.
4 Rieder P, Louis M, Jolliet P, Chevrolet JC. The repeated measurement of vital capacity is a poor predictor of the need for mechanical ventilation in myasthenia gravis. *Intensive Care Med* 1995;**21**:663–8.
5 Black LF. Maximal static respiratory pressures in generalized neuromuscular disease. *Am Rev Respir Dis* 1971;**103**:641–7.
6 Hart N, Polkey MI. Investigation of respiratory muscle function. *Clin Pulm Med* 2001;**8**:180–7.
7 David WS, Doyle JJ. Acute infantile weakness: a case of vaccine-associated poliomyelitis. *Muscle Nerve* 1997;**20**:747–9.
8 Hull HF, Birmingham ME, Melgaard B, Lee JW. Progress toward global polio eradication. *Infect Dis* 1997;**175**(suppl 1):S4–9.
9 Leis AA, Stokic DS, Polk JL, Dostrow V, Winkelmann M. A poliomyelitis-like syndrome from West Nile virus infection. *New Engl J Med* 2002;**347**:1279–80.
10 Goode GB, Shearn DL. Botulism. A case with associated sensory abnormalities. *Arch Neurol* 1982;**34**:55.

11   Griffin JW, Li CY, Ho TW, *et al.* Guillain–Barré syndrome in northern China. The spectrum of neuropathological changes in clinically defined cases. *Brain* 1995;**118**:577–95.
12   Hadden RDM, Cornblath DR, Hughes RAC, *et al.* The Plasma Exchange/ Sandoglobulin Guillain–Barré Syndrome Trial Group. Electrophysiological classification of Guillain–Barré syndrome: clinical associations and outcome. *Ann Neurol* 1998;**44**:780–8.
13   Ho TW, Mishu B, Li CY, *et al.* Guillain–Barré syndrome in northern China. Relationship to *Campylobacter jejuni* infection and anti-glycolipid antibodies. *Brain* 1995;**118**:597–605.
14   Bolton CF. Critical illness polyneuropathy: a useful concept. *Muscle Nerve* 1999;**22**:419–22.
15   Sedgwick EM, Senanayake N. Pathophysiology of the intermediate syndrome of organophosphorus poisoning. *J Neurol Neurosurg Psychiatry* 1999;**62**:201–2.
16   Cavanagh JB, Fuller NH, Johnson HRM, Rudge P. The effects of thallium salts, with particular reference to the nervous system changes. *Q J Med* 1974;**43**:293–319.
17   Greenberg SA. Acute demyelinating polyneuropathy with arsenic ingestion. *Muscle Nerve* 1996;**19**:1611–13.
18   Logina I, Donaghy M. Diphtheritic polyneuropathy. A clinical study and comparison with Guillain–Barré syndrome. *J Neurol Neurosurg Psychiatry* 1999;**67**:433–8.
19   Swift TR, Rivener MH. Infectious diseases of nerve. In: Matthews WB, ed. *Handbook of clinical neurology.* Amsterdam: Elsevier, 1987;179–84.
20   Calderon-Gonzalez R, Rizzi-Hernandez H. Buckthorn neuropathy. *N Engl J Med* 1967;**277**:69–71.
21   Norman M, Elinder G, Finkel Y. Vincristine neuropathy and a Guillain–Barré syndrome: a case with acute lymphatic leukemia and quadriparesis. *Eur J Haematol* 1987;**39**:75–6.
22   Vital C, Vital A, Julien J, *et al.* Peripheral neuropathies and lymphoma without monoclonal gammopathy: a new classification. *J Neurol* 1990;**237**:177–85.
23   Ridley A. Porphyric Neuropathy. In: Dyck PJ, Thomas PK, Lambert EH, Bunge R, eds. *Peripheral neuropathy.* Philadelphia: Saunders, 1984;1704–16.
24   Thadani H, Deacon A, Peters T. Diagnosis and management of porphyria. *Br Med J* 2000;**320**:1647–51.
25   Mitchell G, Larochelle J, Lambert M, *et al.* Neurologic crises in hereditary tyrosinemia. *N Engl J Med* 1990;**322**:432–7.
26   Liyanage Y, Hoch W, Beeson D, Vincent A. The agrin/muscle-specific kinase pathway: new targets for autoimmune and genetic disorders at the neuromuscular junction. *Muscle Nerve* 2002;**25**:4–16.
27   Hughes JM, Blumenthal JR, Merson MH, Lombard GL, Dowell VR, Gangarosa EJ. Clinical features of type A and B food-borne botulism. *Ann Intern Med* 1981;**95**:442–5.
28   Swift TR. Weakness from magnesium-containing cathartics: electrophysiologic studies. *Muscle Nerve* 1979;**2**:295–8.
29   Argov Z, Kaminski HJ, Al-Mudallal A, Ruff RL. Toxic and iatrogenic myopathies and neuromuscular transmission disorders. In: Karpati G, Hilton-Jones D, Griggs RC, eds. *Disorders of voluntary muscle.* Cambridge: Cambridge University Press, 2001;676–88.
30   Lindesmith LA, Baines RD, Bigelow DD, Petty TL. Reversible respiratory paralysis associated with polymyxin therapy. *Ann Intern Med* 1968;**68**:318–27.
31   Senanayake N, Roman GC. Toxic neuropathies in the tropics. *J Trop Geographic Neurol* 1991;**1**:3–15.

32 Mills AR, Passmore R. Pelagic paralysis. *Lancet* 1988;**i**:161–4.
33 Felz MW, Smith CD, Swift TR. A six-year-old girl with tick paralysis. *N Engl J Med* 2000;**342**:90–4.
34 Nicolle MW, Stewart DJ, Remtulla H, Chen R, Bolton CF. Lambert–Eaton myasthenic syndrome presenting with severe respiratory failure. *Muscle Nerve* 1996;**19**:1328–33.
35 Braun NM, Arora NS, Rochester DF. Respiratory muscle and pulmonary function in polymyositis and other proximal myopathies. *Thorax* 1983;**38**:616–23.
36 Keunen RWM, Lambregts PCLA, Op de Coul AAW, Joosten EMG. Respiratory failure as initial symptom of acid maltase deficiency. *J Neurol Neurosurg Psychiatry* 1984;**47**:549–52.
37 Trend P, Wiles CM, Spencer GT. Acid maltase deficiency in adults: diagnosis and management in 5 cases. *Brain* 1985;**108**:845–60.
38 Mohamed SD, Chapman RS, Crooks J. Hypokalaemia, flaccid quadruparesis, and myoglobinuria with carbenoxolone. *Br Med J* 1966;**1**:1581–2.
39 Newman JH, Neff TA, Ziporin P. Acute respiratory failure associated with hypophosphatemia. *N Engl J Med* 1977;**296**:1101–3.
40 Mastaglia FL, Ojeda VJ. Inflammatory myopathies. *Ann Neurol* 1985;**17**:215–27,317–23.
41 Sitwell LD, Weinshenker BG, Monpetit V, Reid D. Complete ophthalmoplegia as a complication of acute corticosteroid- and pancuronium-associated myopathy. *Neurology* 1991;**41**:921–2.
42 Sander HW, Golden M, Danon MJ. Quadriplegic areflexic ICU illness: selective thick filament loss and normal nerve histology. *Muscle Nerve* 2002;**26**:499–505.
43 De Vere R, Bradley WG. Polymyositis: its presentation, morbidity and mortality. *Brain* 1975;**98**:637–66.
44 Dalakas MC, Karpati G. Inflammatory myopathies. In: Karpati G, Hilton-Jones D, Griggs RC, eds. *Disorders of voluntary muscle*. Cambridge: Cambridge University Press, 2001;636–59.
45 Pendersen J. The effect of nasotracheal intubation on the paranasal sinuses. *Acta Anaesthesiol Scand* 1991;**35**:11–13.
46 Azar I. The response of patients with neuromuscular disorders to muscle relaxants — a review. *Anaesthesiology* 1984;**61**:173–87.
47 Absalon A, Pledger D, Kong A. Adrenocortical function in critically ill patients 24 h after a single dose of etomidate. *Anaesthesia* 1999;**54**:861–7.
48 Lichtenfeld P. Autonomic dysfunction in the Guillain–Barré syndrome. *Am J Med* 1971;**50**:772–80.
49 Ropper AH, Wijdicks EFM. Blood pressure fluctuations in the dysautonomia of Guillain–Barré syndrome. *Arch Neurol* 1990;**47**:706–8.
50 Winer JB, Hughes RAC. Identification of patients at risk of arrhythmia in the Guillain–Barré syndrome. *Q J Med* 1988;**68**:735–9.
51 Hazard P, Jones C, Benitone J. Comparative clinical trial of standard operative tracheostomy with percutaneous tracheostomy. *Crit Care Med* 1991;**19**:1018–24.
52 Friedman Y, Fildes J, Mizock B, *et al*. Comparison of percutaneous and surgical tracheostomies. *Chest* 1996;**110**:480–5.
53 Ciaglia P. Percutaneous dilatational tracheostomy – results and long term follow-up. *Chest* 1992;**101**:464–7.
54 The Acute Respiratory Distress Syndrome Network. Ventilation with lower tidal volumes as compared with traditional tidal volumes for acute lung injury and the acute respiratory distress syndrome. *N Engl J Med* 2000;**342**:1301–8.

55 Maynard N. Post-operative feeding. *Br Med J* 1991;**303**:1007–8.
56 Wilmore DW. Catabolic illness – strategies for enhancing recovery. *N Engl J Med* 1992;**325**:695–702.
57 Pingleton S. Nutritional management of acute respiratory failure. *JAMA* 1987;**257**:3094–9.
58 Deitch EA. The role of intestinal barrier failure and bacterial translocation in the development of systemic infection and multiple organ failure. *Arch Surg* 1990;**125**:403–4.
59 Detsky AS. Parenteral nutrition – is it helpful? *N Engl J Med* 1991;**325**:573–5.
60 Freeman J. Association of intravenous lipid emulsion and coagulase negative staphylococcal bacteremia in neonatal intensive care units. *N Engl J Med* 1990;**323**:301–8.
61 Stellato TA. Endoscopic intervention for enteral access. *World J Surg* 1992;**16**:1042–7.
62 Dive A, Miesse C, Galanti L, *et al.* Effect of erythromycin on gastric motility in mechanically ventilated critically ill patients: a double-blind, placebo-controlled study. *Crit Care Med* 1995;**23**:1356–62.
63 Davies AR, Froomes PR, French CJ, *et al.* Randomized comparison of nasojejunal and nasogastric feeding in critically ill patients. *Crit Care Med* 2002;**30**:586–90.
64 Atkinson S, Sieffert E, Bihari D. A prospective randomised, double-blind, controlled clinical trial of enteral immunonutrition in the critically ill. *Crit Care Med* 1998;**26**:1164–72.
65 Van den Berghe G, Wouters P, Weekers F, *et al.* Intensive insulin therapy in critically ill patients. *N Engl J Med* 2001;**345**:1359–67.
66 Cook D, Guyatt G, Marshall J, *et al.* A comparison of sucralfate and ranitidine for the prevention of upper gastrointestinal bleeding in patients requiring mechanical ventilation. *N Engl J Med* 1998;**338**:791–7.
67 Kollef M. The prevention of ventilator-associated peneumonia. *N Engl J Med* 1999;**340**:627–34.
68 Fagon J-Y. Nosocomial pneumonia in patients receiving continuous mechanical ventilation. *Intensive Care Med* 1989;**139**:877–84.
69 Ruiz-Santana S, Garcia Jimenez A, Esteban A, *et al.* ICU pneumonias: a multi-institutional study. *Crit Care Med* 1987;**15**:930–2.
70 Tuck RR, McLeod JG. Autonomic dysfunction in Guillain–Barré syndrome. *J Neurol Neurosurg Psychiatry* 1981;**44**:983–90.
71 Tripathi M, Kaushik S. Carbamezapine for pain management in Guillain–Barré syndrome patients in the intensive care unit. *Crit Care Med* 2000;**28**:655–8.
72 Pandey CK, Bose N, Garg G, *et al.* Gabapentin for the treatment of pain in Guillain–Barré syndrome: a double-blinded, placebo-controlled, crossover study. *Anesth Analg* 2002;**95**:1719–23.
73 The Guillain–Barré Syndrome Study Group. Plasmapheresis and acute Guillain–Barré syndrome. *Neurology* 1985;**35**:1096–104.
74 Raphael J-C, Chevret S, Hughes RAC, Annane D. Plasma exchange for Guillain-Barré syndrome. In: Cochrane Collaboration. *Cochrane Library*. Issue 2. Cochrane Database of Oxford: Update Software, 2001.
75 van der Meché FGA, Schmitz PIM, Dutch Guillain–Barré Study Group. A randomized trial comparing intravenous immune globulin and plasma exchange in Guillain–Barré syndrome. *N Engl J Med* 1992;**326**:1123–9.
76 Plasma Exchange/Sandoglobulin Guillain–Barré Syndrome Trial Group. Randomised trial of plasma exchange, intravenous immunoglobulin, and combined treatments in Guillain–Barré syndrome. *Lancet* 1997;**349**: 225–30.

77 Hughes RAC, Raphael J-C, Swan AV, van Doorn, PA. Intravenous immunoglobulin for Guillain–Barré syndrome. In: Cochrane Collaboration. *Cochrane Library*. Issue 3. Oxford: Update Software, 2001.

78 Hughes RAC, van der Meché, FGA. Corticosteroid treatment for Guillain–Barré syndrome. In: Cochrane Collaboration. *Cochrane Library*. Issue 4. Oxford: Update Software, 2002.

79 van Doorn PA, Van Koningsveld R, Schmitz PIM, van der Meché FGA, Visser LH, Meulstee J. Randomized trial on the additional effect of methylprednisolone on standard treatment with intravenous immunoglobulin in Guillain–Barré syndrome. *Neuromusc Dis* 2002;**12**: 781–2.

80 Gajdos P, Chevret S, Clair B, Tranchant C, Chastang C. Clinical trial of plasma exchange and high-dose intravenous immunoglobulin in myasthenia gravis. *Ann Neurol* 1997;**41**:789–96.

81 Gajdos P, Chevret S, Toyka K. Plasma exchange for myasthenia gravis. In: Cochrane Collaboration. *Cochrane Library*. Issue 4. Oxford: Update Software, 2002.

82 Cosi V, Lombardi M, Piccolo G, Erbetta A. Treatment of myasthenia gravis with high dose intravenous immunoglobulin. *Acta Neurol Scand* 1991; **84**:81–4.

83 Arsura E, Bick A, Brunner NG, Grob D. Effects of repeated doses of intravenous immunoglobulin in myasthenia gravis. *Am J Med Sci* 1988; **295**:438–43.

84 Arsura E. Experience with intravenous immunoglobulin in myasthenia gravis. *Clin Immunol Immunopathol* 1989;**53**:S170–9.

85 Panegyres PK, Squier M, Mills KR, Newsom-Davis J. Acute myopathy associated with large parenteral dose of corticosteroid in myasthenia gravis. *J Neurol Neurosurg Psychiatry* 1993;**56**:702–4.

86 Palace J, Newsom-Davis J, Lecky B, Myasthenia Gravis Study Group including Hughes RAC. A randomized double-blind trial of prednisolone alone or with azathioprine in myasthenia gravis. *Neurology* 1998;**50**: 1778–83.

87 Mastaglia FL, Phillips BA, Zilko P. Treatment of inflammatory myopathies. *Muscle Nerve* 1997;**20**:651–64.

88 Dau PC. Plasmapheresis in idiopathic inflammatory myopathy. Experience with 35 patients. *Arch Neurol* 1981;**38**:544–52.

89 Dau PC. Plasma exchange in polymyositis and dermatomyositis. *N Engl J Med* 1992;**327**:1030–1.

90 Miller FW, Leitman SF, Cronin ME, *et al*. Controlled trial of plasma exchange and leukapheresis in polymyositis and dermatomyositis. *N Engl J Med* 1992;**326**:1380–4.

91 Jann S, Beretta S, Moggio M, Adobbati L, Pellegrini G. High-dose intravenous human immunoglobulin in polymyositis resistant to treatment. *J Neurol Neurosurg Psychiatry* 1992;**55**:60–2.

92 Dalakas MC, Illa I, Dambrosia JM, *et al*. A controlled trial of high-dose intravenous immune globulin infusions as treatment for dermatomyositis. *N Engl J Med* 1993;**329**:1993–2000.

93 Esteban A, Alia I. Clinical management of weaning from mechanical ventilation. *Intensive Care Med* 1998;**24**:999–1008.

94 Senanayave N, Johnson MK. Acute polyneuropathy after poisoning by a new organophosphate insecticide. *N Engl J Med* 1982;**306**:155–7.

95 Moore D, House I, Dixon A, *et al*. Thallium poisoning. *Br Med J* 1993;**306**: 1527–9.

96 Donofrio PD, Wilbourne AJ, Albers JW, Rogers L, Salanga V, Greenberg HS. Acute arsenic intoxication presenting as Guillain–Barré like syndrome. *Muscle Nerve* 1987;**10**:114–20.

97 Greenberg C, Davies S, McGowan T, Schorer A, Drage C. Acute respiratory failure following severe arsenic poisoning. *Chest* 1979;**76**:596–8.
98 Beattie AD, Briggs JD, Canavan JSF, Doyle D, Mullin PJ, Watson AA. Acute lead poisoning. Five cases resulting from self-injection of lead and opium. *Q J Med* 1975;**44**:275–84.
99 Vernay D, Dubost JJ, Thevent JP, Sauvezie B, Rampon S. "Choreé fibrillaire de Morvan" followed by Guillain–Barré syndrome in a patient receiving gold therapy. *Arthritis Rheum* 1986;**29**:1413–4.
100 Brust JCM, Hammer JS, Challenor Y, Healton EB, Lesser R. Acute generalized polyneuropathy accompanying lithium poisoning. *Ann Neurol* 1979;**6**:360–2.
101 Johnston SRD, Burn DJ, Brooks DJ. Peripheral neuropathy associated with lithium toxicity. *J Neurol Neurosurg Psychiatry* 1991;**54**:1019–20.
102 Mueller JM, Flaherty MJ. Vincristine-induced quadriparesis. *South Med J* 1978;**71**:1310–11.
103 McLeod JG. Peripheral neuropathy associated with lymphomas, leukemias, and polycythemia vera. In: Dyck PJ, Thomas PK, eds. *Peripheral neuropathy*. Philadelphia: Saunders, 1993;1591–8.
104 Hughes RAC, Cameron JS, Hall SM, Heaton J, Payan JA, Teoh R. Multiple mononeuropathy as the initial presentation of systemic lupus erythematosus – nerve biopsy and response to plasma exchange. *J Neurol* 1982;**228**:239–47.
105 Christie AB. Diphtheria. In: Weatherall DJ, Ledingham JGG, Warrell DA, eds. *Oxford textbook of medicine*. Oxford: Oxford University Press, 1987, 5.164–5.
106 Heath JW, Ueda S, Bornstein MB, Daves GD, Raine CS. Buckthorn neuropathy in vitro: evidence of a primary neuronal effect. *J Neuropathol Exp Neurol* 1982;**41**:204–20.
107 Argov Z, Mastaglia FL. Drug-induced neuromuscular disorders in man. In: Walton J, ed. *Disorders of voluntary muscle*. 1988;981–1014.
108 Senanayake N, Román GC. Disorders of neuromuscular transmission due to natural environmental toxins. *J Neurol Sci* 1992;**107**:1–13.
109 Warner TT, Mossman S, Murray NMF. Hypokalaemia mimicking Guillain–Barré syndrome. *J Neurol Neurosurg Psychiatry* 1993;**56**:1134–5.
110 Dalakas MC. Polymyositis, dermatomyositis, and inclusion-body myositis. *N Engl J Med* 1991;**325**:1487–98.
111 Danon MJ, Carpenter S. Myopathy with thick filament (myosin) loss following prolonged paralysis with vecuronium during steroid treatment. *Muscle Nerve* 1991;**14**:1131–9.
112 Gould DB, Sorrell MR, Lupariello AD. Barium sulfide poisoning. *Arch Intern Med* 1973;**132**:891–4.

12: Acute visual loss

SHIRLEY H WRAY

Acute visual loss is the presenting symptom of an ocular stroke. A retinal stroke may be due to a central retinal artery occlusion (CRAO) or a branch retinal artery occlusion (BRAO). A stroke of the optic nerve due to infarction causes ischaemic optic neuropathy, termed anterior ischaemic optic neuropathy (AION) or posterior ischaemic optic neuropathy (PION).

Central retinal artery occlusion

Clinical signs and symptoms

Sudden blindness with persistent loss of visual acuity and visual field is the major symptom of a CRAO. Eye pain is atypical but, when present, suggests occlusion of the ophthalmic artery.

Central retinal artery occlusion is diagnosed ophthalmoscopically. What is seen depends on how soon after the occlusion the examination is made. If the fundus is examined within the first few minutes whilst the occlusion persists, the striking finding is the presence of segmentation of the blood column, boxcar segmentation, with slow "streaming" of flow in the retinal veins. Blood in the arterial branches is dark and a few arterioles may show segmentation (clear areas alternating with areas where the cells appear clumped together), but nowhere is this so obvious as in the veins.

Ophthalmoscopy is rarely performed, however, within the first hour and later inspection of the fundus will show surprisingly little. Typically the disc shows mild pallor and the arteries are only slightly attenuated. Gentle digital pressure on the globe may nevertheless elicit segmentation of the blood column, indicating the presence of a slow but not completely arrested circulation. Total obstruction posterior to the lamina should be suspected when the retinal arteries on the disc start

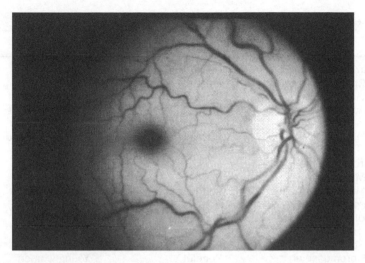

Figure 12.1 Central retinal artery occlusion with opacification of the retina and a macula cherry-red spot

to pulsate at a touch indicating very low retinal diastolic pressure. With the passage of time, typically after an hour or more, the characteristic fundus changes are seen. The ischaemic retina takes on a white ground glass appearance and the normal red colour of the choroid showing through at the fovea accentuates the central cherry-red spot at the macula (Figure 12.1). Within days of the acute event, the retinal opacification, the cherry-red spot, and the nerve fibre layer disappear and optic atrophy of the primary type develops.

Pathogenesis

There are five principal causes of CRAO.

1 Embolic obstruction.
2 Occlusion *in situ* in association with atheromatous disease when the narrowed arterial lumen becomes obliterated by superimposed thrombosis or haemorrhage.
3 Inflammatory endarteritis, such as giant cell arteritis,[1] thromboangiitis obliterans,[2] and polyarteritis nodosa with involvement of the choroidal and retinal arteries.[3]

Table 12.1 Sources of emboli

	Type	Patient age
Cardiac valves		
Rheumatic disease	Platelet/calcium*	Any age
Lupus	Platelet	Young women
Acute or subacute endocarditis	Marasmic	Damaged heart
Floppy mitral valve	Platelet	Any age; mostly women
Cardiac chamber		
Myxoma	Myxoma	Any age
Mural thrombus	Platelet/clot	Older adult
Carotid artery		
Ulcerated plaque	Platelet/cholesterol ester	Older adult
Stenosis	Platelet	Older adult
Fibromuscular dysplasia	Platelet	Young women
Other		
Amniotic	Debris?*	Young women
Long bone fractures	Fat*	Any age
Chronic IV drug users	Talc*	Any age
Disseminated intravascular coagulopathy*	Not known	Any age
Antiphospholipid antibody(s)	Not known	Young adult

From Burde[9] with modification, courtesy of the publishers; *J Clin Neuro-ophthalmol* 1989;**9**:185–9.
*Produces retinal infarction; no amaurosis fugax.

4 Simple angiospasm, a rare cause that may be the mechanism of CRAO associated with Raynaud's disease[4] or with migraine.[5]

5 Arterial occlusion that occurs hydrostatically with either (a) the high intraocular pressure of glaucoma, (b) the low retinal blood pressure of carotid stenosis or the aortic arch syndrome, or (c) severe hypotension.

The pathogenesis of a CRAO may be evident if examination shows: a retinal embolus (Table 12.1), hypertension, atrial fibrillation, and/or disease of other arteries, notably the ophthalmic, temporal, or ipsilateral internal carotid artery (ICA).

Table 12.2 Types of amaurosis fugax*

	Type I	Type II	Type III	Type IV
Onset	Abrupt	Less rapid	Abrupt	Abrupt
Visual loss	All or partial	All or partial	Total or progressive contraction of visual fields	Resembles type I or II
Length	Seconds or minutes	Minutes or hours	Minutes	Any length
Recovery	Complete	Complete	Usually complete	Complete
Pain	No	Rare	Often Vasopasm (migraine) ophthalmic artery or central retinal artery	No
Mechanism	Embolus Arteritis	Hypoperfused carotid/ ophthalmic occlusive disease	Visual loss may spare fixation	Anticardiolipid antibodies or idiopathic
Unusual features	Vision may black out completcly	Loss of contrast vision Photopsias Sunlight provoked		Alternating between eyes

*Based on 850 personal cases.[11]

Most occlusions of the CRAO occur in the region of the lamina cribrosa, regardless of the cause.[6] In patients under the age of 40, retinal arterial occlusions are less likely to be caused by ipsilateral carotid stenosis and more likely by cardiac embolism from rheumatic valvular disease, bacterial endocarditis, or cardiac myxoma[7,8] (Table 12.1[9]), or be attributable to a hypercoagulable state or vasospasm.[10] In older patients, transient monocular blindness, type I or II (Table 12.2[9,11]), as a premonitory symptom suggests an embolic cause or giant cell arteritis (GCA). The source of the embolus may be cardiac[12] or intra-arterial from atheromatous ulceration of the aorta, ipsilateral ICA, or from the stump of a thrombosed ICA following a dissection.

Trauma is also an important cause. Compression of the globe may be self-inflicted in circumstances involving heavy alcohol use with or without drug consumption followed by stupor.[13] Iatrogenic CRAO has been reported in patients undergoing surgery where prolonged pressure to the orbit has occurred inadvertently in association with a period of hypotension during anaesthesia[14,15] or as a complication of patient positioning for spinal surgery.[16]

Diagnosis

The diagnosis of CRAO is usually straightforward. The cause of a CRAO is, however, broad and varies with the age and sex of the patient and the existence of known medical conditions. Giant cell arteritis in persons aged 50 years or older is especially critical to diagnose and a high Westergren ESR suggests the diagnosis.

The differential diagnosis of acute persistent monocular visual loss includes a number of other ophthalmic emergencies: ischaemic optic neuropathy (AION and PION), acute occlusion of the central retinal vein, detachment of the macula, acute closed angle glaucoma, sudden vitreous or macular haemorrhage, as well as factitious visual loss.

Emergency treatment

There is no definitive treatment of CRAO. Both medical and surgical approaches are disappointing.[17-19] The standard therapy includes ocular massage, anterior chamber paracentesis, topical medications to lower the intraocular pressure, intravenous or oral acetazolamide, and inhalation of a mixture of 95% oxygen and 5% carbon dioxide (carbogen). The efficacy of these treatments has not been proven.[20]

Nevertheless, in cases that have been blind for less than 24 hours, gratifying recovery of vision has been reported in eyes treated six, eight, and twelve hours after the event.[21] For this reason, take the following emergency steps.

1   Place the patient flat and give firm ocular massage to lower intraocular pressure and help dislodge the embolus into the peripheral retinal circulation.

2   Have the patient rebreathe into a paper bag to build up carbon dioxide.

3   Give a bolus of intravenous acetazolamide 500 mg to lower intraocular pressure.

4   Refer the patient immediately to an ophthalmologist for an emergency anterior paracentesis. After surgery consider intravenous heparin therapy and, if there is a suspicion of vasospasm, give an intravenous bolus of methylprednisolone.

Other medical therapies proposed include sublingual nitroglycerine, oral warfarin sodium (coumadin), calcium channel blocking agents, vasodilators, antiplatelet agents, intravenous heparin, urokinase or tissue plasminogen activator (tPA), and intra-arterial urokinase or tPA. Schmidt et al.[22] reported that five of 14 patients with CRAO had improvement of visual acuity, visual field, or both following intra-arterial urokinase infusion. In a further five patients, no improvement occurred with this therapy. In these five patients, visual acuity was impaired preoperatively for more than seven hours.

Systemic thrombolytic agents were used in a pilot study involving three consecutive patients with acute CRAO.[18] The selection of the thrombolytic agent, tPA or anistreplase, was at the discretion of the internist. Patients were treated in the hospital emergency department with cardiovascular monitoring. Intravenous heparin sodium and oral coumadin were given as adjuvant therapy after thrombolytic infusion. All three patients noted subjective improvement within several hours of treatment. The best achieved visual acuity was recorded within 96 hours of therapy (Table 12.3[18]). Nevertheless, whilst the results of these pilot studies are encouraging, outside of a randomized clinical trial, the use of superselective fibrinolytic therapy for CRAO cannot be recommended on the basis of current evidence.[23]

Another therapy, early hyperbaric oxygen no later than eight hours after the beginning of visual symptoms, is reported to have a beneficial effect on visual outcome in patients with retinal artery occlusion. However, further large scale prospective controlled studies are needed to confirm this.[24]

Table 12.3 Clinical summary of thrombolytic therapy for three male patients

Patient no./ age (yr)	Pretreatment visual acuity	Time to therapy*	Thrombolytic agent	Adjunctive therapy	Post-treatment visual acuity
1/56	Hand motion	5·5	Anistreplase	Intravenous heparin, aspirin	20/60+
2/74	Light perception	4·0	Tissue plasminogen activator	Intravenous heparin, warfarin,	20/400
3/61	Hand motion	2·75	Tissue plasminogen activator	Intravenous heparin, warfarin	20/25

Data from Mames et al.[18]
*Time to initiation of thrombolytic therapy in hours.

Associated cardiovascular disease

Heart disease is frequently present in patients with embolic CRAO, particularly patients under the age of 40. In a retrospective study 30% of younger and 23% of older patients had cardiac valvular disease as a source of the embolus.[8] In a prospective study 56% of patients under age 50 had a potential cardiac source of embolus, compared with 24% in the older age group. Aortic stenosis was the commonest finding and, in the majority, the aortic valve disease was not of haemodynamic significance.[25] These data emphasise the importance of a careful cardiac assessment, especially in younger patients, and echocardiography.

CRAO may also be a consequence of disease *in situ*. Potentiation of atheroma in the ophthalmic or central retinal artery by hypertension may be associated. Patients should be designated hypertensive if the diastolic pressure is 100 mmHg or greater or if they are taking antihypertensive drugs. Most of these patients require a clinical cardiac assessment, an electrocardiogram, and total blood cholesterol (desirable < 200 mg/dl) and low-density lipoprotein (LDL) cholesterol values (desirable < 130 mg/dl).

Prognosis

The prognosis for visual recovery in CRAO is extremely poor. A total of 58% of eyes are blind and only 21% of eyes retain useful vision.

Associated major artery disease

Ophthalmic artery

Ophthalmic artery occlusion mimics a CRAO clinically and produces opacification of the infarcted retina. The typical cherry-red spot may be absent or extremely indistinct due to coexisting infarction of the choroid.[26–28] Visual loss is typically severe and permanent, with most eyes having no light perception or only bare perception of light.[29] There may be associated eye pain and pupillary dilatation from concurrent ischaemia to the ciliary ganglion or iris sphincter. The eye may be hypotonic. The retinal vessels are markedly constricted and the optic disc may or may not be swollen. Over time, most patients develop a characteristic fundus appearance characterised by optic atrophy, arterial attenuation, and diffuse pigmentary changes.

The pathogenesis of ophthalmic artery occlusion is much the same as that of ICA occlusion. The artery may be occluded: firstly, by a thrombus originating in the artery itself; secondly, by a thrombus propagated from an occluded ICA; thirdly, by an embolus from a distant site, most often the heart,[29] the common carotid artery, or the extracranial portion of the ICA; or, fourthly, by an extrinsic process that compresses the vessel, for example tumour or aneurysm. When only the proximal portion of the ophthalmic artery is occluded, there may be no ocular symptoms or signs because collateral channels from branches of the external carotid artery usually provide sufficient blood supply to the orbital and ocular vessels normally supplied by the ophthalmic artery. When the occlusion is more extensive, visual loss and typical ophthalmoscopic signs are present. Rarely, in isolated cases of ophthalmic artery occlusion, vision recovers from light perception vision to 20/30 or from an acuity of counting fingers at 6 inches (15 cm) to 20/50 with the restoration of normal retinal and choroidal blood flow.[28]

Diagnosis Fundus fluorescein angiography is diagnostic in CRAO or ophthalmic artery occlusion provided that:

- a timed transit is obtained within hours or days of the event
- a wide angle lens is used on the fundus camera
- the optic disc is photographed in the centre of the picture.

In isolated acute CRAO the choroidal circulation of the eye is normal and the delay is in the filling of the branches of the central retinal artery. In acute occlusion of the ophthalmic artery there is delayed filling in both the choroidal and retinal circulation.

Orbital colour Doppler imaging is, however, the diagnostic procedure of choice for establishing embolism as the cause of CRAO when no emboli are visible in the retinal circulation. This non-invasive technology enables prompt differentiation of embolic disease from arterial occlusion caused by intrinsic atherosclerosis, vasospasm, or vasculitis from giant cell arteritis. Clearly, recognition of emboli has important management implications for these patients.[30]

Emergency treatment The emergency treatment of ophthalmic artery occlusion is the same as for an acute CRAO.

Temporal artery

Occlusion of the central retinal artery occurs in 5–10% of elderly patients over the age of 60 with giant cell arteritis in the absence of classic cranial and systemic arteritic symptoms. Risk of blindness in the fellow eye is extremely high and all cases warrant an immediate Westergren ESR (<50 years of age: males 0–15 mm/h, females 0–20 mm/h; >50 years of age: males 0–20 mm/h, females 0–30 mm/h) and fibrinogen level (200–400 mg/dl) which, if elevated, indicate the need for high dose corticosteroid therapy and a temporal artery biopsy. Prednisone (60–80 mg per day) is the drug of choice. The dose should be regulated by the symptoms and the ESR and tapered slowly to a maintenance dose of 7·5–10 mg per day. Immediate corticosteroid therapy is advisable even when a clinical index of suspicion for giant cell arteritis is high in spite of a normal ESR and pending a temporal artery biopsy.

Diagnosis The diagnosis of giant cell arteritis is confirmed by biopsy of the temporal artery. Involvement of the vessel may be segmental and the diagnosis missed unless serial sections of a long biopsy specimen are performed. Dramatic response of headache, when present, to a trial of corticosteroids can confirm the diagnosis. There is usually no improvement in vision.

Internal carotid artery

The presence of ICA disease has varied among different series.[25,31] Clinical features of value in predicting a potentially operable carotid lesion on angiography have included increasing age, a localised carotid bruit, and cholesterol emboli in retinal branches. No operable lesions have been found in patients under 50 who did not have either a carotid bruit or cholesterol emboli. Twenty years ago, Wilson and colleagues found 12 of 18 patients had carotid irregularities or stenosis on angiography.[23] Ten years later, Merchut and associates,[31] grouping CRAO and BRAO together, found 29 of 34 (85%) patients had an abnormal ICA on arteriography, of which 12 had occlusion or severe stenosis and 17 had plaques, ulcers, or stenosis of less than 60%. In five of 34 patients (15%) the angiograms were normal.

Diagnosis Auscultation of the neck, eyes, and head for a bruit is very important, the higher the pitch the tighter the carotid stenosis. High pitched bruits that fade into diastole are diagnostic of a haemodynamically significant (70%) stenosis. The most widely used tests to evaluate the carotid artery are carotid non-invasive studies which combine carotid duplex Doppler with colour flow imaging at the bifurcation of the common carotid artery, with anterior transcranial Doppler insonation of flow in the intracranial (siphon portion) of the internal carotid artery, the ophthalmic artery, and through the transtemporal window the middle, anterior, and posterior cerebral artery stems. When the stenotic lesion at the origin of the internal carotid artery is narrow enough to produce a pressure drop across it (haemodynamically significant is > 70% stenosis), it can be identified by these methods with highly significant specificity and confirmed by magnetic resonance angiography or CT angiography. It is not certain, however, if CRAO is more common in these haemodynamically significant stenoses as opposed to those that are not. What is certain is that the rate of stroke is higher significantly in patients with such haemodynamically significant lesions.[32]

Ipsilateral headache or neck pain with tinnitus preceding CRAO is highly suggestive of ICA dissection and early diagnosis is imperative to reduce the risk of hemispheric stroke by artery to artery embolism.[33]

Associated antiphospholipid antibodies

CRAO is also associated with elevated levels of antiphospholipid antibodies (APA).[34–39] Among patients with systemic lupus erythematosus, persistently positive tests for APA, especially lupus anticoagulant and anticardiolipid antibody (aCL), characterise a subset of patients with thrombotic tendency.[38] In particular, the presence of aCL has been found to be an independent risk factor for ischaemic stroke, especially among young patients,[39] and an association between transient monocular blindness and elevated levels of APA, especially aCL, has been suggested (for review see Donders *et al.*[40]).

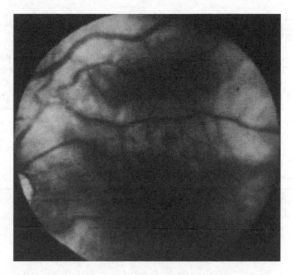

Figure 12.2 Branch retinal artery occlusion with impaction of two emboli in the artery. The retina shows an arcuate band of infarction

The primary antiphospholipid syndrome and factor V Leiden mutation, as well as other forms of thrombophilia, should be considered in the differential diagnosis of unexplained retinal vascular occlusions. The coexistence of severe thrombophilic disorders may carry a particularly high risk for thrombotic manifestations.[41]

Branch retinal artery occlusion

Clinical signs and symptoms

The impaction of an embolus in the central retinal artery usually produces sudden and permanent loss of a sector of the visual field with retinal infarction corresponding to the vascular territory of the arteriole (Figure 12.2). Frequently, however, retinal emboli are asymptomatic and detected at a routine eye examination. A history of amaurosis fugax (transient monocular blindness) is the most common preceding visual symptom (Table 12.4). A history of a transient cerebral ischaemic attack is rare.

Table 12.4 Preceding vascular events in occlusion of branch and central retinal arteries

	Retinal artery occlusion	
Preceding event	**Branch*** **n = 68**	**Central†** **n = 35**
Amaurosis fugax	12 (18)	4 (11)
Transient cerebral ischaemia	8 (12)	1 (3)
Stroke	2 (3)	4 (11)
Ischaemic heart disease	15 (22)	2 (6)
Claudication	5 (7)	2 (6)

Based on data in Wilson et al.[25]
Numbers in parentheses are percentages.
*43 male, 25 female patients; mean age 55.
†23 male, 12 female patients; mean age 36.

Pathogenesis

Branch retinal artery occlusion, like CRAO, is an ophthalmoscopic diagnosis. The appearance of a retinal embolus can provide specific information about the embolic material and its possible source. The commonest emboli that lodge within retinal vessels are cholesterol, platelet-fibrin, and calcific emboli. Less common varieties include tumour emboli from cardiac myxoma and metastatic neoplasms, fat emboli from fractures of long bones, septic emboli, talc emboli, and miscellaneous emboli of depo drugs, silicone, or air that occur after injections in the region of the face or scalp (Table 12.1).

Cholesterol emboli are bright yellowish, glinting lipid structures that reflect the ophthalmoscopic light beam. They are named Hollenhorst plaques (Figure 12.2), after Hollenhorst who demonstrated that these plaques were cholesterol crystals that arose from ulcerating atheromatous plaques in the aorta or carotid arteries.[42,43] Cholesterol emboli also produce focal opacification in an arteriole in which they become impacted.[25] In an eye with a history of transient visual loss but without visible retinal emboli this sign suggests that an embolus may have been present at one time. Patients in whom Hollenhorst plaques are seen have significantly reduced life expectancy, usually from concurrent cardiac disease.[44] Bruno *et al.*[45] suggest that these emboli are a marker of systemic atherosclerosis associated with hypertension, cigarette smoking, and bilateral carotid disease, and that asymptomatic retinal cholesterol embolism is an independent risk factor for stroke.[46]

Diffuse disseminated atheroembolism from disease of the aorta is a rare condition closely related to atherosclerosis. Cholesterol-rich atheromatous emboli break off from unusually fragile plaques in the aorta and its major branches and occlude arteries in the brain, retina, kidney, bowel, and other organs. The diagnosis of diffuse disseminated atheroembolism deserves serious consideration in all patients in middle age or late life with headache, stroke, transient monocular blindness, elevated ESR, hypertension, or cholesterol emboli in the retina. Early diagnosis is important because anticoagulation seems to increase the risk for serious, even fatal embolisation in these patients.

Calcific emboli are characteristically matt white and non-scintillating and somewhat wider than the blood column. They may be dislodged by the surgical manipulation of calcified heart valves at the time of valvulotomy or occur spontaneously from rheumatic valvular vegetations and from other disorders of the heart and great vessels that predispose to the formation of calcium.[47-50] Unlike Hollenhorst plaques and platelet-fibrin emboli, calcific emboli tend to lodge permanently in the blood vessels, occasionally resulting in the development of collateral vessels forming shunts around the embolic blockage. Patients with these emboli are at significant risk for stroke, heart attack, and death.[51]

Circulating microemboli that pass through the retina, so-called migrant pale emboli, are composed of platelets and associated with thrombocytosis. Emboli that occur after myocardial infarction fall into the category of fibrin plugs. They are especially frequent in patients who have neurological complications after open heart surgery. From the description of Fisher[52] and Ross Russell,[53] platelet-fibrin emboli appear as dull, grey-white plugs that resemble a long white worm slowly passing through the retinal arteries. They become temporarily impacted at bifurcations and then pass on, gradually fragmenting, and resolve over time.

Diagnosis

The diagnosis of a BRAO is made by ophthalmoscopic examination.

Emergency treatment

The emergency treatment of a patient with BRAO is similar to that for an acute CRAO. Anterior paracentesis and/or medication to lower intraocular pressure are the most common therapeutic approaches. Anticoagulation is advisable in patients with atrial fibrillation. However, it is likely that in many instances the retinal artery occlusion results from lipid, cholesterol, or calcific emboli rather than from fibrin-platelet thrombi. Consequently these emboli cannot be expected to respond to anticoagulant therapy.

Associated cardiac and vascular disease

A patient with a visible retinal embolus, even though suffering no visual loss, should be investigated urgently because of the risk of a stroke. Arrhythmias are the most common cause of cardiac related embolic retinal vascular disease and they may be the most common cause of all emboli to the brain. Abnormal heart rhythms most likely to produce emboli are chronic atrial fibrillation (AF), paroxysmal AF, and the abnormal rhythms that develop in patients with disturbances of cardiac conduction.

In patients with calcific retinal emboli, the investigative work up should focus on the heart valves (Table 12.5). Two-dimensional echocardiogram studies may reveal thickened, calcified valve leaflets or a tight calcified annulus. Transoesophageal echocardiography (TEE) may facilitate cardiac evaluation of patients with suboptimal transthoracic scans such as those with obesity or emphysema. Compared with transthoracic echocardiography (TTE), a transoesophageal study is more sensitive for detection of prosthetic valve dysfunction, atrial thrombus and other masses, atrial septal defects (especially of the sinus venous type), aortic dissection, and infective endocarditis.

The diagnostic yield of TTE and TEE echocardiography in identifying potential sources of emboli in patients with retinal

Table 12.5 Clinical findings in occlusion of branch and central retinal arteries

	Retinal artery occlusion	
Clinical finding	Branch* n = 68	Central[†] n = 35
Hypertension	17 (25)	20 (57)
Carotid bruits	12 (18)	5 (14)
Visible retinal embolus	46 (68)	4 (11)
Cardiac valvular abnormality	23 (34)	6 (17)

Based on data in Wilson et al.[25]
Numbers in parentheses are percentages.
*68 patients.
[†]35 patients.

ischaemia or embolism is significant. In a prospective study of 73 consecutive cases TTE was performed in 83·6% of patients, TEE was performed in 5·5% of patients, and both TTE and TEE were performed in 11·0% of patients. Ophthalmological diagnoses consisted of amaurosis fugax ($n = 28$), asymptomatic cholesterol embolism to the retina ($n = 34$), and branch or central retinal artery occlusion ($n = 11$). Echocardiography identified a potential cardiac or proximal aortic source for embolism in 16 of 73 (21·9%) patients, including eight who also had either atrial fibrillation or internal carotid artery stenosis. Thus, eight of 73 (11·0%) patients had lesions detected only by echocardiography. The most commonly identified lesions were proximal aortic plaque of more than 4 mm thickness ($n = 7$, 9·6%) and left ventricular ejection fraction of less than 30% ($n = 6$, 8·2%). TEE was particularly helpful in identifying prominent aortic plaques.[54]

To rule out ipsilateral ICA disease as a source of emboli, urgent investigations should include oculopneumoplethysmography, carotid ultrasonography and Doppler studies, and neuroimaging screening with a magnetic resonance angiography of the neck and brain and/or CT angiography.

Hyperhomocysteinaemia, defined by the 95th percentile (plasma homocysteine level 15·8 micromoles/L) and not homozygosity, for the MTHFR C677T mutation is now a recognised risk factor for retinal artery occlusion as well as for cardiovascular disease. Mean plasma folate levels are significantly lower in these patients compared with normal control subjects (5·6 +/− 2·3 ng/ml vs, 6·3 +/− 2·5 ng/ml; $p = 0.04$),[55] and both these blood tests are indicated in young ocular and cerebral stroke patients.

Prognosis

Savino *et al.*[44] reported that patients with retinal infarcts and visible emboli showed a shortened survivorship compared to age and sex matched controls (59% versus 75% over nine years) and that a visible retinal embolus predicted a dramatic reduction in survivorship (44%). When no embolus was visible, more patients survived. Death was found to be related in most cases to cardiac infarction.

Ischaemic optic neuropathy

Ischaemic optic neuropathy (ION) is due to infarction of the optic nerve and presents with sudden painless persistent loss of visual acuity, a visual field defect that is classically altitudinal or arcuate but which may be central, and an afferent pupil defect.[56] There is no significant sex predilection and the average age ranges from 57 to 69 years, with a peak range of 60–69 years.[57]

The critical regions of damage in both non-arteritic and arteritic anterior ischaemic optic neuropathy (AION) are the prelaminar, laminar, and immediate retrolaminar portions of the optic nerve which receive their blood supply from terminal branches of the ophthalmic artery, the lateral and medial posterior ciliary arteries, and from the pial circulation. In AION the ischaemic microvascular process may be solely or partially retrolaminar.[58] Lessell[59] suggests that the border zone that determines the site of infarction is between the lamina cribrosa and the centripetal branches of the pial vessels in the retrobulbar segment of the optic nerve. Besides vascular anatomical considerations, the best documented anatomical correlation is with cup–disc ratios. The discs at risk[60] have small cup–disc ratios[61] and cross-sectional areas,[62] which imply that the optic nerve fibres are crowded within the scleral canal. This crowding is probably a contributing factor in the pathogenesis of non-arteritic AION.[63] A small cup–disc ratio

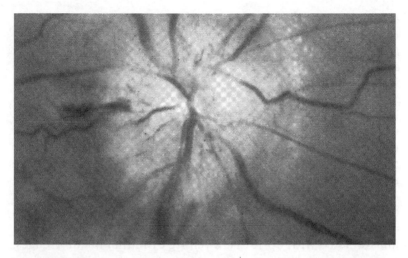

Figure 12.3 Anterior ischaemic optic neuropathy with pale swelling of the optic disc and flame shaped peripapillary haemorrhages

may be a risk factor for development of AION in association with the use of sildenafil citrate.[64]

Clinical signs and symptoms

The loss of vision in ischaemic optic neuropathy is usually painless, although some patients (approximately 8%) report discomfort behind and around the eye at the time of visual loss.[65] Visual acuity (VA) data for the initial loss of vision indicate that 31–52% of patients have a VA better than 20/64, whereas 35–54% have a VA worse than 20/200.[57,65,66] Altitudinal field defects comprise the most common pattern of visual field loss in 58–80% of cases.[56,65–68]

In acute AION, the optic disc is swollen with the swelling being either diffuse (75% of cases) or focal (25% of cases[57]). The disc may be pale or hyperaemic. Single or multiple flame shaped haemorrhages are present in the peripapillary region and a few soft exudates (Figure 12.3). As disc oedema begins to subside, optic atrophy develops and optic disc cupping similar to that seen in glaucoma may occur.

Some cases of AION may be associated with other signs of ocular ischaemia, such as choroidal infarction, retinal emboli, or iris or anterior chamber neovascularisation. The finding of iris neovascularisation in conjunction with AION in the absence of diabetic retinopathy or evidence of giant cell arteritis strongly suggests concomitant and causative ipsilateral carotid occlusive disease.

Posterior ischaemic optic neuropathy (PION) due to ischaemia of the retrobulbar portion of the optic nerve occurs in many settings, both arteritic and non-arteritic.[56,69–75] This results in clinical signs and symptoms of ischaemic optic neuropathy with acute visual loss, a field defect, a relative afferent pupillary defect but with, initially, a normal appearing optic disc. In such cases, optic disc pallor usually develops within four to six weeks. Thus, PION is distinguishable from AION by signs of optic nerve dysfunction unassociated with optic disc swelling or retinal haemorrhages.

Pathogenesis

Ischaemic optic neuropathy occurs in two forms, non-arteritic (median age 56 years) and arteritic (median age 74 years).

Non-arteritic ischaemic optic neuropathy

The non-arteritic form, AION or PION, may occur in patients with carotid artery disease and may be the initial manifestation of an ICA occlusion.[76] Rarely, patients with ICA disease experience the simultaneous occurrence of cerebral infarction and ipsilateral ischaemic optic neuropathy. This combination is called the opticocerebral syndrome.[77] Three patients described by Bogousslavsky[77] had AION and cerebral signs. Other patients reported had ICA occlusion or severe stenosis, acute hemispheric stroke, and simultaneous monocular blindness caused by PION in the ipsilateral eye.[78] No patient gained improvement in vision in the affected eye and all patients developed optic atrophy.

The pathogenesis of AION in the setting of disease of the ipsilateral ICA is multifactorial. In some cases, optic nerve infarction results from reduced blood flow secondary to carotid occlusion, poor collateral blood supply, and local changes in the pial circulation of the optic nerve. In other cases AION or PION may be due to embolism to multiple posterior ciliary arteries, pial vessels, or both.[79,80] In the majority of cases, however, non-arteritic AION is a disease of small vessels and not directly related to carotid disease but rather reflects shared risk factors, such as hypertension, diabetes mellitus, or cigarette smoking.[66,81-83]

Perioperative non-arteritic AION is also the result of multiple factors and occurs in the setting of various surgical interventions. The two most important factors in conjunction with surgery are hypotension and blood loss (for review see Williams et al.[84]). Severe anaemia alone may not cause AION, but even a short episode of hypotension in an already anaemic patient may predispose to AION induced visual loss.[85]

Loss of vision after a severe spontaneous haemorrhage is usually bilateral but it may affect both eyes asymmetrically or be unilateral. The severity ranges from mild or transient blurred vision in one eye to irreversible total blindness in both eyes. The visual loss often occurs at the time of haemorrhage but it may, in rare instances, be delayed beyond 10 days. Most patients are debilitated and over 40 years of age. Many have intercurrent systemic illnesses but they do not necessarily have risk factors for atherosclerosis. Visual loss typically follows repeated haemorrhage although visual loss can occur after a single massive bleed.[86] Ophthalmoscopy typically shows the characteristic changes of AION but the discs can appear normal initially when infarction of the optic nerve(s) occurs in the midorbital portion.[87] About 50% of patients who lose vision after an acute bleed experience some recovery of vision, but only 10–15% recover completely.

Clinical features that profile patients at risk of PION (infarction of the optic nerve posterior to the lamina cribrosa) include middle aged men (mean age of 50 years) who undergo spine surgery, blood loss ranging from 2000 to 16 000 ml with a drop in haematocrit from 9·5% to 19% (mean 14%), and intraoperative systemic hypotension in all patients. Prevention or immediate correction of hypovolaemic hypotension can reduce the incidence of PION.

Anterior ischaemic optic neuropathy occurring in chronic uraemic patients on dialysis has some common risk factors, including hypotension and anaemia. Uraemic children can be affected. What is striking, in the three published paediatric cases, is that they all had polycystic kidney disease.[88]

Arteritic ischaemic optic neuropathy

In arteritic AION or PION, constitutional symptoms of giant cell arteritis may be absent and acute visual loss is the herald symptom. The stroke to the optic nerve is caused by inflammatory occlusion of the short posterior ciliary arteries that supply the immediate retrolaminar and laminar portions of the optic disc. The inflammation may also produce sectorial areas of choroidal ischaemia.

In some cases of arteritic AION or PION, the constitutional symptoms of giant cell arteritis are insidious. They include fatigue, anorexia, weight loss, and alterations in mental status, including depression and memory impairment. Severe persistent headache is present in 40–90% of patients with or without tenderness over the temporal arteries or scalp, intermittent claudication of the masseters, and facial swelling. Severe systemic manifestations include respiratory tract symptoms, myocardial infarction, and gastrointestinal complications due to generalised vasculitis.

Acute visual loss is usually unilateral but it may be bilateral and simultaneous or the second eye may be affected days, weeks, or even months after the first eye, particularly if corticosteroid treatment is not begun immediately or is stopped while the disease is still active. Episodes of transient monocular visual loss may precede persistent visual loss caused by AION and occasionally transient visual loss may be induced by exertion or changes in posture. The appearance of the ischaemic optic disc in giant cell arteritis resembles that of non-arteritic AION.

Giant cell arteritis causing PION must also be suspected in acutely blind elderly patients with a normal appearing optic disc in the affected eye due to interruption of blood flow to the retrolaminar optic nerve. Infarction in these cases may even affect the intracranial portion and in most cases of giant cell arteritis-associated PION, histopathological examination reveals inflammatory occlusion of the ophthalmic artery and short posterior ciliary arteries.[68]

Ocular ischaemia from polyarteritis nodosa (PAN) is rare but PAN can produce ischaemia of a variety of ocular structures, including the retina, choroid, and optic nerve. In one patient, all three structures were affected. The patient, a 70 year old woman with hand and foot numbness, suddenly lost vision in the right eye from a CRAO and then developed a left AION and bilateral triangular areas of pigment epithelial disturbance caused by choroidal infarction – the triangular sign of Amalric. Initially, giant cell arteritis was suspected because of the combination of bilateral ocular ischaemia in an elderly patient with an elevated ESR and CRP. However the patient's peripheral neuropathy made this less likely, and a multiple mononeuropathy was demonstrated by EMG and nerve conduction velocity studies. Biopsy specimens from her sural nerve and biceps muscle showed a necrotising vasculitis with fibrinoid necrosis consistent with PAN.[89] Treatment of PAN consists primarily of corticosteroids with the addition of cyclophosphamide therapy if there is significant visceral organ involvement, continued progression of disease, or both. Bilateral ocular ischaemia AION is also reported in Takayasu arteritis.[90]

Diagnosis

The diagnosis of ischaemic optic neuropathy is based on the visual symptoms and signs. The investigations indicated in all cases are a complete blood count, ESR, fibrinogen level, and carotid non-invasive studies, including transorbital Doppler evaluation. A cardiac evaluation, including two-dimensional transthoracic echocardiogram, Holter monitor, and magnetic resonance angiography of the head and neck and/or CT angiography are indicated when ischaemic optic neuropathy is thought to be embolic. In non-arteritic ischaemic optic neuropathy tests should also be directed towards the detection of associated systemic vascular disease such as hypertension, diabetes mellitus, and hyperlipidaemia or a variety of coagulopathies, for example, those caused by decreased concentrations of protein C, protein S, or antithrombin III.[91] In giant cell arteritis-associated ischaemic optic neuropathy with a high ESR and fibrinogen level, a temporal artery biopsy is mandatory.

Emergency treatment

Both medical and surgical treatment has been proposed for the treatment of non-arteritic ischaemic optic neuropathy but, to date, no therapy is of significant benefit. Numerous drugs have been tried including anticoagulants, sub-Tenon's injections of vasodilators, intravenous noradrenaline (norepinephrine), thrombolytic agents, and corticosteroids. Johnson et al.[92] reported that a combination of levodopa and carbidopa (Sinemet) prompted visual recovery in patients with non-arteritic AION of more than six months' duration. These results have not been confirmed. Haemodilution has also been described as improving visual function in longstanding non-arteritic AION[93] and in AION of less than two weeks' duration when combined with pentoxifylline.[94] Further verification of this potentially beneficial treatment is required. Direct surgical intervention by optic nerve sheath decompression has been shown in a multicentred randomised trial to be ineffective and possibly visually harmful.[57] This type of surgery is no longer used in the United States.

The emergency treatment of choice in giant cell arteritis-associated AION or PION is high dose prednisone (60–80 mg per day) pending a temporal artery biopsy. Because of the risk to the second eye, this treatment is also recommended in suspected cases of giant cell arteritis in spite of a normal ESR or fibrinogen level. Corticosteroids in non-arteritic ischaemic optic neuropathy are of questionable value although they are frequently used when the second eye becomes involved. Embolic ischaemic optic neuropathy when symptomatic of ipsilateral ICA disease should be managed according to the severity of the carotid artery disease. (For additional guidance with regard to the management of retinal embolic disease, see "Branch retinal artery occlusion", the section "Emergency treatment".)

Prognosis

The prognosis for recovery of vision is poor, particularly in patients with the arteritic form of ischaemic optic neuropathy. The long term clinical course in non-arteritic ischaemic optic neuropathy is not well documented. In one follow up study of 205 patients, there was a slightly greater incidence of stroke and myocardial infarction than expected but no greater mortality.

Management of acute visual loss

Loss of vision is a common complaint in the emergency department. It may represent a permanent vision threatening disorder. A logical and organised approach to the history and the physical examination is key to the diagnosis. The physician must pay meticulous attention to the following.

- A detailed medical history and the tempo of evolution of visual loss and associated symptoms.
- Visual acuity, pupil reflexes, dilated fundoscopic examination.
- Blood pressure, heart rate and rhythm, palpation of the temporal arteries, and auscultation of the heart, neck, eyes, and head.
- Immediate blood tests: complete blood count, prothrombin time, partial thromboplastin time, platelet count, ESR, fibrinogen level, fasting blood sugar, cholesterol, triglyceride, and blood lipids. A test for antiphospholipid antibodies (anticardiolipin antibody and lupus anticoagulant) and measurement of protein C, protein S, and antithrombin III are recommended in unexplained cases of ocular strokes. In these patients a plasma homocysteine and folate levels should be checked.
- Non-invasive investigations:

  - Carotid non-invasive studies; useful tests give information about the presence of a haemodynamic lesion (Doppler ultrasonography and oculoplethysmography), analyse the bruit to determine the residual lumen diameter (phonoangiography), or image the artery with ultrasound (B-scan ultrasonography).
  - Two-dimensional transthoracic and transoesophageal echocardiography.

- Invasive investigations are required in selected patients:

  - A temporal artery biopsy.
  - A carotid arteriogram if the patient is a candidate for endarterectomy after non-invasive screening by magnetic resonance angiography and/or CT angiogram of the neck and brain.
  - A timed fundus fluorescein angiogram, particularly in cases of central retinal artery occlusion when occlusion of the ophthalmic artery is suspected, in cases of anterior ischaemic optic neuropathy of possible embolic origin, or in giant cell arteritis-associated ischaemic optic neuropathy.

Emergency treatment in central retinal artery occlusion is designed to lower intraocular pressure and dislodge the embolus. In impending central retinal artery occlusion, heparin is useful. Urgent systemic corticosteroids are needed when central retinal artery occlusion or ischaemic optic neuropathy is due to giant cell arteritis. In other situations, treatment is directed towards preventing recurrence or involvement of the other eye by reducing or eliminating risk factors.

References

1   Cullen JF. Occult temporal arteritis. *Trans Ophthalmol Soc UK* 1963;**83**:725–36.
2   Gresser EB. Partial occlusion of retinal vessels in a case of thromboangitis obliterans. *Am J Ophthalmol* 1932;**15**:235–7.
3   Goldsmith J. Periarteritis nodosa with involvement of the choroidal and retinal arteries. *Am J Ophthalmol* 1946;**29**:435–46.
4   Anderson RG, Gray EB. Spasm of the central retinal artery in Raynaud's disease. *Arch Ophthalmol* 1937;**17**:662–5.
5   Katz B. Migrainous central retinal artery occlusion. *J Clin Neuro-Ophthalmol* 1986;**6**:69–75.
6   Hayreh SS. Pathogenesis of occlusion of the central retinal vessels. *Am J Ophthalmol* 1971;**72**:998–1011.
7   Cogan DG, Wray SH. Vascular occlusions in the eye from cardiac myxomas. *Am J Ophthalmol* 1975;**80**:396–403.
8   Appen RE, Wray SH, Cogan DG. Central retinal artery occlusion. *Am J Ophthalmol* 1975;**79**:374–81.
9   Burde RM. Amaurosis fugax, an overview. *J Clin Neuro-Ophthalmol* 1989;**9**:185–9.
10 Greven CM, Slusher MM, Weaver RG. Retinal arterial occlusions in young adults. *Am J Ophthalmol* 1995;**120**:776–83.
11 Wray SH. Extracranial internal carotid artery disease. In: Bernstein EF, ed. *Amaurosis fugax*. New York: Springer Verlag, 1988;72–80.
12 Zimmerman LE. Embolism of central retinal artery, secondary to myocardial infarction with mural thrombosis. *Arch Ophthalmol* 1965;**73**:822–6.
13 Jayam AV, Hass WK, Carr RE, Kumar AJ. Saturday night retinopathy. *J Neurol Sci* 1974;**22**:413–18.
14 Givner I, Jaffe N. Occlusion of the central retinal artery following anesthesia. *Arch Ophthalmol* 1950;**43**:197–207.
15 Hollenhorst RW, Svien HJ, Benoit CF. Unilateral blindness occurring during anesthesia for neurosurgical operation. *Arch Ophthalmol* 1954;**52**:819–30.
16 Wolfe SW, Lospinuso MF, Burke SW. Unilateral blindness as a complication of patient positioning for spinal surgery. *Spine* 1992;**17**:600–5.
17 Brown GC. Retinal arterial obstructive disease. In: Schachat AP, Murphy RP, eds. *Retina*, 2nd edn. St Louis: CV Mosby, 1994:1361–77.
18 Mames RN, Shugar JK, Levy N, *et al.* For the CRAO Study Group. Peripheral thrombolytic therapy for central retinal artery occlusion. *Arch Ophthalmol* 1995;**113**:1094.
19 Mangat HS. Retinal artery occlusion. *Surv Ophthalmol* 1995;**40**:145–56.
20 Atebara NH, Brown GC, Carter J. Efficacy of anterior chamber paracentesis and carbogen in treating acute nonarteritic central retinal artery occlusion. *Ophthalmology* 1995;**102**:2029–35.
21 Stone R, Zink H, Klingele T, Burde RM. Visual recovery after central retinal artery occlusion: two cases. *Ann Ophthalmol* 1977;**9**:445.
22 Schmidt D, Schumacher M, Wakhloo AK. Microcatheter urokinase infusion in central retinal artery occlusion. *Am J Ophthalmol* 1992;**113**:429–34.
23 Beatty S, Eong KG. Local intra-arterial fibrinolysis for acute occlusion of the central retinal artery: a meta-analysis of the published data. *Br J Ophthalmol* 2000;**84**:914–16.
24 Beiran I, Goldenberg I, Adir Y, Tamir A, Shupak A, Miller B. Early hyperbaric oxygen therapy for retinal artery occlusion. *Eur J Ophthalmol* 2001;**11**:345–50.

25 Wilson LA, Warlow CP, Ross Russell RW. Cardiovascular disease in patients with retinal arterial occlusion. *Lancet* 1979;**i**:292–4.

26 Burde RM, Smith ME, Black JT. Retinal artery occlusion in the absence of a cherry red spot. *Surv Ophthalmol* 1982;**27**:181–6.

27 Brown GC, Magargal LE, Sergott R. Acute obstruction of the retinal and choroidal circulations. *Ophthalmology* 1986;**93**:1373–82.

28 Duker JS, Brown GC. Recovery following acute obstruction of the retinal and choroidal circulations. *Retina* 1988;**8**:257–60.

29 Rafuse PE, Nicolle DA, Hutnik CML, *et al.* Left atrial myxoma causing ophthalmic artery occlusion. *Eye* 1997;**11**:25–9.

30 Foroozan R, Savino PJ, Sergott RC. Embolic central retinal artery occlusion detected by orbital color Doppler imaging. *Ophthalmology* 2002;**109**:744–7.

31 Merchut MF, Gupta SR, Naheldy MH. The relation of retinal artery occlusion and carotid artery stenosis. *Stroke* 1988;**19**:1239–42.

32 Kistler JP, Furie KL. Carotid endarterectomy revisted. *N Engl J Med* 2000;**342**:1743–5.

33 Mokhtari F, Massin P, Paques M, *et al.* Central retinal artery occlusion associated with head or neck pain revealing spontaneous internal carotid artery dissection. *Am J Ophthalmol* 2000;**129**:108–9.

34 Englert H, Hawkes CH, Boey ML, *et al.* Dego's disease: association with anticardiolipin antibodies and the lupus anticoagulant. *Br Med J* 1984;**289**:576.

35 Glueck HI, Kant KS, Weiss MA, *et al.* Thrombosis in systemic lupus erythematosus: relation to the presence of circulatory anticoagulants. *Arch Intern Med* 1985;**145**:1389–95.

36 Shalev Y, Green L, Pollack A, *et al.* Myocardial infarction with central retinal artery occlusion in a patient with antinuclear antibody-negative systemic lupus erythematosus. *Arthritis Rheum* 1985;**28**:1185–7.

37 Jonas J, Kolbe K, Volcker, HE, *et al.* Central retinal artery occlusion in Sneddon's disease: association with antiphospholipid antibodies. *Am J Ophthalmol* 1986;**102**:37–40.

38 Asherson RA, Khamashta MA, Gil A, *et al.* Cerebrovascular disease and antiphospholipid antibodies in systemic lupus erythematosus, lupus-like disease, and the primary antiphospholipid syndrome. *Am J Med* 1989;**86**:391–9.

39 The Antiphospholipid Antibodies in Stroke Study (APASS) Group. Anticardiolipin antibodies are an independent risk factor for first ischemic stroke. *Neurology* 1993;**43**:2069–73.

40 Donders RC, Kappelle LJ, Derksen RH, *et al.* Transient monocular blindness and antiphospholipid antibodies in systemic lupus erythematosus. *Neurology* 1998;**51**:535–40.

41 Dori D, Beiran I, Gelfand Y, *et al.* Multiple retinal arteriolar occlusions associated with coexisting primary antiphospholipid syndrome and factor V Leiden mutation. *Am J Ophthalmol* 2000;**129**:106–8.

42 Hollenhorst RW. The ocular manifestations of internal carotidarterial thrombosis. *Med Clin North Am* 1960;**4**:897–908.

43 Hollenhorst RW. Significance of bright plaques in the retinal arterioles. *JAMA* 1961;**178**:123–9.

44 Savino PJ, Glaser JS, Cassady J. Retinal stroke: is the patient at risk? *Arch Ophthalmol* 1977;**95**:1185–9.

45 Bruno A, Russell PW, Jones WL, *et al.* Concomitants of asymptomatic retinal cholesterol emboli. *Stroke* 1992;**23**:900–2.

46 Bruno A, Jones WL, Austin JK, *et al.* Vascular outcome in men with asymptomatic retinal cholesterol emboli: a cohort study. *Ann Intern Med* 1995;**122**:249–53.

47 D'Cruz IA, Cohen HC, Prabhu R, *et al*. Clinical manifestations of mitral-annulus calcification, with emphasis on its echocardiographic features. *Am Heart J* 1977;**94**:367–77.
48 Guthrie J, Fairgrieve J. Aortic embolism due to myxoid tumour associated with myocardial calcification. *Br Heart J* 1963;**25**:137–40.
49 diBono DP, Warlow CP. Mitral-annulus calcification and cerebral or retinal ischemia. *Lancet* 1979;**ii**:383–5.
50 Stefensson E, Coin JT, Lewis WR III, *et al*. Central retinal artery occlusion during cardiac catheterization. *Am J Ophthalmol* 1985;**9**:586–9.
51 Howard RS, Ross Russell RW. Prognosis of patients with retinal embolism. *J Neurol Neurosurg Psychiatry* 1987;**50**:1142–7.
52 Fisher CM. Observations of the fundus oculi in transient monocular blindness. *Neurology* 1959;**9**:333–47.
53 Ross Russell RW. Observations on the retinal blood-vessels in monocular blindness. *Lancet* 1961;**ii**:1422–8.
54 Mouradian M, Wijman CA, Tomasian D, Davidoff R, Koleini B, Babikian VL. Echocardiographic findings of patients with retinal ischemia or embolism. *J Neuroimaging* 2002;**12**:219–23.
55 Weger M, Stanger O, Deutschmann H, *et al*. The role of hyperhomocysteinemia and methylenetetrahydrofolate reductase (MTHFR) C677T mutation in patients with retinal artery occlusion. *Am J Ophthalmol* 2002;**134**:57–61.
56 Boghen DR, Glaser JS. Ischemic optic neuropathy. The clinical profile and natural history. *Brain* 1975;**98**:689–708.
57 The Ischemic Optic Neuropathy Decompression Trial Research Group. Optic nerve decompression surgery for nonarteritic anterior ischemic optic neuropathy (NAION) is not effective and may be harmful. *JAMA* 1995;**273**:625–32.
58 Onda E, Cioffi GA, Bacon DR, *et al*. Microvasculature of the human optic nerve. *Am J Ophthalmol* 1995;**120**:92–102.
59 Lessell S. Nonarteritic anterior ischemic optic neuropathy. *Arch Ophthalmol* 1999;**117**:386–8.
60 Burde RM. Optic disc risk factors for nonarteritic anterior ischemic optic neuropathy. *Am J Ophthalmol* 1993;**116**:760–4.
61 Beck RW, Savino PJ, Repka MX, *et al*. Optic disc structure in anterior ischemic optic neuropathy. *Ophthalmology* 1984;**91**:1334–7.
62 Mansour AM, Schoch D, Logani S. Optic disc size in ischemic optic neuropathy. *Am J Ophthalmol* 1988;**106**:587–9.
63 Doro S, Lessell S. Cup–disc ratio and ischemic optic neuropathy. *Arch Ophthalmol* 1985;**103**:1143–4.
64 Pomeranz HD, Smith KH, Hart WM Jr, Egan RA. Sildenafil-associated nonarteritic anterior ischemic optic neuropathy. *Ophthalmology* 2002;**109**:584–7.
65 Rizzo JF 3rd, Lessell S. Optic neuritis and ischemic optic neuropathy. Overlapping clinical profiles. *Arch Ophthalmol* 1991;**109**:1668–72.
66 Repka MX, Savino PJ, Schatz NJ, Sergott RC. Clinical profile and long-term implications of anterior ischemic optic neuropathy. *Am J Ophthalmol* 1983;**96**:478–83.
67 Hayreh SS, Podhajsky P. Visual field defects in anterior ischemic optic neuropathy. *Doc Ophthalmol Proc Ser* 1979;**19**:53–71.
68 Ellenberger C Jr, Keltner JL, Burde RM. Acute optic neuropathy in older patients. *Arch Neurol* 1973;**28**:182–5.
69 Hayreh SS. Posterior ischemic optic neuropathy. *Ophthalmologica* 1981;**182**:29–41.
70 Cullen JF, Duvall J. Posterior ischemic optic neuropathy (PION). *Neuro-ophthalmology* 1983;**3**:15–19.

71 Isayama Y, Takahashi T, Inoue M, *et al.* Posterior ischemic optic neuropathy: III. Clinical diagnosis. *Ophthalmologica* 1983;**187**:141–7.

72 Rizzo JF 3rd, Lessell S. Posterior ischemic optic neuropathy during general surgery. *Am J Ophthalmol* 1987;**103**:808–11.

73 Sawle GV, Sarkies NJC. Posterior ischemic optic neuropathy due to internal carotid artery occlusion. *Neuro-ophthalmol* 1987;**7**:349–53.

74 Shimo-Oku M, Miyazaki S. Acute anterior and posterior ischemic optic neuropathy. *Jpn J Ophthalmol* 1984;**28**:159–70.

75 Perlman JI, Forman S, Gonzalez ER. Retrobulbar ischemic optic neuropathy associated with sickle cell disease. *J Neuro-ophthalmol* 1994;**14**:45–8.

76 Mori S, Suzuki J, Takeda M. A case report of internal carotid occlusion with ischemic optic neuropathy as initial symptom. *Jpn Rev Clin Ophthalmol* 1983;**77**:1530–3.

77 Bogousslavsky J, Regli F, Zografos L, *et al.* Optico-cerebral syndrome: simultaneous hemodynamic infarction of optic nerve and brain. *Neurology* 1987;**37**:263–8.

78 Newman NJ. Cerebrovascular disease. In: Miller NR, Newman NJ, eds. *Clinical neuro-ophthalmology,* vol 3, 5th edn. Baltimore: Williams and Wilkins, 1998, 3449.

79 Lieberman MF, Shahi A, Green WR. Embolic ischemic optic neuropathy. *Am J Ophthalmol* 1978;**86**:206–10.

80 Portnoy SL, Beer PM, Packer AJ, *et al.* Embolic anterior ischemic optic neuropathy. *J Clinic Neuro-ophthalmol* 1989;**9**:21–5.

81 Guyer DR, Miller NR, Auer CI, *et al.* The risk of cerebrovascular and cardiovascular disease in patients with anterior ischemic optic neuropathy. *Arch Ophthalmol* 1985;**103**:1136–42.

82 Moro F, Doro D, Mantovani E. Anterior ischemic optic neuropathy and aging. *Metab Pediatr Syst Ophthalmol* 1989;**12**:46–57.

83 Chung SM, Guy CA, McCrary JA 3rd. Nonarteritic ischemic optic neuropathy. The impact of tobacco use. *Ophthalmology* 1994;**101**: 779–82.

84 Williams EL, Hart W Jr, Tempelhoff R. Postoperative ischemic optic neuropathy. *Anesth Analg* 1995;**80**:1018–29.

85 Brown RH, Schauble JF, Miller NR. Anemia and hypotension as contributors to perioperative loss of vision. *Anesthesiology* 1994;**80**: 222–6.

86 Kamei A, Takahashi Y, Shiwa T, *et al.* Two cases of ischemic optic neuropathy after intestinal hemorrhage. Presented at the VIIIth International Neuro-Ophthalmology Symposium, Winchester, England, 1990, June 13–29.

87 Johnson MW, Kincaid MC, Trobe JD. Bilateral retrobulbar optic nerve infarctions after blood loss and hypotension: a clinicopathologic case. *Ophthalmology* 1987;**94**:1577–84.

88 Dunker S, Hsu HY, Sebag J, Sadun AA. Perioperative risk factors for posterior ischemic optic neuropathy. *J Am Coll Surg* 2002;**194**:705–10.

89 Hsu CT, Kerrison JB, Miller NR, Goldberg MF. Choroidal infarction, anterior ischemic optic neuropathy, and central retinal artery occlusion from polyarteritis nodosa. *Retina* 2001;**21**:348–51.

90 Malik KP, Kapoor K, Mehta A, *et al.* Bilateral anterior ischemic optic neuropathy in Takayasu arteritis. *Indian J Ophthalmol* 2002;**50**:52–4.

91 Bertram B, Remky A, Arend O, *et al.* Protein C, protein S and antithrombin III in acute ocular occlusive disease. *German J Ophthalmol* 1995;**4**:332–5.

92 Johnson IN, Gould TJ, Krohel GB. Effect of levodopa and carbidopa on recovery of visual function in patients with nonarteritic anterior ischemic

optic neuropathy of longer than six months' duration. *Am J Ophthalmol* 1996;**121**:77–83.

93 Haas A, Uyguner I, Sochor GE, *et al*. Non-arteritic anterior ischemic optic neuropathy. Long-term results after hemodilution therapy. *Klin Monatsbl Augenheilkd* 1994;**205**:143–6.

94 Wolf S, Schulte-Strake U, Bertram B, *et al*. Hemodilution therapy in patients with acute anterior ischemic optic neuropathy. *Ophthalmology* 1993;**90**:21–6.

13: Criteria for diagnosing brain stem death

MD O'BRIEN

The traditional criteria of cardiac and respiratory arrest for the certification of death are appropriately used in the huge majority of cases, but the development and widespread use of cardiac resuscitation and artificial ventilation in the late 1960s created a need to redefine the criteria of death in the very small numbers of patients in apnoeic coma, who could be maintained on a ventilator for days or weeks, a need made more pressing by the demand for organs for transplantation.[1]

Twenty years ago, many such patients were ventilated until asystole supervened, by which time the brain had often liquefied. Over several years the concept that apnoeic coma, caused by irreversible destruction of the brain stem, was incompatible with life led to the establishment of criteria to diagnose brain stem death. Brain stem death equates with death of the brain as a whole but not, of course, with death of the whole brain. Wijdicks[2] has reviewed the brain death criteria throughout the world, obtaining information from 80 countries. Practice guidelines for brain death in adults were present in 70 countries and these were associated with legal standards, relating to organ transplantation, in 55 countries. The criteria varied considerably, many countries including the United States, require death of the whole brain, while many others follow the United Kingdom criteria for brain stem death. There were major differences in the requirement for apnoea testing. Forty one countries required an apnoea test with specified P_{CO_2} targets, 20 countries required disconnection from the ventilator only which may result in inadequate respiratory centre stimulation, and nine countries had no apnoea test requirement.

Brain stem death can be ascertained clinically at the bedside with absolute reliability and without the use of special techniques such as EEG, evoked responses, neuroimaging or blood flow measurements, provided that the appropriate protocol is rigorously followed. If these criteria are met, life support systems may be withdrawn with the confidence that recovery cannot occur. Organs may then be removed for transplantation and better use made of intensive care facilities. Relatives should be kept fully informed at each stage in this process.

If ventilation is maintained, cardiac asystole usually occurs within a few days and nearly always within a week or two. However, there are a number of well-documented patients who have filled the criteria for brain stem death, but who have maintained vital organ function on a ventilator for extended periods. Shewmon identified 175 patients from his own experience and in a search of the literature who survived more than one week.[3] Of these, there was sufficient information for a detailed analysis in 56 patients, 17 survived for two months, seven for six months and four for over a year. There was a single patient whose vital organs except the brain were still functioning at the time of the report after 10 years. However, in this patient multimodal evoked potentials showed no intracranial response, magnetic resonance angiography showed no intracranial blood flow and neuroimaging showed that the entire cranial cavity was filled with disorganised membranes, proteinaceous fluids and ghost-like outlines of the former brain. It is clear that this patient had been dead for many years, but there is still widespread misunderstanding of the concept of brain stem death and confusion in the minds of relatives. Further confusion arises over the differentiation of brain stem death from the persistent vegetative state, which has been discussed by Cranford[4] and Jennett.[5] Patients in the persistent vegetative state have a functioning brain stem and breathe spontaneously. They may show apparent sleep–wake cycles. This state may persist for years, but these patients do not fulfil the criteria for brain stem death and cannot be certified as dead. In the United Kingdom, withdrawal of medical support or stopping feeding requires judicial approval.

The diagnosis of brain stem death requires preconditions that are of critical importance. Examples in the medical literature claiming survival after brain stem death have failed to fulfil the preconditions. Only when the cause of the brain damage has been established and is known to be irreversible should the tests of brain stem function be carried out. These are tests of reflex function of the brain stem. Although the oculocephalic reflex (doll's eye movement) was not part of the United Kingdom code,[1] it is worth doing because it is simple and easy to elicit. If the oculocephalic reflex is present, there is no need to proceed further. The pupil light reflex should be elicited with a bright light; the light from an ophthalmoscope is not sufficient. Similarly, the corneal and gag reflexes should be sought with adequate stimuli, which need to be relatively coarse compared with those used in a conscious patient. In addition, motor responses should be sought by adequate stimulation in the trigeminal nerve territory and in the limbs. Ice cold water irrigation of the tympanic membrane should not elicit any eye movement. Tonic deviation of either eye during this test indicates some residual brain stem function. These are all straightforward bedside tests and should not create any difficulties. The tests for spontaneous ventilation with blood gas analysis and specific P_{CO_2} targets is usually carried out by an anaesthetist, who should be available together with the appropriate equipment in all intensive care units where these problems are likely to arise.

The criteria have been set out in a form suitable for reproduction and inclusion in a patient's notes (Box 13.1).[6] The background to the concept of brain stem death, the historical aspects, and its validation has been fully discussed by Pallis.[7,8]

References

1. Conference of Medical Royal Colleges and the Faculties in the United Kingdom. Diagnosis of Brain Stem Death. *BMJ* 1976;2:1187–8.
2. Wijdicks EFM. Brain Death Worldwide. *Neurol* 2002;58:20–5.
3. Shewmon DA. Chronic "Brain Death", Meta-analysis and Conceptual Consequences. *Neurol* 1998;1538–45.
4. Cranford RE. Discontinuation of ventilation after brain stem death, policy should be balanced with concern for the family. *BMJ* 1999;318:1754–5.
5. Jennett B. Discontinuation of ventilation after brain stem death, brain stem death defines death in law. *BMJ* 1999;318:1755.
6. O'Brien MD. Criteria for diagnosing brain stem death. *BMJ* 1990;301: 108–9.
7. Pallis C. ABC of Brain Stem Death. London: British Medical Association, 1983.
8. Pallis C. Brain stem death. In: Vinken PJ, Bruyn GW, Klawans HL, eds. *Handbook of clinical neurology*. New York: Elsevier, 1990, pp 441–96.

Assessment form

Patient's name .... Ward ....

Date of birth .... Hospital number ....

	Assessor A	Assessor B	Assessor A	Assessor B
Name				
Status				

If a patient in deep coma, requiring mechanical ventilation, is thought to be dead because of irreversible brain damage of known cause, an assessment of brain stem function should be made according to the following guidelines. These follow the Department of Health recommendations in "Cadaveric organs for transplantation – a code of practice, including the diagnosis of brain death", 1983 (London: HMSO).

Two assessments should be made by two doctors once the preconditions have been met. Diagnosis should not normally be considered until at least six hours after the onset of coma or, if anoxia or cardiac arrest was the cause of the coma, particularly in children, until 24 hours after the circulation has been restored, and then only if the preconditions have been satisfied.

(1) Two medical practitioners, who have expertise in this field, should assure themselves that the preconditions have been met before the examination.

(2) It is often convenient for the examination to be performed by one assessor and witnessed by the other.

(3) The respirator disconnection test is usually performed by an anaesthetist and witnessed by one of the assessors.

What is the cause of the irremediable brain damage? ....

Why is it irremediable? ....

Start of coma: Time .... Date ....

Preconditions (All answers must be "No") Time ....

Date ....

1 Could primary hypothermia, drugs, or metabolic/ endocrine abnormalities be contributing significantly to the apnoeic coma? (Where appropriate, check plasma and urine for drugs, and plasma pH, glucose, sodium, and calcium.)

2 Have any neuromuscular blocking drugs been administered during the preceding 12 hours?

3 Is the rectal temperature below 35°C? (If so, warm the patient and reassess.)

Examination
Do not proceed until the preconditions have been met.
The answer to all questions must be "No".

		1st A	1st B	2nd A	2nd B
	Time Date				
1	When the head is gently but fully rotated to either side is there conjugate deviation of the eyes in the opposite direction (Doll's head eye movement)?				
2	Do the pupils react to light?				
3	Is there any response to corneal stimulation on either side?				
4	Do the eyes deviate when either ear is irrigated with 50 ml of ice cold water for 30 seconds? (First confirm tympanic membranes visible and intact.)				
5	Is there a gag reflex?				
6	Is there a cough reflex following bronchial stimulation by a suction catheter?				
7	Are there any motor responses within the cranial nerve distribution following adequate stimulation of any somatic area? (Supraorbital and nail bed pressure.)				
8	*Tests for spontaneous ventilation* Are there any spontaneous respiratory movements?				
		CO_2	O_2	CO_2	O_2
	Pre-oxygenate the patient for 10 minutes with 100% oxygen. Record blood gases ($Pa\text{co}_2$ before disconnection must not exceed 5·3 kPa. If not, slow ventilation until $Pa\text{co}_2$ rises to this level). Ventilation with 95% O_2 and 5% CO_2 is an alternative.				
	Disconnect the patient from the ventilator and give oxygen at 6 litres per minute via a suction catheter in the trachea. Wait approximately 10 minutes, then measure blood gases ($Pa\text{co}_2$ must exceed 6·65 kPa at the end of the disconnection period).				
	Is there any spontaneous respiratory movement?				
	Assessors' signatures				

Index

Page numbers in **bold** refer to figures; those in *italics* refer to tables/boxed material. Common abbreviations used as sub entries include: BRAO, branched retinal artery occlusion; CRAO, central retinal artery occlusion; CSF, cerebrospinal fluid; CT, computed tomography; ICP, intracranial pressure; MRI, magnetic resonance imaging; SAH, subarachnoid haemorrhage; TBI, traumatic brain injury.

anaesthesia, status epilepticus
  early stage 171
  refractory 172–3
  see also individual drugs
analgesia *see* pain control
angiospasm, ocular stroke 410
Anopheles mosquitos 329
antibiotic therapy
  "best guess" 322, *322*, 336
  brain abscess 336
  meningitis *322*, 322–4
    CSF drug levels 322–3
    drug choice 323–4
    time-course 324
  minimal bactericidal
      concentration (MIC) 322
  neuromuscular blockade 387
  resistance to 323
  see also individual drugs
anticholinergic drugs, psychosis
    induction 146
anticholinesterases, myasthenia
    gravis 386, 397
anticoagulants, acute ischaemic
    stroke 87–90, **89**
anticonvulsants *see* antiepileptic
    drugs
antidepressant drugs 135–6
antiepileptic drugs
  barbiturates *see* barbiturates
  benzodiazepines *see*
      benzodiazepines
  ideal 163
  pharmacology 162–3
  status epilepticus 168–82, *169*
    failure 182, *182*
    kinetics 162–3
    refractory 172–3
    response to treatment
        161–2
    see also tonic-clonic status
        epilepticus
  tolerance 171–2
  see also individual drugs
antifibrinolytics, subarachnoid
    haemorrhage therapy 267

anti-inflammatory drugs
  bacterial meningitis
      324–5
  corticosteroids *see* steroids
  see also individual drugs
anti-Jo1 antibodies,
    polymyositis 390
antiphospholipid antibodies,
    ocular stroke 418–19
antipsychotic drugs
  acute psychotic disorders
      146, 147–8
  adverse effects
    extrapyramidal symptoms
        122, 138
    neuroleptic malignant
        syndrome 148
    QT prolongation 122
  atypical 123, 138, 148
  delirium management 121,
      122–3
  mania management
      137–8
  see also individual drugs
anxiety disorders 139–41
  adjustment disorder 141
  generalised (GAD) 139
  management 141–2
  panic disorder 139–40
    differential diagnosis 140
  phobias 139
  post-traumatic 140
aortic stenosis, central retinal
    artery occlusion and 415
APACHE scores, TBI outcome
    prediction 59
apolipoprotein E, TBI
    pathophysiology 48
arachadonic acid, TBI
    pathophysiology 46
arboviruses, epidemic
    encephalitis 306–8
arterial occlusion, ocular
    stroke 410
arteritis, acute visual loss 409,
    417, 424, 428–9